Patriarchy and Fertility:
Japan and Sweden, 1880–1960

POPULATION AND SOCIAL STRUCTURE

Advances in Historical Demography

Under the Editorship of

E. A. HAMMEL

Department of Anthropology
University of California, Berkeley

Kenneth W. Wachter with *Eugene A. Hammel* and *Peter Laslett,* Statistical Studies of Historical Social Structure

Nancy Howell, Demography of the Dobe !Kung

Bennett Dyke and *Warren T. Morril* (Editors), Genealogical Demography

J. Dupaquier, E. Helin, P. Laslett, M. Livi Bacci, and *S. Sogner* (Editors), Marriage and Remarriage in Populations of the Past

Ronald F. E. Weissman, Ritual Brotherhood in Renaissance Florence

John C. Caldwell, Theory of Fertility Decline

Carl Mosk, Patriarchy and Fertility: Japan and Sweden, 1880–1960

Patriarchy and Fertility: Japan and Sweden, 1880–1960

CARL MOSK

Department of Economics
University of California
Berkeley, California

1983

ACADEMIC PRESS

A Subsidiary of Harcourt Brace Jovanovich, Publishers
New York London
Paris San Diego San Francisco São Paulo Sydney Tokyo Toronto

ACADEMIC PRESS, INC.
111 Fifth Avenue, New York, New York 10003

United Kingdom Edition published by
ACADEMIC PRESS, INC. (LONDON) LTD.
24/28 Oval Road, London NW1 7DX

Library of Congress Cataloging in Publication Data

Mosk, Carl.
Patriarchy and fertility: Japan and Sweden, 1880-1960.

Includes index.
1. Fertility, Human--Japan--History. 2. Fertility, Human--Sweden--History. 3. Japan--Population--History. 4. Sweden--Population--History. 5. Fertility, Human--Economic aspects--Case studies. 6. Demographic transition--Case studies. I. Title.
HB1061.M67 304.6'32'0952 82-4064
ISBN 0-12-508480-3 AACR2

PRINTED IN THE UNITED STATES OF AMERICA

83 84 85 86 9 8 7 6 5 4 3 2 1

To Sachiyo

Contents

List of Illustrations

List of Tables

Preface

One of the most remarked upon observations in scholarship concerned with human society is that populations experience a decline in fertility when they modernize in their economic and social spheres. Japan and Sweden, the nations studied here, experienced this process of fertility decline during the last century or so. The process by which natality falls from relatively high to relatively low levels is known as the fertility transition, and social scientists in a variety of disciplines, most notably economics, sociology, anthropology, and psychology, have attempted to explain why this process occurs and what connection it bears to economic and social development. Within this general field of inquiry, economists made an especially important contribution during the 1960s and 1970s by developing theoretical models of the household (the unit that makes decisions concerning fertility) and statistical techniques for testing these models. Two major criticisms of these models and their empirical tests can be and have been made: the models are too abstract and they do not give proper weight to institutional and cultural factors that may be important; and the empirical analysis usually is limited to the study of only the early or late phases of the fertility transition and does not encompass the entire process. This book is designed to grapple with both of these problems. For this reason it should be of special interest to economists and sociologists concerned with questions of long-term demographic change.

The scope of this volume is as follows. At its core is an economic theory of the household that is sensitive to cultural and institutional considerations. We shall prove this theory to be broadly applicable to the Japanese and Swedish populations. We shall then show how the theory of the household can explain how and why the fertility transition takes place and shall provide detailed evidence for

Japan and Sweden that is consistent with this explanation. Part I of this volume is devoted to elaborating our theoretical model; Part II to showing that this theory of household behavior provides a reasonable description of Japanese and Swedish households and their evolution during the last century; and Part III to demonstrating that it can account for the Japanese and Swedish fertility transitions.

Inevitably a book of this sort, which concerns long-term economic, social, and demographic change in a country in Asia and a country in Europe, crosses a number of scholarly boundaries, stepping from economics to history, sociology, and Asian and European studies. We hope that it will prove of interest to specialists in these disciplines. It is, however, the work of an economist and economic historian, and this particular imprint is evident throughout the work.

Acknowledgments

Patriarchy and Fertility is the culmination of many years of research and thought. Its origins lie in the work I did for my doctoral dissertation, "Demographic Transition in Japan, 1920–1960," which was accepted at Harvard University in 1976. My interest in combining demographic and economic history into a research topic stemmed from courses and seminars I took with Harvey Leibenstein, Alexander Gerschenkron, and Henry Rosovsky, and from conversations with Simon Kuznets. I entered graduate school with the specific intention of studying Japanese economic history, and I am especially grateful to Henry Rosovsky, Kazushi Ohkawa, and Irene Taeuber for encouraging me in my study of Japan and economic history at Harvard and for helping me arrange funding and institutional affiliations for a year's research effort in Tokyo (1974–1975).

While in Japan I was supported by a research grant from the Ford Foundation, and I conducted my work at two institutions: The Institute of Economic Research at Hitotsubashi University and the Institute of Population Problems at the Ministry of Health and Welfare. I am especially grateful to Professor Mataji Umemura of the Institute of Economic Research for advice and encouragement and to Toshio Kuroda, Kiichi Yamaguchi, Kazumasa Kobayashi, Hidehiko Hama, Yoichi Okazaki, Sumiko Uchino, Shigeru Hayashi, Michiko Yamamoto, Tatsuya Itoh, and Akiko Yajima for assisting me at the Institute of Population Problems. I have especially pleasant memories of conversing with Akiko Yajima, Sumiko Uchino, and Michiko Yamamoto—memories that will remain with me always.

Upon obtaining an appointment at the University of California at Berkeley in 1976, I received research support for the Institute of Business and Economic Research of that university. This support permitted me to carry out further research on Japan and to prepare research proposals that were subsequently funded by the Social Science Research Council, The Japan Foundation, and the National Science Foundation (SOC 78-24407). These three extramural grants were ultimately processed through the Institute of International Studies of the University of California at Berkeley, and I am especially grateful to Cleo Stoker and Karin Beros of the Institute of International Studies for efficiently administering my grants and for helping me prepare the applications. In addition, I received grants from the Center for Japanese Studies of the University of California, Berkeley, and I am grateful to the center for supporting my research.

A considerable number of research assistants were hired on the grants just mentioned, and I wish to acknowledge my debt to them here. They are Simon Pak, Richard Kerner, Irene Kasakova, Charles Salazar, Kaoru Yamaguchi, Sooh-hee Yang, Thomas Paynter, Elizabeth Savoca, John Faris, Marta Gomez, Henry Hayase, Kim Euichul, Thomas Ackley, Christina Allen, Steven Kamin, Deborah Kim, Barbara Mikalson, Ko Nagashima, Akihito Tsukioka, Steven Stoft, and David Wong. I wish to acknowledge a special debt to Simon Pak, who exhibited exceptional energy and dedication in doing the work under considerable pressure of time. In addition, a number of typists prepared drafts of this book and other related papers that emerged out of this project. I wish to thank Nadine Zelinski, Barbara Priest, Lenora Warkentin, Helen Way, Betty Kendall, and Winifred McLeod. Nadine Zelinski and Lenora Warkentin were especially kind to me in setting aside other work to type the final revisions.

Many of my colleagues at Berkeley and Stanford commented on aspects of this research in seminars or in private discussion, and I wish to thank them here. In particular, Eugene Hammel, Kenneth Wachter, Ronald Lee, Carlo Cipolla, Richard Sutch, Jan DeVries, Lovell Jarvis, Pranab Bardhan, Benjamin Ward, Thomas Smith, Paul David, Warren Sanderson, William Skinner, Sheila Johanssen, and Bent Hansen helped me with advice and comment. I am especially grateful to Bent Hansen for providing me with information about Sweden and for encouraging me in my academic endeavors during the last five years. Carlo Cipolla, Albert Fishlow, Kenneth Wachter, Benjamin Ward, Pranab Bardhan, John Rogers, Brinley Thomas, John Quigley, Kalpana Bardhan, Michael Wiseman, and Thomas Smith read portions of or entire early drafts of the book and made helpful suggestions. In particular Ronald Lee made many valuable suggestions on improving the presentation of the theoretical arguments and the statistical findings. None of my colleagues, of course, are responsible for errors that may remain in this book.

PART I

The Thesis

CHAPTER 1

Introduction

1.1. The Purpose

The central concern of this book is the economy and demography of the household within a particular institutional setting, that of a patriarchal stem family system, and the implications of these two household factors for the long-term evolution of fertility*: A model of the household is presented; its applicability to two historical populations, the Japanese and the Swedish, is demonstrated; and its ability to account for the evolution of natality in these two populations over the epoch 1880–1960 is shown. Accomplishment of this task will suggest at least a partial solution to a major problem that has confronted demographic and economic historians during the last decade: why is there such diversity in the long-term evolution of natality associated with modern economic development in the nineteenth and twentieth centuries?

The main purpose of this chapter is to provide some basic detail concerning this question, that is, how and why there is diversity in the evolution of fertility. In the next section the nature of this diversity will be defined in terms of the observed behavior of indices of fertility for a variety of populations in Europe and Asia during the nineteenth and twentieth centuries.

* Throughout the text "fertility" and "natality" are used interchangeably to mean some measure of the birthrate of a population.

1.2. The Problem

Examination of social and economic statistics for a wide range of countries in the postwar period reveals that levels of fertility and mortality tend to fall into two fairly distinct clusters. There are countries — mainly those enjoying relatively high incomes per capita — that have fairly low levels of natality and mortality, and there is a second group of countries — generally with lower average standards of living — for which rates of mortality and especially fertility are considerably higher. Of course the distribution of each of these variables is not perfectly bimodal because there are nations in which intermediate levels of birth and/or death rates obtain. But the data do reveal a pronounced division.

It is well known and has been thoroughly documented that at one time birth and death rates were substantially higher in the countries that presently enjoy low rates. It is clear that these populations experienced transitions in the levels of the vital rates. That is, levels of natality fell during specific epochs in those countries, as did levels of mortality. We commonly call these long-term secular declines the "fertility transition" and the "mortality transition." Taken together, we call the two processes the "demographic transition." During the last half-century or so, demographers, sociologists, and economists have studied these secular movements in levels of vital events; have measured their timing, speed, and duration; have speculated about the possible causes underlying these trends; and have attempted to develop analytical models that can be tested with data. This has produced a flourishing body of literature concerned with the fertility and mortality transitions.

The first recorded transition in natality probably occurred in France, beginning around the end of the eighteenth century, although there is evidence for early fertility decline in Hungary as well.[1] Around 1870–1890 fertility transitions commenced in a considerable number of other European countries, including the Scandinavian countries, Belgium, England and Wales, and Germany. By 1930 almost all of Western Europe enjoyed low levels of fertility; and this pattern of diminished reproduction extended into many areas of Eastern Europe as well. Because Europe initiated the secular decline in fertility, much of the work regarding the description and analysis of fertility transitions has focused on the European experience.

Major advances in research on this topic began about two decades ago at the Office of Population Research at Princeton University, under the direction of Ansley Coale.[2] This has come to be known as the European Fertility Project, and out of it has arisen a large body of writings, both books and articles, as well as a major conference (a summary conference held at Princeton in July 1979).[3] A number of notable achievements have emerged out of this research effort, and it would be useful to mention briefly here the ones that most clearly apply to the problem of diversity in the evolution of natality.

First, a simple and intuitively appealing methodology has emerged from the project, namely, that of the Hutterite indices developed by Coale in the early 1960s and used throughout the publications arising from the project.[4] There are four main indices: an index of overall fertility I_f, an index of marital fertility I_g, an index of nuptiality I_m, and an index of illegitimate fertility I_h. Before giving the formal definitions of these indices, it would be useful to present them in an intuitive fashion. First, I_f and I_g are ratios formed by dividing the births that actually occur to women (all women in the case of I_f; married women in the case of I_g) by those that hypothetically would occur to these women if they were to reproduce at close to "maximal" levels. For a "maximal reproductive" population, Coale selected married Hutterite women from the cohort of 1921 to 1930.[5] Thus we would expect most populations to have values of I_f and I_g substantially less than one, and we would suppose that a population extensively practicing birth control would have a very small value for these indices. The index of marriage I_m is a measure of the proportion of women married, secured by using the Hutterite fertility rates as weights (this choice of weights is convenient because it gives the indices very attractive multiplicative features).

The formal definitions of the indices are as follows:

f_i = births per woman in ith age interval
g_i = births per married woman in ith age interval
h_i = births per nonmarried woman in ith age interval
w_i = number of women in ith age interval
m_i = number of married women in ith age interval
u_i = number of nonmarried women in ith age interval
F_i = births per woman in ith age interval for the standard population (married Hutterites, 1921–1930)

where i runs over the standard seven quinquennial age classes covering an average woman's potential reproductive life ($i = 1$ for 15–19; $i = 2$ for 20–24; . . . ; $i = 7$ for 45–49). Then the indices are[6]

$$I_f = \Sigma f_i w_i / \Sigma F_i w_i$$
$$I_g = \Sigma g_i m_i / \Sigma F_i m_i$$
$$I_h = \Sigma h_i u_i / \Sigma F_i u_i$$
$$I_m = \Sigma F_i m_i / \Sigma F_i w_i$$

The indices have the convenient property that

$$I_f = (I_m I_g) + [(1 - I_m)(I_h)] \qquad (1.1)$$

Note that if $I_h = 0$ (i.e., the level of illegitimate fertility is typically close to zero), then

$$I_f = I_m I_g \tag{1.2}$$

There are a number of reasons why these indices are particularly useful in the study of fertility transitions. First, they are almost completely standardized for age structure (a point discussed in Chapter 3). Second, computation of the indices requires only a minimal input of data (live births classified by legitimacy status and the female population classified by quinquennial age class and marital status). Third, the indices I_f and I_g have an intuitively simple meaning in the sense that comparison to what is, in principle, "maximal" performance tells us to what degree a population is falling short of that maximal performance (presumably mainly, but not exclusively, because of birth control).

The second major finding to emerge from the European Fertility Project concerns levels of the Hutterite indices I_m, I_f, and I_g before the transitions actually began. (It should be noted in this context that the European Fertility Project has endeavored to compute the Hutterite indices for every province in each country of Europe.) Broadly speaking the detailed computations of this project have shown (in an especially striking fashion when presented in the form of maps with shading or colors) that I_m and I_g (and, consequently, I_f) varied considerably throughout Europe *prior* to the fertility transitions of these populations. The diversity in the predecline situations is quite impressive and can largely be understood in terms of two ideas: Hajnal's notion of a (Western) "European" marriage pattern (affecting I_m) and Henry's notion of natural fertility. Let us discuss variations in nuptiality first, and to guide our discussion in a quantitative manner, let us begin by focusing on Table 1.1.

Hajnal imagines a line running across Europe from Trieste to Leningrad; he notes that west of the line nuptiality customs in 1870 were markedly different from those east of this hypothetical boundary. In the western areas men and women tended to wed at advanced ages, and there was a considerable proportion of people single at age 50. In the eastern areas, by contrast, men and (especially) women married at fairly young ages, and there was a far lower proportion of people single at 50. Hajnal notes that this diversity in marriage patterns is associated with variations in mortality rates: death rates tend to be lower in areas witnessing later marriages, whereas areas in which nuptiality occurs early and virtually universally have higher death rates. These points can be gleaned from an examination of Table 1.1, by comparing the percentages in several key quinquennial age classes of men and women who are single (calculated from census figures) with the crude death rates (deaths per 1000 population) and infant mortality rates (deaths of

TABLE 1.1

Fertility, Mortality, and Population Increase for Selected European Countries or Regions Prior to Their Modern Fertility Transitions[a]

Country and approximate date	Fertility										Mortality		
		Nuptiality characteristics											
	Crude birth rate (CBR)	Males (% single)		Females (% single)		Age gap at marriage at wife's age		Hutterite indices			Crude death rate (CDR)	Infant mortality rate (IMR)	Natural rate of increase (NRI)
		25–29	45–49	20–24	45–49	20	25	I_m	I_g	I_h			
Sweden, 1880	30	60	11	82	20	.9	1.7	.41	.70	.05	18	130	12
Norway, 1870[b]	30	54	11	77	18	.7	1.9	.41	.77	—	18	115	12
Denmark, 1870[c]	31	50	9	75	13	.7	1.9	.46	.65	—	20	129	11
Switzerland, 1870[d]	30	30	16	78	17	.6	1.9	.41	.73	—	24	210	6
Italy, 1870[e]	37	—	13	54	12	4.1	4.2	.57	.65	.05	29	—	8
Bulgaria, 1900	41	23	3	24	1	1.2	3.0	.73	.70	—	24	—	17
European Russia, 1897	49	18	3	28	4	—	—	.70	.76	—	36	262	13

[a] Source: Mosk (1979d), Institut International de Statistique (1916); and Kuczynski (1935). Note that dashes indicate data not available.
[b] Percentage single for 1900.
[c] Medians of values for provinces of the country in the cases of Norway, Denmark, and Switzerland.
[d] Mean of values for provinces of the country in the cases of Norway, Denmark, and Switzerland.
[e] Figures for age groups 45–49 actually for age groups 50–54.

children age 0 per 1000 live births). It should be noted that the figures on I_m reflect the figures on the proportion of people single: I_m is low in the western nations and high in the eastern zones. The maps produced by the scholars working on the European Fertility Project reveal that there are gradations as one moves eastward, southward, and northward from France: Hajnal's notion of a sharp line is therefore a bit extreme. A movement eastward, for instance, takes one gradually into regions where marriage occurred earlier and more universally.

Two additional observations not dwelt on by Hajnal can be drawn from Table 1.1, ones that are important to this book and the theory developed herein. The first is that, where nuptiality occurs early, it is especially early for women. Consider the figures on age gaps at marriage, given in the table (see Note 7 for the formulas).[7] Note that the age gaps tend to be larger where marriage takes place at early ages in these regions; females are considerably younger than their spouses. This is decidedly not the case in those areas where matrimony takes place at advanced ages.

The second observation is that nuptiality appears to vary not only with mortality but also with marital fertility. In this context note that areas where marriage occurs early and universally tend to have fairly substantial values for I_g. Where I_g is high (and/or mortality is low), I_m tends to be low. Note that this apparent inversion of I_g and I_m serves to equalize I_f across populations in nineteenth-century Europe (because $I_f \cong I_g I_m$—a point that can be sensed, at least in part, from the figures for crude birth rates (CBRs, births per 1000 population). Were Italy, for example, to have an I_g value as high as that of Norway, the overall CBR would exceed 40 per 1000 population. More generally we can see that the relationship among all three variables (nuptiality, marital fertility, and mortality) tends to equalize the natural rate of increase (NRI, which by definition is the CBR minus the CDR, where CDR is the crude death rate measured as deaths per 1000 population) across these populations. For example, were Russia, at the end of the nineteenth century, to enjoy mortality levels of the sort enjoyed by Sweden in 1880, the NRI would equal 31 per 1000 instead of 13 per 1000. These observations should be kept in mind because they will receive considerable attention in the theoretical and empirical analysis of this book. The point to be made here is that Hajnal's proposition concerning the variation of nuptiality with mortality can be extended to incorporate a third variable, marital fertility, as well.

Now consider the second major component of natality, marital fertility, which is represented in Table 1.1 by I_g. Note that the levels of I_g vary considerably, from .65 to .77, before any of these areas' populations have entered into their fertility transitions. To understand the meaning of this variation, we must consider the distinction advanced by the noted French demographer Henry (1961)—that between natural fertility and parity-specific control. By natural fertility, Henry means the marital fertility that obtains when a couple does not practice "deliberate control"—deliberate control being behavior by which a couple modifies its reproductive practices after achieving a certain number of births, a certain parity. Thus Henry refers to deliberate control as parity-specific control. (Chapter 3 and Appendix 7 develop these notions further and provide examples; in particular, Chapter 3 characterizes the fertility transition as the increase in an index of parity-specific control.) It should be noted that Coale's Hutterite indices are based quite explicitly on the natural fertility concept. The Hutterite women of the cohort of 1921 to 1930 did not practice, to the best of our knowledge, parity-specific control: they were a natural fertility population. Moreover, their lactation practices and relatively high fecundity meant that their level of natural fertility was exceptionally high. And here we arrive precisely at the point where we can posit a thesis as to why I_g varies before there is any parity-specific control: because fecundity, the presence of postpartum sexual taboos, and lactation practices vary among populations, one would expect I_g to vary as a consequence.

The third major theme of the European Fertility Project consists in describing the fertility transition itself. The two major points to be made in this context can be simply stated: the fertility transition and its parameters —duration, speed, and timing—should be gauged in terms of levels and movements in the index I_g (not I_f, I_m, or I_h); and there is considerable diversity in the transition experience in terms of the parameters of the transition (i.e., the various facets involving I_g) and the other related components of natality (e.g., I_m and I_f).

To illustrate these points, consider Fig. 1.1, which gives values of I_f, I_g, and I_m for two European countries, Sweden and Italy, during (and to some extent before) their transitions. Note that I_m actually increases for both countries, which tends to increase the overall fertility I_f (recall that $I_f \cong I_g I_m$). That overall fertility in fact falls to low levels is due strictly to the precipitous and irreversible declines in I_g. Thus the transitions can be dated from the period at which I_g begins its irreversible decline (irreversible until it reaches a floor at low levels; no statement is intended about fluctuations in I_g after the transition in marital fertility to a low level is achieved). The speed of decline can also be characterized in terms of how long it takes I_g to fall to low levels once it begins its decline. Figure 1.1 suggests that the transition was more rapid in Sweden than in Italy. Note the diversity in timing and duration between these two countries and also the difference in the speed at which and extent to which I_m increases. The universality of decline in I_g as the hallmark of the transition coupled with the associated regional diversities are basic observations of the European Fertility Project and have been

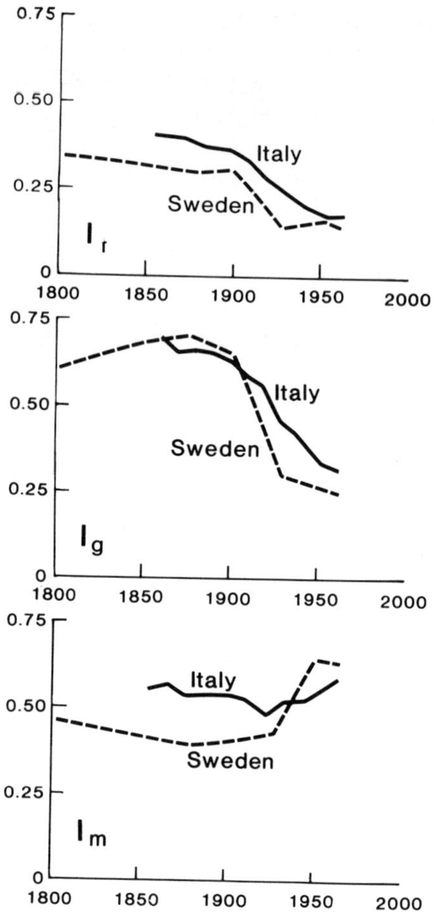

Fig. 1.1. Hutterite indices, Sweden and Italy.

essential to its spirit from its very inception. For example, Coale (1973:63) writes:

> The strong difference from region to region in the conditions under which fertility declines was first noticed in W. Leasure's research on his doctoral dissertation, a study of change in fertility in Spain [see Leasure (1963)]. . . . When Spain is divided into the standard regions that are used by Spanish statistical authorities, regions delineated in part because they once constituted different kingdoms, and differ in language and traditions, analysis of variance shows that over 90 percent of the total variance in marital fertility is between regions and less than 10 percent within. Similar results have been found by Knodel in Germany.

Thus a careful study of regionality, at the provincial level, has been a major emphasis of the European Fertility Project all along.

The diversity of transitions uncovered by the European Fertility Project is fascinating, and it is clear that robust treatment and theory of fertility transitions should cope both with the question of why I_g declines, and how and why the diversity occurs and its implications for the process of the transition. One approach to this question would be to contrast systematically the experience of two regions within Europe. Presumably their fertility transitions would have to be rather different, and this contrast would capture the process of diversity. But would diversity captured in this way be enough? Would it not be better to expand the geographical scope of the inquiry to strengthen the contrast between the populations under examination? In this section we should like to suggest why the inclusion of Eastern Asia immeasurably broadens the range of potential comparisons. Before this case is argued, it will be useful to discuss briefly the notion of Eurasia.

A number of scholars have noted that a historical perspective that encompasses Eurasia is useful in understanding the dynamics of modern economic and social development. In a provocative and stimulating historical synthesis, McNeill (1963) argues that the notion of a balance of power and exchange of cultural and technological developments among the four great civilizations of the Eurasian land mass—European, Chinese, Indian, and Moslem—provides a fascinating way of understanding the expansion of civilization throughout history. (It should be noted that, in terms of the cultural identity of modern societies in the world today, almost all societies are either located within this great land mass or have cultures partially derivative of the Eurasian cultures.) Jones (1981) picks up this theme in a recent book that attempts to explain why industrialization began in Europe as opposed to elsewhere in Eurasia. And Lewis (1978), concentrating on the period 1870–1914, shows how the two great migration streams from Eurasia in the eighteenth and nineteenth centuries—a European migration largely to more temperate climates (e.g., North America and Australia) and an Asiatic migration (mainly Chinese and Indian) largely to tropical climates (e.g., Southeast Asia and Africa)—were instrumental not only in settling and providing labor for these frontier regions hitherto sparsely settled and largely removed from the great economic and social advances occurring within Eurasia but also in determining the factoral terms of trade and standards of living of these frontier regions into which these migration flows were directed.

Granted, then, that the idea of formulating comparisons among several areas and/or countries within Eurasia has a tradition within the literature, why does it seem especially reasonable to discuss fertility within this context? Why, for example, should we not compare a European experience with that of a population in a temperate or tropical area of fairly recent settlement, like the United States or Canada? To see the problems attendant on

TABLE 1.2

Fertility, Mortality, and Population Increase for Selected Asian Countries or Regions Prior to Their Modern Fertility Transitions[a]

Country and approximate date	Fertility										Mortality		Natural rate of increase (NRI)
	Crude birth rate (CBR)	Nuptiality characteristics						Hutterite indices			Crude death rate (CDR)	Infant mortality rate (IMR)	
		Males (% single)		Females (% single)		Age gap at marriage at wife's age							
		25–29	45–49	20–24	45–49	20	25	I_m	I_g	I_h			
Central Asia, 1897	—	—	—	—	.4	—	—	.89	.53	—	—	—	—
Central Asia, 1970	—	—	—	—	2	—	—	.72	.64	—	—	—	—
Korea, 1925[b]	45	12	2	3	1	3.4	4.1	.88	.52	.11	35	—	10
Korea, 1960	36	37	.2	49	.1	.6	3.7	.66	.72	.00	12	—	24
Japan, 1925	36	25	2	30	2	2.5	4.1	.70	.55	.05	20	167	16
Taiwan, 1915[c]	43	27	5	13	.5	—	—	.79	.60	—	29	191	14
Taiwan, 1930[c]	45	17	4	14	.7	—	—	.78	.67	—	22	151	23

[a] Sources: Mosk (1979d); Nihon. Sōrifu Tōkeikyoku; United Nations (1973). Note that dashes indicate data not available.

[b] Actual rate of population increase (between 1920–1924), not natural rate. Crude death rate calculated as difference between crude birth rate and rate of population increase.

[c] Percentage single for age groups 45–49 is actually for 35 years of age and over.

such an approach, it is useful to consider the distinction, made a number of years ago by Simon Kuznets, between the demographic and economic experiences of open and closed countries. By an "open" country Kuznets means one with a substantial frontier, such as the areas of temperate and tropical settlement in the nineteenth century. It has been convincingly shown for the United States (by Yasuba, 1962) that the existence of a substantial frontier encouraged early marriage and consequently high overall fertility. That is to say, a population mainly derivative of Europe in terms of its rules and attitudes concerning inheritance and the like was able, in the presence of a substantial frontier, virtually to ignore constraints on nuptiality that helped to hold down natality in Europe. As the American frontier was settled, fertility tended to fall toward European levels; much of this decline could be explained by an increase in marriage ages to European levels, due to increased costs and diminished opportunities for young men to acquire land. A comparison between a frontier open nation and a closed one from which the open nation drew many of its numbers (e.g., European emigration to the United States) tells us something about the impact of the frontier; but it does not tell us much about diversity of fertility transitions in areas of dense and long-established settlement. It would seem better to compare closed populations with one another, or open populations with one another. We are therefore drawn back to the notion of comparisons within Eurasia.

If we restrict our investigation to regions of Eurasia, we are almost forced to concentrate on Europe and East Asia because many Eurasian populations outside of these regions (e.g., Islamic and Indian populations) have yet to complete (or in many instances even commence) fertility transitions. But if we restrict ourselves to comparisons between zones of Europe and zones of East Asia, do we have sufficient diversity of experience in the evolution of fertility?

Table 1.2 suggests that in this case we do have such diversity. A perusal of this table covering regions of Northeast Asia reveals that marriage occurred extremely early for both sexes and virtually universally before the transitions in these areas. Age gaps at marriage were quite large compared with those in nineteenth-century Western Europe, whereas levels of I_g (marital fertility) appear to have been very low by the same comparison (see Table 1.1). Also note in Table 1.2 that I_g appears to rise in these populations over time and I_m (nuptiality) appears to fall before the transition in I_g begins. This pattern can be seen most clearly in the Korean series illustrated in Fig. 1.2. Before I_g begins its irreversible decline around the late 1950s in Korea, the index actually reveals a pronounced and sustained secular increase. The national Japanese series, also represented in Fig. 1.2, does not extend back in a fully reliable manner before 1920. However Chapter 5 will present

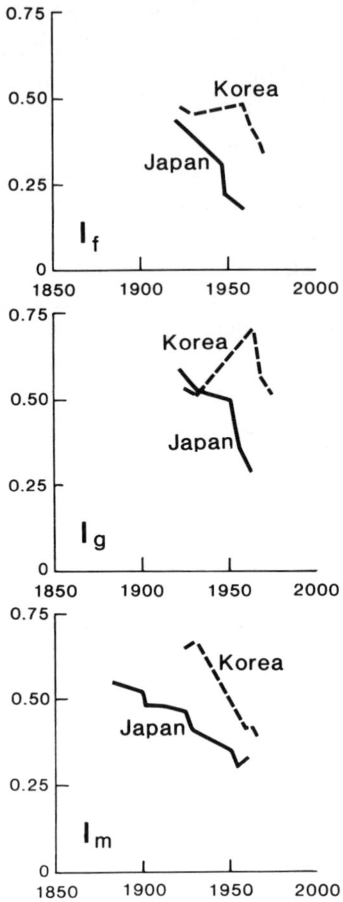

Fig. 1.2. Hutterite indices, Japan and Korea.

regional data for Japan that suggests I_g rose substantially in Japan before World War I.

Thus it would appear that a comparison between the experience of Western European and East Asian populations is eminently reasonable. Coale (1979:22–23) has remarked on the great interest inherent in such an approach:

> When we extend our purview from the experience of populations in Western Europe and overseas areas settled by Western Europeans to Russia and the central Asian republics especially, and to populations of Chinese culture, the variety of changes in fertility that are seen to accompany modernization is much extended . . . in spite of the unifying concept that the demographic transition promised, it becomes more complex—and more interesting—the more it is studied.

The only problem concerns the lack of systematic work on Asia equivalent to the European Fertility Project. Irene Taeuber, author of a celebrated general work on Japanese population (Taeuber, 1958), had been at work on a major project concerning the Chinese population, which would have included systematic work on other populations in Northeast Asia as well. Unfortunately Taeuber died (in the early 1970s) in the midst of her research project, so the synthesis she had conceived of remains unachieved. (See Hårm, 1976, for a discussion of Taeuber's data tape, and Orleans, 1976, for a bibliography of works on Chinese population, which includes many of Taeuber's articles containing her preliminary results from the project.) Cho and Kobayashi (1979) have edited a book containing papers on various East Asian populations. Unfortunately the analyses in that volume are not tied together thematically and methodologically like the publications that have emerged from the European Fertility Project. General far-reaching comparisons between European and Asian populations are thus beyond the resources of any scholar at the moment.

1.3. The Approach

The central aim of this study is to develop an economic and demographic model of the household that, among other things, can account for the evolution of natality in a variety of populations (the model can definitely be applied to a much wider variety of concerns, but this study will concentrate on its implications for fertility). In particular, the model is applicable to populations in which a patriarchal stem family system prevails. This system characterized a considerable number of the regions of Eurasia in the nineteenth and twentieth centuries and, as shown in Chapter 4, was in place during that time in Japan and Sweden. In fashioning a model of the household that accounts for levels and trends of natality in these two populations, this study implicitly deals with the question of how and why diversity occurs in the evolution of natality. Although this theory probably does not account for all of the diversity in the evolution of natality observed for Eurasia, it does offer one hypothesis that, with suitable modification, can be extended to other regions of Eurasia and the rest of the world as well.

The organization of this book is as follows. The next chapter lays out the model of the household and demonstrates that this can be fruitfully applied to an analysis of trends in and levels of natality. The discussion focuses around a simple, basic equation that captures the essence of the theory behind this study. Part II (Chapters 3–4), begins the empirical work, with a systematic comparison of aggregate economic and social development in Japan and Sweden and shows that this particular comparison is unusually-worthwhile. Chapter 4 provides a good deal of evidence about the institutional rules governing household behavior and the economic and demographic operation of the household in Japan and Sweden and demonstrates the applicability of the theory of the household for Japanese and Swedish populations. Finally, Part III (Chapters 5–8) shows that this theory can account empirically for the evolution of natality in Japan and Sweden over the period 1880–1960. Thus the third part of this volume especially contributes an explanation for the diversity of evolutions in natality associated with economic development in the nineteenth and twentieth centuries.

Notes to Chapter 1

1. On Hungary, see Demeny (1968).
2. For a fairly detailed discussion of the history of this project, see Haines (1978).
3. See, among others, Demeny (1968) on Austria–Hungary, Leasure (1963) on Spain, Livi-Bacci (1971, 1977) on Portugal and Italy, Knodel (1974) on Germany, Lesthaeghe (1977) on Belgium, Van de Walle (1974) on France, and Coale *et al.* (1979) on Russia.
4. See Coale (1965) for the first presentation of this methodology.
5. The age-specific marital fertility rates of these Hutterite women (F_i) are .330 for 15–19; .550 for 20–24; .502 for 25–29; .447 for 30–34; .406 for 35–39; .222 for 40–44; and .061 for 45–49 where the rates are given per woman in each age group.
6. A fifth Hutterite index I_m^* is another index for the proportion of women married computed in the European Fertility Project. Using the variable definitions from the text, the formula for this index is $I_m^* = \Sigma(m_i/w_i)F_i/\Sigma F_i$.
7. Age gaps at marriage (at exact age of wife x) have been calculated using the following method (on the basis of census figures only):

(1) Beginning with data on married males 15–54 and females 15–49 by quinquennial age classes, cumulate the column of married females to obtain cumulated married females less that 20, less than 25, etc; do the same for males. Denote CMF_x as the cumulated married females to age x and CMM_x as cumulated married males to age x.

(2) Match the cumulated figures CMF_{20}, CMF_{25}, . . . , CMF_{50} against the cumulated male column. In the general case CMF_x lies between CMM_y and CMM_{y+5}, and usually between CMM_x and CMM_{x+5} (i.e., $x = y$). It is possible that there might be no match if $CMF_x > CMM_y$ for all y (e.g., if CMF_{50} were to exceed CMM_{55}). In this case no estimate is obtained.

(3) Calculate the gap as a ratio. In the general case, where $CMM_y \leq CMF < CMM_{y+5}$, the estimated age gap at marriage for exact age x of wife is

$$AG_x = \frac{CMF_x - CMM_y}{CMM_{y+5} - CMM_y} 5 + (y - x)$$

For almost all cases $y = x$, so the formula usually reduces to

$$AG_x = \frac{CMF_x - CMM_x}{CMM_{x+5} - CMM_x} 5$$

I am grateful to Simon Kuznets for suggesting this technique to me.

CHAPTER 2

The Argument

2.1. Introduction

This chapter will set forth a theory of the household in a population that adheres to a patriarchal stem family system, and this will be applied to the problem of explaining levels of and trends in natality in such a population. The discussion is organized along the following lines. The next section presents the basic thesis. Section 2.3 then advances a simple mathematical model that captures the essence of that thesis. Section 2.4 provides some possible modifications of and amplifications to the model of the household and confronts possible objections to this approach. Section 2.5 considers the implications of our model of the household for natality before the fertility transition, and Section 2.6 considers the same during the transition. Finally in Section 2.7 this approach for analyzing the household and fertility is compared with other approaches, and mention is made of some of the major contributions that have been advanced in this field by economists and sociologists.

2.2. Brief Statement of the Thesis

The basic theory concerns the operation of a peasant household that controls a fixed amount of land and arrives at its own decisions about production and consumption, subject to institutional rules and exogenous constraints (e.g., the operation of external labor markets and the general level of health prevailing in the surrounding community).

Institutional Rules

The relevant institutional rules governing the patriarchal stem family system are twofold: (a) Labor tasks are differentiated on the basis of sex; and (b) One son inherits the land when the patriarch, the household head, dies or retires. The surviving parent(s) continue to reside with the heir, but the other children leave.

Decision Making

Decision making in the household is characterized as follows: (a) The patriarch makes decisions for the household subject to bargaining with household members. The patriarch's principal motivations in decision making are his own welfare and continuation of the family line on the land. (b) The patriarch has leverage over his children; specifically he arranges jobs and/or marriages for them, grants them bequests, and allocates consumption goods to them. Because the patriarch has leverage, he secures labor services from his offspring (i.e., he controls their labor services during a certain period of their lives). We may summarize and slightly amplify on these two points with the following scheme.

Household member	Motivation	Control instruments	Constraints
Patriarch	Maximize his income and continue his family	Bequests and dowries; arrangements of marriages and jobs	Children can leave home
Son	Maximize his income and marry young enough to continue his family	Working for or denying work effort to patriarch	Alternative forms of employment available to him
Daughter	Maximize her income by marrying a male with earning power, and ensure her old-age security by marrying at a sufficiently young age	Working for or denying work effort to patriarch	Alternative forms of employment available to her

With these assumptions about decision making, subject to the institutional rules previously elaborated, we can derive some simple and useful properties of household behavior.

Economic–Demographic Adjustment

Adjustment mechanisms that involve demographic variables adjusting to a combination of economic and demographic variables through a process of maximization are now described. Specifically the patriarch has three demographic instruments over which he exercises choice: the length of interbirth intervals, the age of his wife when they marry, and whether or not to cease reproduction altogether at some point through terminal abstinence. Variables that are exogenous to the household when the head goes about making his decisions are the age at which *he* is able to marry, the general state of health of the community, the sex ratio of births, and the capacity to work as a function of age.

The model can now be formulated as a problem in constrained maximization. To maximize his own welfare and to perpetuate the family line, the patriarch adopts a strategy of natural fertility by which he regulates birth intervals and determines his bride's age at marriage so as to secure the maximum economic value from her at marriage. This will be subject to their meeting the constraint (on reproduction) that there will always be at least a certain number of male workers on the land at all times (technically, the total household capacity to produce a given amount of work at all times). The patriarch obtains the future flow of male labor supply for his household from his current flow of births. Meeting the constraint on internal household labor supply guarantees that his lineage will continue into the future as a production unit. The logic of this argument can be broken into three parts.

(a) The patriarch looks for two things in a bride: economic value (dowry, skills) and a capacity to produce surviving children (a diminishing function of her age across the relevant ages at marriage). The patriarch maximizes the age of his bride (and thus maximizes her economic value) subject to her providing sufficient reproductive value to meet the constraint on the internal male labor supply.

(b) A natural fertility strategy dominates over one of terminal abstinence because the latter requires a more youthful bride than the former (i.e., greater reproductive value in the early years of marriage) and, consequently, loss of economic value. Moreover natural fertility ensures a steady flow of children who can provide labor services and serve as substitutes for older children who might die or prove incompetent (insurance motive).[1]

(c) The patriarch regulates birth intervals (through lactation practices and postpartum sexual taboos) so that each year of reproductive life yields the maximum possible number of surviving children (this is necessary if the patriarch is to maximize the age of his bride). If birth intervals are too short, infants may die in unnecessarily high proportions; if birth intervals are too protracted, periods of reproductive life will be wasted (i.e., used inefficiently). (See Appendix 8 for a discussion of the literature on this point.

Contemporary surveys of women in Africa and Indonesia suggest couples behave precisely in this way.)

In brief, efficiency in a demographic strategy for a peasant household, which adheres to a patriarchal stem family system and consequently operates under a constraint on total household labor supply, requires that the patriarch select a natural fertility strategy with optimum birth intervals so that the economic value of his bride is maximized.

Two assumptions about the exogenous variables that constrain maximization deserve mention. First, a man marries relatively late because he must await the death or retirement of his father before he acquires sufficient assets to found a new line. Second, the age schedule of mortality and morbidity depends on community health conditions; the worse health is, the higher are the risks of death. An important implication of this second point is that when conditions governing health are relatively poor (as in premodern Japan) the optimal level of natural fertility is relatively low; thus a man tends to marry a youthful bride with little dowry but sufficient reproductive value guaranteed through her youth. When health conditions are relatively good (as in premodern Sweden), a man tends to wed an older bride with a larger dowry because the optimal level of natural fertility is very high.

This completes a brief overview of this simplified model of the household. It is formalized in the next section using a basic mathematical equation, and this equation is used to derive the model's analytical properties. Now we turn to the equilibrium properties of aggregate populations.

Aggregate Relationships

Health conditions are positively related to income, and mortality is negatively related to income. Hence levels of natural fertility rise as income per head increases; and nuptiality will adjust to this process, that is, the age at marriage of females increases with the rising trend in income.

Undermining Influences

The theory emphasizes two structural changes in accounting for the disappearance of both the household behavior described by the economic–demographic adjustment mechanism sketched out in the preceding analysis and the associated aggregate demographic properties (including the end of the regime of natural fertility). These changes are as follows: (a) the expansion of education, which offers job certification independent of the patriarch; and (b) the growth of labor markets, which offer alternatives to the children and diminishes the patriarch's control. The result of these two structural shifts is that the costs of patriarchal leverage rise and the benefits from patriarchal leverage fall; this new balance of costs and benefits encourages parity-specific control (i.e., the ending of the practice of natural fertility).

This completes a brief overview of the thesis of this book. Now we can turn to a more formal presentation of the model of household behavior.

2.3. The Basic Equation

This section summarizes the essence of the economic–demographic model using a simple mathematical equation. Some analytical properties of this equation will be derived and some examples given. All functions for which a derivative is defined are assumed to be differentiable in their ranges of definition.

We begin with definitions for the following variables:

A_m = age at marriage of patriarch, household head
A_f = age at marriage of patriarch's wife
a_m = age of patriarch
a_f = age of patriarch's wife
$B(a_m)$ = births at age a_m for patriarch
$p(x)$ = probability of survival to age x
$\bar{p}(a_m)$ = probability that patriarch will survive from age A_m to a_m [$\bar{p}(a_m) = p(a_m)/p(A_m)$]
l = measure of weighted combination of length of postpartum sexual taboos and lactation, infanticide, etc.
h = measure of community health conditions
$s(l)$ = component of $p(x)$ that depends only on length of birth intervals prevailing in an individual's family of origin
$p^*(x, h)$ = component of $p(x)$ that depends only on age and health conditions of community [$p(x) = s(l)p^*(x, h)$]
$n(x)$ = Hutterite natural fertility schedule (a function of the age of the mother, x) (See discussion in Chapter 1)
$M(l, h)$ = component of natural fertility schedule that depends on the population's health conditions h and on l (For convenience this is indexed so that $M(l, h) \leq 1$)
l^* = value of l that maximizes $s(l)M(l, h)$
$w(x)$ = capacity to work as a function of age x (males only)
$c(x)$ = consumption as a function of age x (males only)
$W(a_m)$ = total capacity to work in household (i.e., all male labor controlled by patriarch) as a function of patriarch's age a_m (males only)

$CW(a_m)$ = total children's capacity to work in household (i.e., all male children's labor controlled by patriarch) as a function of patriarch's age a_m (males only)

$CC(a_m)$ = total children's consumption in household as a function of patriarch's age a_m (males only)

With these definitions we can proceed to a formal presentation of the model.

The basic condition for perpetuation of the family line as an economic unit is that total (male) work capacity controlled by the patriarch be above a critical minimum W^*. Let x be the patriarch's age, $A_m \leq x \leq a_m$. Then when the patriarch reaches a_m the total male work capacity stemming from year x is

$$w(a_m - x)B(x)p(a_m - x)$$

because males born when the patriarch is age x survive to the time when he is age a_m with probability $p(a_m - x)$ and, if they survive to that time, they will be age $a_m - x$ and will contribute labor capacity units $w(a_m - x)$. We can then express the total household work capacity controlled by the patriarch as a function of the patriarch's age a_m (assuming the sex ratio of births is 1:2) as

$$W(a_m) = w(a_m)\overline{p}(a_m) + \tfrac{1}{2} \int_{A_m}^{a_m} w(a_m - x)B(x)p(a_m - x)\, dx \qquad (2.1)$$

where $w(a_m)p(a_m)$ is the labor flow deriving directly from the patriarch and

$$CW(a_m) = \tfrac{1}{2} \int_{A_m}^{a_m} w(a_m - x)B(x)p(a_m - x)\, dx \qquad (2.2)$$

is the labor flow deriving from the patriarch's male children. The basic condition of the model, then, is

$$W(a_m) = w(a_m)\overline{p}(a_m) + \mathrm{CW}(a_m) \geq W^* \qquad (2.3)$$

for all a_m. To proceed further, we shall consider the term $CW(a_m)$ in greater detail.

The key to the analysis of $CW(a_m)$ is the decomposition of the various terms in the integral. First, we write the survival probability as a product of the terms $s(l)$, which reflects the survivorship of infants aged 0 (taken as a function of l), and $p^*(x, h)$, which depends on age x and the health conditions of the community h. That is,

$$p(x) = s(l)p^*(x, h) \qquad (2.4)$$

We also assume that $ds/dl > 0$ and $\partial p^*(x, h)/\partial h > 0$. Note that by definition $\partial p^*(x, h)/\partial x \leq 0$. Part (A) of Fig. 2.1 shows graphically that the effect of

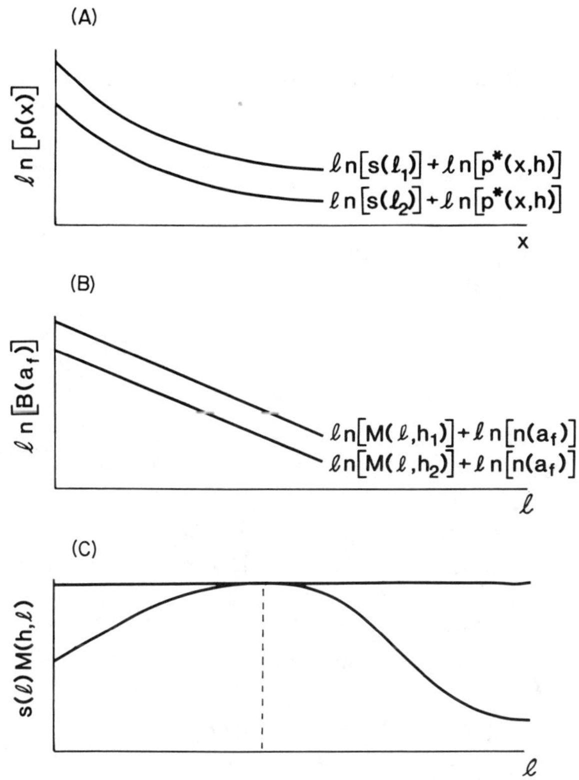

Fig. 2.1. Graphs of decompositions used in analysis of the basic equation. (A) Decomposition of $p(x)$: $l_1 > l_2$. (B) Decomposition of $B(a_f)$: $h_1 > h_2$. (C) Maximization of $s(l)\ M(h, l)$.

changing l is to shift survivorship up and down on a semilogarithmic scale.

Now let us decompose fertility $B(x)$. Given that we have natural fertility

$$B(a_f) = n(a_f)M(l,\ h) \tag{2.5}$$

where $n(a_f)$ is the (maximal) Hutterite natural fertility schedule; $M(l, h)$ a shift factor representing the effects of both the practices designed to lengthen birth intervals (e.g., lactation, postpartum sexual taboos) and the community health conditions h; and $dn(a_f)/da_f < 0$, $\partial M(l, h)/\partial l < 0$, and $\partial M(l, h)/\partial h > 0$. Equation (2.5) represents $B(a_f)$ as a function of the wife's age. We can rewrite it as a function of the patriarch's age because $a_f = a_m - (A_m - A_f)$, hence

$$B(a_f) = B[a_m - (A_m - A_f)] = n[a_m - (A_m - A_f)]M(l,\ h) \tag{2.6}$$

In Part (B) of Fig. 2.1 these relationships are shown on a semilogarithmic scale.

With these substitutions, let us return to the childhood component of Eq. (2.2). We can rewrite this as

$$CW(a_m) = \tfrac{1}{2} \int_{A_m}^{a_m} w(a_m - x)n[x - (A_m - A_f)]M(l, h)s(l)p^*(h, a_m - x)\, dx \tag{2.7}$$

And consequently we can take out the terms that do not depend on x from the integral, arriving at

$$CW(a_m) = [\tfrac{1}{2}M(l, h)s(l)] \int_{A_m}^{a_m} w(a_m - x)n[x - (A_m - A_f)]p^*(h, a_m - x)\, dx \tag{2.8}$$

Now consider the term $M(l, h)s(l)$. Recall that h is an exogenous variable, but l is an endogenous variable subject to choice. The assumption is that the patriarch chooses $l = l^*$ such that $s(l)M(l, h)$ is at a maximum (i.e., maximizes reproductive capacity subject to the constraint of community health conditions). Note that $ds(l)/dl > 0$ and $\partial M(l, h)/\partial l < 0$ so that a maximum or minimum must exist. In accordance with Part (C) of Fig. 2.1, we impose the additional second-order condition that $\partial^2 s(l)M(l, h)/\partial l^2 < 0$ so that in fact we have a maximum. Also note that, if h increases, the curve given in Part (C) of Fig. 2.1 shifts upward for *all* values of l because $\partial M/\partial h > 0$, and consequently, if h increases, the value of $s(l)M(l, h)$ at the maximum value of $l = l^*$ must increase. ($l = l^*$ will in general vary with h.) This is shown graphically in Part (C) of Fig. 2.1.

Now let us turn to Eq. (2.8), assuming that l^* has been chosen so that $\tfrac{1}{2}M(l^*, h)s(l^*) = k$ is a maximum. Then the remaining instrument available to the patriarch in formulating his strategy for perpetuation of the family line is A_f. The assumption is that, to maximize his wife's economic value, the patriarch maximizes A_f subject to the condition that

$$W(a_m) = w(a_m)\bar{p}(a_m) + \tfrac{1}{2}k \int_{A_m}^{a_m} w(a_m - x)n[x - (A_m - A_f)]p^*(h, a_m - x)\, dx \geq W^*$$

or (2.9)

$$CW(a_m) = \tfrac{1}{2}k \int_{A_m}^{a_m} w(a_m - x)n[x - (A_m - A_f)]p^*(h, a_m - x)\, dx \geq W^* - w(a_m)\bar{p}(a_m)$$

Examples worked out subsequently will show how to select the maximal ("cut-off") value for A_f, given values for k, A_f, and schedules for $w(x)$, $n(a_f)$, and $p^*(h, x)$.

Before turning to the examples, however, it would be useful to derive some other implications of this model of the household economy. The first concerns the balance between consumption and production units, a principal concern of theories of the peasant household going back to the classic work by Chayanov (1966). It can be seen that the total number of (male) consumption units under the patriarch's control, as a function of the patriarch's age a_m, is

$$C(a_m) = c(a_m)\overline{p}(a_m) + \tfrac{1}{2} \int_{A_m}^{a_m} c(a_m - x)B(x)p(a_m - x)\, dx$$
$$= c(a_m)p(a_m) + CC(a_m) \tag{2.10}$$

and thus the ratio of total (male) consumers to total (male) producers is

$$\frac{C(a_m)}{W(a_m)} = \frac{c(a_m)\overline{p}(a_m) + CC(a_m)}{w(a_m)\overline{p}(a_m) + CW(a_m)} \tag{2.11}$$

In this model, A_f and l are selected to meet the condition on the labor equation, and consumption simply adjusts to this. For this reason, the extent to which labor capacity is actually utilized (i.e., its intensity as measured in terms of hours worked per work unit) may well vary substantially over the life cycle of the household as the ratio C/W changes (it would be expected first to rise and then fall as the children grow from being consumers only to being both workers and consumers). It should also be noted that the model could be reformulated to take into account males and females, assuming specialization of labor tasks by sex. However, this would complicate the mathematics and not contribute significantly to the analysis undertaken here, so I hew to the simple and highly stylized version in the preceding equations.

The second implication of Eq. (2.3) concerns the relationship between health h and variables l and A_f subject to decision making. Differentiating Eq. (2.9) (incorporating the decompositions of mortality and natural fertility here) with respect to h and letting $k(l, h) = s(1)M(l, h)$, we have

$$\frac{\partial W(a_m)}{\partial h} = w(a_m)\frac{\partial \overline{p}(a_m)}{\partial h} + \frac{1}{2}\left[\frac{\partial k(l^*, h)}{\partial h}\right]$$
$$\cdot \left\{\int_{A_m}^{a_m} w(a_m - x)n[x - (A_m - A_f)]p^*(h, x)\, dx\right\}$$
$$+ \frac{1}{2}k(l^*, h)\left\{\int_{A_m}^{a_m} w(a_m - x)n[x - (A_m - A_f)]\frac{\partial p^*}{\partial h}\, dx\right\} \tag{2.12}$$

where

$$\frac{\partial k(l^*, h)}{\partial h} = \left(\frac{\partial s(l^*)}{\partial l^*}\frac{\partial l^*}{\partial h}\right)M(l^*, h) + s(l^*)\left(\frac{\partial M}{\partial h} + \frac{\partial M}{\partial l^*}\frac{\partial l^*}{\partial h}\right)$$

Note that l^* is a function of h in the sense that it maximizes $k(l, h)$ for each value of h. As h increases, $K(l, h)$ increases (i.e., the curve in Part (C) of Fig. 2.1 is shifted upward for all values of l). Thus even though we may have $\partial l^*/\partial h < 0$ (and, consequently, $(\partial s/\partial l^*)(\partial l^*/\partial h) < 0$), the overall sum for $\partial k/\partial h$ previously given must be positive. Because $\partial M(l, h)/\partial h > 0$, $\partial p^*(h, x)/\partial h > 0$ and the other terms in the equation are positive it follows that $\partial W(a_m)/\partial h > 0$. Thus if we consider households in two separate communities with different levels of health h_1 and h_2, we can ask how their demographic structures would differ. The household in the community with poorer h would have to bring in a younger bride to keep $W(a_m) \geq W^*$ $[\partial W(a_m)/\partial A_f = \partial W/\partial n \; \partial n/\partial A_f < 0]$. This result would be even stronger if, as is plausible, $w(x)$ is sensitive to h conditions (i.e., if maturation and diminution of work capacity in middle age are sensitive to health conditions).

Now we can proceed with some illustrative examples.

Example I Let us assume the following age schedules for $w(x)$ and $n(a_f)$:

$$w(x) = \begin{cases} 0, & x < 10 \\ \frac{1}{2}, & 10 \leq x < 15 \\ \frac{3}{4}, & 15 \leq x < 25 \\ 1, & 25 \leq x < 45 \\ \frac{3}{4}, & 45 \leq x < 55 \\ \frac{1}{2}, & 55 \leq x < 60 \\ 0, & 60 \leq x \end{cases}$$

and

$$n(a_f) = \begin{cases} 0, & a_f < 15 \\ .5 - .5/30(a_f - 15), & 15 \leq a_f < 45 \\ 0, & 45 \leq a_f \end{cases}$$

These schedules are graphed in Parts (A) and (B) of Fig. 2.2. According to the work schedule the patriarch begins "partial retirement" at age 45. We are thus especially interested in this crucial age when his work capacity begins a pronounced diminution. (Because of the shape of the fertility and work schedules—the latter remaining flat from ages 45 to 55—we need worry only about $CW(45)$. This is admittedly a bit artificial but allows us to concentrate on one age for the analysis.) Assume a simple age-specific death schedule in which $\frac{1}{3}$ of all infants die and there is no further mortality until age 60. Thus $p(45) = 1$ and $W(45) = (\frac{3}{4})(1) + CW(45)$. We assume different values for optimal levels of $s(l)M(l, h)$ and then compute the optimal A_f, the wife's age at marriage, under the condition that $W(45) \geq 1$ (i.e., $CW(45) \geq .25$) and the assumption that the husband marries at age 30. We then have

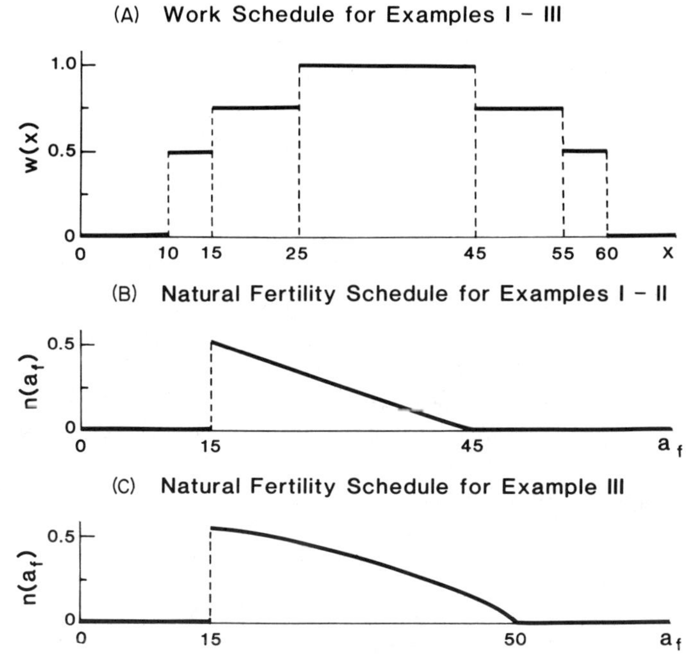

Fig. 2.2. Work schedule and natural fertility schedules for Examples I–III.

$$CW(45) = (\tfrac{1}{2})(\tfrac{2}{3})(\tfrac{1}{2})[s(l)M(l,\ h)]\left[\int_{A_f}^{A_f+5} n(x)\ dx\right]$$

(the first $\frac{1}{2}$ represents the sex ratio, the second $\frac{1}{2}$ the worker units, and the $\frac{2}{3}$ the survivorship rate); because, if the husband marries at age 30 and his children do not begin to provide work units until age 10, it is only from the fertility of the first five years of marriage that child work units useful to the patriarch at age 45 can come. Gathering together all of the constants into a general term k, we have

$$CW(45) = k \int_{A_f}^{A_f+5} [.5 - (.017)(x - 15)]\ dx$$

$$\cong k[3.6 - (.085)A_f]$$

We set $CW(45)$ equal to .25 and arrive at

$$A_f = \frac{3.6k - .25}{k(.085)} = 42.2 - \frac{2.94}{k}$$

The accompanying tabulation gives the results for reasonable values of $s(l)M(l, h)$. It should be noted that these derivations and computations have been approximated (rounded off) in the preceding discussion.

$s(l)M(l, h)$	k	A_f
.7	.11	15.5
.8	.13	19.7
.9	.15	22.7
1.0	.17	24.8

Example II Let us assume the same schedules for $w(x)$ and $n(a_f)$ used in Example I and that mortality by age is as follows: the infant death rate is $\frac{1}{3}$, and there is no further mortality until age 45, when the probability of death is .3 (i.e., $p(45) = .7$). Assume no further mortality until age 60. Assume also that the patriarch marries at age 25 and that $s(l)M(l, h) = .8$. Then we impose the condition as in Example I that $W(45) = (.7)(.75) + CW(45) \geq 1$. Thus $CW(45) = .47$, and we compute

$$CW(45) = k_1 \int_{A_f}^{A_f+5} [.5 - (.017)(x - 15)]\, dx$$

$$+ k_2 \int_{A_f+5}^{A_f+10} [.5 - (.017)(x - 15)]\, dx$$

where the constants k_1 and k_2 incorporate worker units at a rate of $\frac{3}{4}$ and $\frac{1}{2}$, respectively. The first integral works out to $k_1(3.6 - .085A_f)$, and the second integral to $k_2(3.2 - .085A_f)$. Approximating our computations to the nearest tenth, we have

$$\begin{aligned} CW(45) &= k_1 3.6 + k_2 3.2 - (k_1 + k_2)(.085)A_f \\ &= 1.14 - .028A_f = .47 \end{aligned}$$

and thus $A_f = 23.9$. This second example suggests how considerations of the patriarch's own mortality (i.e., the level of adult mortality) might tend to push downward ages at marriage for females.

Example III Again let us assume the same work schedule as in Examples I and II and approximate the natural fertility schedule with a logarithmic assumption [see Fig. 2.2, Part (C)].

The natural fertility schedule we adopt is

$$n(a_f) = \begin{cases} 0, & a_f < 15 \\ \ln\left(2 - \dfrac{a_f}{50}\right), & 15 \leq a_f < 50 \\ 0, & 50 \leq a_f \end{cases}$$

We make the same mortality assumptions as in Example I and also suppose the patriarch marries at age 30. Again we concentrate on $CW(45)$ and the condition $W(45) \geq 1$ (i.e., $CW(45) \geq .25$). Collecting together the constants as in Example I into a single constant k we have

$$CW(45) = k \int_{A_f}^{A_f+5} \ln\left(2 - \frac{x}{50}\right) dx$$

Letting $u = 2 - x/50$, we have

$$k \int_{A_f}^{A_f+5} \ln\left(2 - \frac{x}{50}\right) dx = -50k \int_{2-(A_f/50)}^{2-[(A_f+5)/50]} \ln(u)\, du$$

$$= -50k[u \ln(u) - u] \Big|_{2-(A_f/50)}^{2-[(A_f+5)/50]} = .25$$

Various approximations to $\ln(u)$ (e.g., using a Taylor series expansion) will yield approximations for A_f.

This completes the group of examples. Although the examples and Eq. (2.3) on which they rest are certainly stylized, they do provide a useful mathematical framework for understanding the basic logic of the model developed here. Now let us turn to a discussion of some qualifications of and amplifications to the theory of the household.

2.4. The Economics of the Peasant Household

At various points in the previous two sections, some assumptions or assertions about peasant households were made that require more detailed discussion. One was the assumption of a fixed amount of land; a second concerned the reliance on family labor, which is implicit in the basic equation; a third concerned the impact of the ratio of consumers to workers in determining work effort; and a fourth involved the shape of the work schedules used in the analysis.

First let us consider the issue of land. It is not necessary to assume that the amount of land is absolutely constant, and no direct use of such an assumption is made in the mathematical derivations. The point of the assumption is that the household does not consider the adjustment of the amount of land it cultivates, compared with its family size and composition, a *major* part of its strategy for perpetuation of the family line and maximization of welfare (as households in Russia during the late nineteenth and early twentieth centuries may have done, through some collective reorganization of village land or through market mechanisms; see Chayanov, 1966). The possibility of renting land (or leasing it to others) is an option that

Japanese and Swedish peasant households did adopt (in adjusting the land they cultivated to their internal household labor supplies), and this process can be interpreted as an efficient adjustment of the household to its changing position in the life cycle (e.g., when labor capacity increases, the household may attempt to rent land to bolster the marginal and average productivity of household labor). The distinction between land held in long-term tenancy agreements (according to which a household holds land for years or even through generations) and land directly owned by the household is important for some social issues but is irrelevant to the analysis. The point of Eq. (2.3) is that the household perpetuates itself through time as a production unit; land per se is not directly involved in the analysis. It would be useful to develop a class of models that would incorporate land into them (e.g., one could make W^* depend on land size L), but this would take us away from the principal concerns of this work.

Second, let us clarify the issue of reliance on family labor. There are a number of reasons for believing that this assumption is a reasonable strategy for perpetuation of the family line and maximization of the patriarch's welfare. First, because output per head is relatively poor and the chance of crop failure considerable in most agrarian peasant economies, households opt for a "safety first" strategy by avoiding the hiring of outside labor, relying almost exclusively on family labor.[2] For, if the family brings in an outside member as a domestic servant or a hired hand on a short-term contract, the family must pay out wages to him or her regardless of whether or not the crop fails.[3] And if the harvest is poor, payment of wages may drive the household into debt and force it to relinquish land. In the case where family members alone constitute the household labor force, the final output is simply divided after the harvest. Moreover, family members share in the output, so their incentive to produce is correspondingly greater and their supervision costs are lower than for paid employees. Second, family members share a common socialization, which facilitates teamwork in production. Finally, the intensity of labor input varies considerably with the seasons, and the timing of these spurts is not perfectly predictable; so that arranging for short-term contracts entails considerable risk, whereas hiring workers on long-term contracts involves paying them for idle periods. Thus households concerned with maintaining their hold on the land (whether the household owns the land or holds it by customary right through a tenancy agreement is of little consequence here) and unable to amass considerable stores of goods and food-stuffs because of low and fluctuating yields, opt for a strategy that attempts to guarantee a family labor supply sufficient to meet the demand for labor throughout the year. Because status typically attaches to the control of land and labor when these are almost the only means of generating income and because there are few other means of enhancing

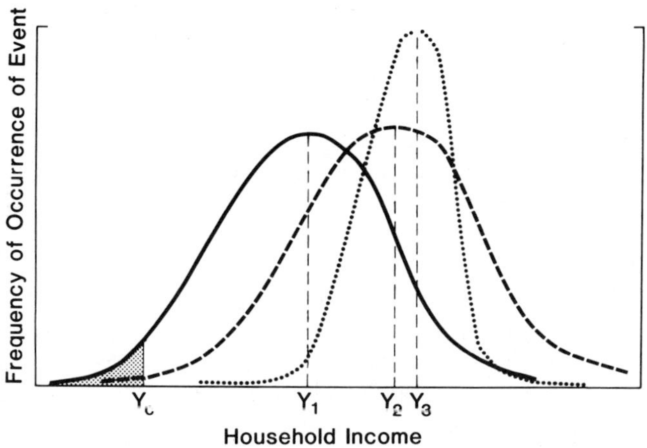

Fig. 2.3. Household income in peasant economy under different assumptions about its mean and distribution and cut-off income Y_c.

status (income being too low for conspicuous consumption), the reliance on family labor also tends to ensure efficiently the perpetuation of the status of the patriarch and his household over time.

The logic of the safety first principle underlying these arguments is captured graphically by Fig. 2.3, which shows the distribution of a typical household's income at various levels of the mean of that income Y_1, Y_2, and Y_3 in a peasant economy. The point to bear in mind is the relationship between the distribution of income and a lower bound for income (cut-off income) Y_c. If the household falls below Y_c, it finds itself in serious straits and may have to sell off assets or dissolve itself altogether as an agricultural enterprise in order to purchase food for consumption and seed for the next year's planting. Note that, even if the distribution remains unchanged, a shift in the mean (from Y_1 to Y_2) will substantially reduce the probability of falling short of Y_c and presumably will encourage the household head to take greater risks, including the hiring of paid workers. Moreover it is likely that, as agricultural productivity improves and average household income increases, the variance of household income decreases (the movement from Y_1 to Y_3 and the associated distributions as drawn in Fig. 2.3), further reducing the probability of falling below Y_c.

However, the obvious objection to the preceding argument concerning family labor is that the long-term opportunity costs of relying on the labor of children are greater than the benefits the patriarch secures. For children are net consumers for many years after birth before their contributions to a household's output exceeds their demand on household resources. If the present discounted value of the net benefits is calculated (using a positive interest rate), the net costs during the early years (discounted only slightly) will usually be found to outweigh the more heavily discounted net benefits later on.

This computation, however, assumes a perfect capital market. It also assumes that if the patriarch has fewer children, he invests as savings the resources he would have allocated to an additional child and that he later expends that income flow on hired labor. There are two objections to this line of reasoning.

First, capital markets are not perfect in such an environment. In a low or moderate-income setting, with widely fluctuating yields, few farmers ever find themselves in a position where they can set themselves up as financial intermediaries, borrowing money and being prepared to pay back loans with interest at some future time, because the risk of a short-term economic shortfall is so great. Should their own harvest fail, could they pay back their lenders? Moreover, costs of transportation and information are so considerable in a peasant economy that the size of most rural markets (in a low- or moderate-income setting) is fairly limited, discouraging urban merchants from entering these village markets as financial intermediaries. Moreover, even if there were one or two farmers in a village whose income and wealth were considerable (who could theoretically establish themselves as local bankers), how great would their gains be compared with bearing the considerable costs of establishing a banking operation to acquire funds for investment? Even if the going interest rates were fairly low, in a low-income rural setting having scant demand for industrial products would the opportunities for returns through investment exceed these rates? Also, because the harvest tends to be either good or bad for all farmers in a locality, if the crop failed for one of the lenders, it would probably fail for most of them, and consequently, the village banker would have to liquidate his assets rapidly to make payments. In short, capital markets in the typical peasant economy are far from perfect.

Second, there are the advantages that family labor has compared with paid labor. In addition to those benefits already outlined, family labor is preferable for another reason; the patriarch can pay a family member considerably less than the wage an equivalent hired worker would command. For the patriarch enjoys a monopoly in the placement of sons and daughters in jobs and marriages and this permits him to extract labor services from his wife and children at a cost equal to the consumption he foregoes by supporting the family worker in the household.[4] If this is substantially below the market wage (and in Chapter 4 evidence will be produced for Japan that supports this thesis), then he earns a considerable rent, a rent he would forego by saving in some other form and hiring labor at the market wage later.

In sum, the assumption of a strategy based on family labor does seem reasonable as a stylization of behavior in the peasant household. This is not to say that peasant households strictly relied on household labor in Japan and Sweden. For example, Chapter 4 reveals that Japanese farm families did use servants and hired laborers (although not on a significant scale) to adjust their labor supply over the life cycle (i.e., when their internal labor supply was scanty, they occasionally hired in labor; when it was adundant, they sent it out to work in other households' fields). But the possibility of such life cycle adjustments does not vitiate the basic logic of the demographic strategy as a means of securing an internal household labor force. (See Chapter 4 for a discussion of some of these points.) It would be useful to extend the formal model to the case in which one allows a mixed strategy (e.g., reliance on both internal household labor and hired labor). This considerably complicates the analysis, however, and proper development of this question requires a separate study.

The third issue to be considered here concerns variations in hours worked per work unit (i.e., unit of potential work capacity). In line with our previous notation, let C and W indicate the household's total number of consumers and workers, respectively. These are calculated by adjusting each household member for sex and age status and then summing to secure household totals.[5] As previously noted, the consumer–worker ratio (C/W) is computed by dividing C by W.

Now consider the life cycle of a patriarchal stem family. Part (A) of Fig. 2.4 captures this in terms of the C, W, and C/W variables. At the beginning of the life cycle depicted here (duration of the household's existence equal to zero), the son who assumes the headship has just secured control, thus being permitted to wed. His wife enters the household and his brothers and sisters depart, leaving him with his wife and aged parent(s). Initially his children would not provide labor, but they would consume (though they constitute a relatively small drain on the resources for consumption when they are very young). Thus C rises gradually over time as the number of offspring increase and they age, and W remains approximately constant until the eldest of the children reaches about age 10; then W rises sharply, more rapidly than C. As a result, the C/W ratio rises to a peak (at the point where W commences to rise) and then falls. Now consider hours worked per worker unit (*WHPW*) and hours worked by the husband (*WHH*). These are graphed in Part (B) of Fig. 2.4. Both rise to a peak at the point where the eldest child begins making substantial labor contributions (as does the variable *WHW*, hours worked by the wife, which is not graphed in the figure) and then decline. Because the father eventually begins to relinquish his tasks (i.e., his potential work capacity W declines), the *WHH* variable presumably falls more rapidly than the *WHPW* variable. In short, Fig. 2.4 captures the adjustment of hours worked by work unit as the household proceeds through its life cycle.

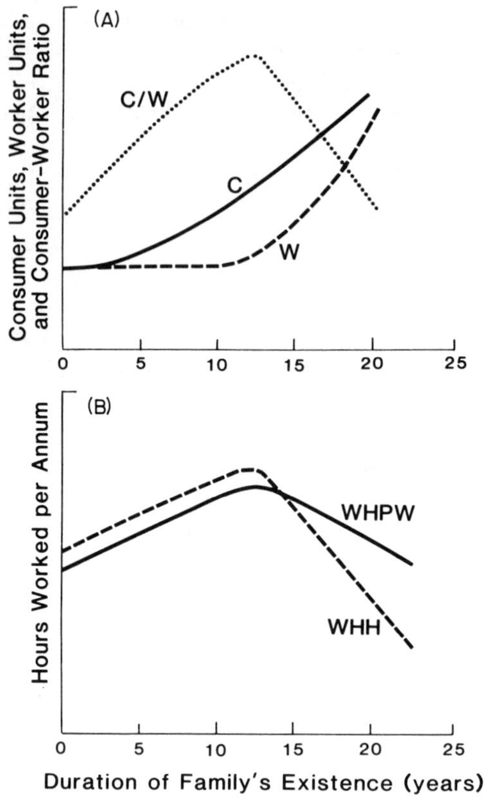

Fig. 2.4. Life cycle of peasant family in patriarchal stem family system: *C, W, C/W,* and hours worked.

The fourth and final issue to be taken up concerns the work schedules discussed in Section 2.3 of this chapter. For instance, consider the schedules utilized in Examples I–III and depicted in Part (A) of Fig. 2.2. Such a schedule is reasonable for the male heir to the land but would probably not adequately describe the work capacity (controlled by the patriarch) of the noninheriting son. In the case of such a son who leaves the household at a definite point, the work capacity controlled by the patriarch falls to zero when the son departs. An example of such a work schedule would be

$$w(x) = \begin{cases} 0, & x < 10 \\ \frac{1}{2}, & 10 \le x < 15 \\ \frac{3}{4}, & 15 \le x < 25 \\ 0, & 25 \le x \end{cases}$$

However, combining a schedule such as this with the schedule for heirs used in Examples I–III of Section 2.3 would not affect the results secured there but would complicate the discussion, therefore these refinements have been omitted from Section 2.3.

2.5. The Premodern Demographic Regime

The goal of this section is to show how the theory of the peasant household previously developed can be extended to a model of aggregate economic and demographic equilibrium for a population. A "premodern demographic regime" may be defined as the complex of nuptiality patterns, natural fertility levels, and mortality prevailing in an aggregate population before the onset of parity-specific control. Sections 2.2 and 2.3 have shown how these variables interlock in a model of household behavior. Now let us consider their interrelationship in an aggregate setting by touching on two issues: First, the relationship of aggregate levels of mortality and natural fertility to aggregate income per head; and second, the operation of marriage markets.

There is a considerable body of literature relating the material standard of living of a population to the average level of mortality prevailing in that population. Although there is some debate as to the extent to which income per head alone—as distinct from public health and medicine (which may or may not depend on the standard of living narrowly defined)—shapes mortality, it is generally agreed that income is an important determinant of levels of mortality. McKeown (1976), for example, places considerable weight on income per head, and especially food consumption, in accounting for the European mortality declines. And although Preston (1976) argues that income per head plays a more limited role than McKeown suggests, he also acknowledges that it is significant. It should be noted that Preston relies mainly on data for countries for the years 1930 and 1960 in drawing his inferences, whereas McKeown is mainly concerned with the period before 1930. Thus it is possible to reconcile these two positions, at least to a degree, by noting that Preston's information mainly relates to the epoch after antibiotics were developed (the scope of the medical contribution to mortality decline was presumably widened significantly by the introduction of antibiotics). In any event, the literature does support the idea that the standard of living is an important determinant of the death rate. For most causes of death, the connection between the standard of living and mortality, once the independent impact of public health and medical technology is removed, runs through the average state of personal health for members of the population; the health conditions improving as income levels are enhanced. Hence it is a reasonable inference that average levels of health and mortality for aggregate populations depend on income per capita for these populations, as well as on independent conditions like medical and public health technology and environmental circumstances like climate. It is, of course, possible that an association between income per capita and health might involve causation running the other way. Although there probably are some effects of health on productivity and the proportion of population that supplies labor, it is unlikely that association between income and health runs primarily in this direction.

The literature also supports the claims made in Sections 2.2 and 2.3 concerning the determinants of levels of natural fertility, although this is a complex issue that requires a more lengthy discussion than can be devoted to it here. For this reason, discussion of the latter issue is relegated to Appendix 8. Now because the state of health is a factor that shapes natural fertility levels and because income per head influences health conditions, it follows that natural fertility levels and mortality are both influenced by levels of income per capita for aggregate populations. In particular, if a population experiences a secular increase in income per head, we would expect its mortality level to drop and its level of natural fertility to increase.

The second issue to be touched on here is the operation of marriage markets. Two points are important. (a) The demand-driven model proposed in Sections 2.2 and 2.3 is reasonable on theoretical grounds as an approximation for aggregate populations. (b) Taking into consideration the size of marriage markets does not unduly affect the analysis.

On the first point, the question is that if the patriarch controls the marriage of his daughter, does he not also determine the age at which she weds, and consequently is not a supply-driven explanation more appropriate for aggregate populations? This objection would be cogent were it not for the bargaining that the model supposes takes place within the household. If the nuptials of a daughter are not arranged when she is at a "marriageable age" (i.e., within the range of ages that are in demand in the local marriage market), she may eventually find herself in a position where her father is unable to arrange a match for her at all. She could, however, withhold her labor services to her own household in retaliation. In consequence, patriarchs must seriously consider in their decision making the nature of demand conditions within the marriage market for their daughters. One would expect the supply considerations to lead to a variation in marriage ages about optimal levels, but a demand-driven thesis of the sort presented in Eq. (2.3) does seem to capture the essence of the situation as a first approximation.

On the second point, the question is: If marriage markets are relatively small within a peasant economy because of the substantial costs of search and information, could a dearth of marriageable partners in a given period so delay the marriages of eligible persons as to distort the pattern of observed ages at marriage in comparison to what one would expect on the basis of the model of optimal marriage ages? This problem has been studied through simulation experiments. Mosk (1981b) shows that, whereas mean ages at marriage turn out to be slightly higher in the simulations than in analytical calculations of optimal levels, the differences are not vast and the systematic relationship of levels of nuptiality to mortality and natural fertility is not distorted.[6]

Finally, let us formalize the preceding arguments. Let

y = income per capita
A_f = average age at marriage of females
M = average level of natural fertility
d = death rate

The logic of the preceding arguments is that for aggregate populations

$$M = G(y), \qquad \text{with } \frac{dG}{dy} > 0 \tag{2.13}$$

$$d = H(y), \qquad \text{with } \frac{dH}{dy} < 0 \tag{2.14}$$

and

$$A_f = J(M, d), \qquad \text{with } \frac{\partial J}{\partial M} > 0 \text{ and } \frac{\partial J}{\partial d} < 0 \tag{2.15}$$

Now note that

$$\frac{dA_f}{dy} = \frac{\partial J}{\partial M}\frac{dG}{dy} + \frac{\partial J}{\partial d}\frac{dH}{dy} \tag{2.16}$$

and that $dA_f/dy > 0$ because both $\partial J/\partial M$ and $\partial G/\partial y$ exceed zero and both $\partial J/\partial d$ and $\partial H/\partial y$ are less than zero.

The relationships laid out in Eqs. (2.13)–(2.16) represent the essential aggregate relationships to be taken up in the aggregative empirical analysis of Chapters 5–8 in Part III. That analysis, however, will also attempt to capture directly the effects of health with a variety of proxies. In any event Eqs. (2.13)–(2.16) will be useful to us in our later analysis and provide us with a useful summary of the arguments of this section. Now let us direct our attention to the problem of the undermining of the premodern demographic regime associated with modern economic development.

2.6. Structural Shift to a Modern Demographic Regime

In this section, using the concept of the costs of and benefits from economic leverage over children, we shall demonstrate how modernization undermines both the rationale for natural fertility and the effective operation of the patriarchal stem family system. That is, a general thesis will be sketched concerning the fertility transition. Moreover the question of the timing of the transition will be discussed, both in terms of why the Swedish transition occurred earlier than the Japanese fertility decline and also in connection with the diffusion of parity-specific control within each country taken separately. The emphasis in this section is on the analysis of the decline in marital fertility, although some issues relating to the evolution of nuptiality that occurs concomitantly with the diffusion of parity-specific control will also be briefly considered.

Although a number of the arguments used here have appeared in the literature before, the concept of the costs of and benefits from leverage provides an original and useful method for integrating the various points and carrying out the analysis.

Modernization undermines natural fertility and the patriarchal stem family system for several reasons. First, it increases the costs of maintaining economic leverage over children; second, it lessens the benefits from this leverage; and third, it changes the relative bargaining position of household members and thus changes the way decisions are fashioned within the family (i.e., undermines the patriarch's power). Let us first begin with increase in the costs of leverage.[7] Three factors of crucial importance in this process are the expansion of education, shifts in the structure of the labor force, and the development of intersectoral gaps in wages and income.

The expansion of education is probably the most important factor in increasing the costs of leverage, for it concerns the patriarch's ability to arrange both jobs and marriages. The idea is that, as the educational attainment of the population improves, employers begin to rely heavily on education as a means of screening persons for jobs, especially for positions where the firm makes significant investments in training employees and hopes for low turnover.[8] Utilizing family connections and recommendations as to the diligence and abilities of candidates from household heads whom the employer knows is a reasonable and efficient strategy for recruiting personnel when more standardized measures of potential productivity are unavailable. However, when significant levels of educational achievement become widely diffused throughout the population, an alternative and more efficient method of recruitment emerges.

In a society in which patriarchal stem families are prevalent, the initial effect of this shift toward education as a screening device will be on the costs of leverage over *sons;* because job opportunities for women outside household labor are initially restricted to short-term work periods, which are expected to terminate when the woman marries and enters the patriarchal family of her husband. Also, structural shifts in the demand for labor, especially an increase in the proportion of employees hired by large firms in the industrial and service sectors, will accentuate the costs incurred by the patriarch in placing sons; firms whose size precludes the concentration of hiring decisions in one person's hands tend to eschew reliance on family connections more thoroughly than those firms whose labor force is minuscule. Thus the expansion of education and its role in the placement of persons in jobs clearly affect the costs of leverage over sons; and those sons who do not expect to inherit the land have a special incentive in demanding more schooling from their father in exchange for their labor contributions.

Women are affected in an indirect way by this process. On the one hand, as we have just seen, the initial impact of educational expansion on jobs for which women qualify outside the household is meager. But as sons bargain for more education and reduce their work effort on the farm (or other family enterprises), the demand for daughters is enhanced, because the patriarch can continue to extract income flow and work services from them as they mature. Thus, one short-term effect of the process by which education reshapes the family system is a reduction in female infanticide and a related improvement in the care of female offspring (reducing the risks of their perishing in infancy or childhood). In the longer run, because women bear the principal responsibility for rearing children within the patriarchal system and because the educational achievement of the adult who spends the bulk of the time with the small child strongly affects that child's subsequent educational performance, prospective grooms and their parents (concerned with the educational costs they will have to bear in order to equip their sons or grandsons for future job placements) begin to take the educational characteristics of women into account in selecting brides. Therefore, the long-term effect of the expansion of education is to increase the costs of arranging marriages and thus the patriarch's costs of leverage over daughters.

Moreover educational performance requires substantial time inputs from children and youth, involving both hours in school and hours devoted to homework. The expansion of education reduces the effective hours of labor time the patriarch can extract from his children; they work fewer hours as children and adults and, as a consequence of reduced work during childhood, they learn fewer of the specific farm skills that help render them superior to hired hands as workers. In sum, as significant educational performance becomes a prerequisite for jobs (and, with a lag, for marriage), costs of leverage over both sons and daughters are increased.

The second factor increasing leverage costs concerns shifts in the composition of the labor force. As the industrial sector expands and the associated economies of scale in industrial production encourage an increase in average firm size, the practice of relying on education for job placement gains ground. Also, in households where the head is himself an employee and his family is not employed in the firm, the ability of the patriarch to form connections that facilitate the placement of children is reduced; furthermore, the father cannot testify to the diligence and ability of his children at the industrial labor he himself performs, thus reducing the value of his recommendation. The reduction of the patriarch's bargaining position within the household further increases the costs of extracting services from offspring (because the children can demand more for their services).

Third, as will be demonstrated in Chapter 3, modern economic growth is associated with differentials in output per worker between sectors (at least in countries like Japan and Sweden). To the extent that these differentials involve wages and income as well as productivity and to the extent that status hinges on conspicuous consumption and hence on income, the growing productivity differentials cause the relative social status of a typical farm household head to fall in comparison to workers in the industrial and service sectors. The widening gap in social status diminishes the ability of a patriarch in the rural sector to maintain effective connections involving jobs with his relatives and associates who occupy more respected positions in the cities. Moreover as the gap in income increases, the opportunity cost to the patriarch of relying on his farm output for the major portion of his income increases. But if he decides to work full time in a factory and maintain his farm with the labor of his wife and children and his own off-time labor input (evenings and weekends), he reduces his own influence over the management of his farm compared with his wife who gains influence and consequently suffers a reduction in influence on that account.

In short, modernization tends to increase the costs of leverage over offspring and (associated with the process) to reduce the bargaining position of the patriarch relative to his sons, his daughters, and his wife.

Now let us turn to the benefits from economic leverage over children (the demand for their income and labor services). The three factors that are most salient here are mechanization, the structure of the labor force, and income per head. Mechanization, and the substitution of reproducible capital for labor, tends to diminish the reliance of farmers (and the owners of small shops) on labor-intensive techniques of production, and hence on family labor. It also increases the requirements of skill and education needed for production, and hence diminishes the utility of child labor. Because efficient operation of tractors and harvesters also typically involves the need for regular work, unbroken by constantly recurring periods of idleness this tends to diminish the utility of both the patriarch's wife, who has domestic household responsibilities (cooking, cleaning, etc.) that break up her workday, and children, who are being educated at school. As income per head rises and the risk of financial ruin stemming from one or two poor production periods is diminished, household heads find themselves increasingly able to hire workers and lend and borrow in capital markets. Transportation and communication costs tend to decline with economic development, and this also encourages household heads to enter capital markets and simultaneously to turn to the market for wage laborers rather than to family members to meet their demand for workers. Furthermore, as the standard of living improves, so does life expectancy and health; and as the vigor and physical stamina of older people improve, the need diminishes for the patriarch and his wife to rely on their sons and daughters or hired help as they reach middle age. Finally, as the composition of the labor force is transformed, the proportion of household heads who run their own enterprises falls, which reduces the proportion relying on wives and children for labor services in production. In sum, economic growth tends to diminish the demand for family labor within the population as a whole.[9]

By now, the implications of these arguments for marital fertility should be clear. The impact of modernization is to reduce substantially—and indeed, for the bulk of the population, probably completely eliminate—the *purely economic advantages* of children. The patriarch's ability to extract income and labor from his children is severely hampered, and the costs he bears to extract these benefits are significantly increased; at the same time, his desire to extract labor services is limited. An eldest son may still offer a purely economic advantage, but as income differentials between the sectors widen, eldest sons of farmers and entrepreneurs may also opt for industrial employment. Indeed the thrust of this argument is that the flow of economic benefits passing from children to parents in a patriarchal stem family setting is reversed by the process of modernization, and this undermines the natural fertility regime. The benefits of continuing the family name and heritage, and personal satisfaction to the parents, make children of lower parity a net asset to most parents regardless of the purely economic considerations. However the net economic costs of children, coupled with the reduced satisfaction and contribution to family lineage that children of higher parity offer relative to lower parity offspring, brings desired fertility down substantially below natural fertility. Assuming rationality of behavior on the part of decision makers, they should adopt parity-specific control.

Note that the thesis hinges on two related but logically separate effects stemming from modernization. The first is the response of the institution of the patriarchal stem family system to the evolution of labor and capital markets, a response exemplified by the dissipation of the patriarch's power

TABLE 2.1
Aspects of Modernization and Their Relationship to the Costs of and Benefits from Economic Leverage over Children in a Stem Family System, Natural Fertility, and Infant Mortality[a]

Variable	Net benefits (benefits minus costs) from leverage over		Benefits from leverage over		Change in labor force structure		Increase in real income and wages				Expansion of education	
	Sons	Daughters	Sons	Daughters	Decline in dependence on agriculture	Decline in importance of family-run enterprises	Income	Male wages	Female wages	Female/male differential	Males	Females
Costs of leverage over sons	−						+				+	
Costs of leverage over daughters		−					+					+
Benefits from leverage over sons	+	−		+	−	−	−	+		−	+	
Benefits from leverage over daughters	−	+	−		−	−	−		+	+		+
Natural fertility		+			+		+				+	+
Infant mortality[b]		−				−	−				−	−

[a] + indicates that the effect is positive; − indicates the effect is negative.
[b] The effect of infant mortality on fertility is not represented in this table. See the text for a discussion of this.

over decision making (i.e., a change in the bargaining positions of household members). The second effect concerns the changes in the costs of and benefits from economic leverage over children as realized *within* the institutional rules of the patriarchal stem family system, as well as the nuclear family system that emerges out of the breakup of the stem family system.

It is useful at this juncture to summarize the argument with Table 2.1. For simplicity of presentation, possible complications arising from interaction of all the different effects suggested here will be ignored; thus attention will be restricted to those effects that are *unambiguously* positive or negative. The implication of the table is that the factors promoting parity-specific control are manifold and that there is little that unambiguously counteracts their influence.

The role of infant mortality should be noted here in regard to these points. If parents have a target number of surviving children, the drop in infant mortality occasioned by improvements in food intake, better education, and the diffusion of public health services (as transportation costs drop) should work to reduce desired marital fertility. But it may also increase natural fertility (for reasons outlined earlier); hence, in the absence of a target, the effect of the drop in infant mortality is uncertain. The argument does not assume a target exists but rather that couples weigh the costs and benefits of an additional birth in considering whether or not to cease childbearing at some point. For example, in the face of an infant death, many couples may attempt to avert future births to avoid going through such an experience again. In short, a replacement effect, which assumes a definite target, may not be operating. In any event we are not assuming a target exists, and thus the impact of infant mortality is ambiguous within our model.

The arguments previously outlined concern the general reasons underlying the fertility transition in societies characterized by a patriarchal stem family system. They do not tell us about the timing of the decline relative to economic growth nor about the speed and duration of the transition. Let us first take up the issue of timing, concentrating on the contrast between Japanese and Swedish cases. The issue is as follows: Why did the Swedish transition occur relatively early compared with the Japanese transition? (The contrast in timing can be gleaned from the figures in Chapter 1. It will receive more detailed attention in Chapter 3.)

Three explanations that suggest themselves on the basis of the preceding theoretical arguments and empirical evidence that appears in Chapter 3 are (1) the difference in levels of per capita income in 1870; (2) the associated difference in premodern demographic regimes; and (3) the initial factor proportions in agriculture, which shaped the process of technological progress in the two countries by encouraging early mechanization in Sweden.

Because income levels were initially higher in Sweden and factor proportions favored mechanization of agriculture almost as soon as modern economic development commenced, the reliance on family labor dropped off quickly. And because the premodern demographic regime in Sweden involved late marriage for females and the accumulation of a dowry, a Swedish woman entered marriage with considerable job experience, skill, and resources, enhancing her position vis-à-vis her husband. Thus the expansion of education and job opportunities outside household production had an early impact on women in Sweden, encouraging them to resist their subordinate position within the patriarchal stem family system by pursuing opportunities in the labor market, whether single, married, or divorced. This raised the patriarch's costs of leverage over children (within the stem family system) by weakening his power and increasing the opportunity cost of children incurred by his wife. In short, the institution of the patriarchal stem family system and household production that relied on family labor both collapsed at an early point in the case of Swedish modern economic growth. By the same token, they declined much later in the case of Japanese modern economic growth.

The final issue concerning the marital fertility transition is the speed and duration of fertility decline. Because of the universal impact of education on a population whose government pursues a policy of compulsory education, the gap between desired marital fertility and natural fertility probably differs little among various subpopulations of that country. Certainly the gap may initially become more pronounced in urban than in rural populations, but the leads and lags with regard to the emergence of the gap are probably not extreme. In any event we would expect the costs of adopting fertility regulation to be the greatest for those subpopulations that commence the transition; consequently, their declines should be the most protracted. Populations that commence the transition later on benefit from contact with the innovators. They also face lower psychological, social, and perhaps economic costs of regulating fertility and, consequently, enjoy more rapid transitions. Although fertility differentials between subgroups during the transition may undoubtedly emerge, the implication of the preceding discussion is that the universal impact of education and the differential cost of control will mute these fertility differentials.

Once marital fertility has reached low levels, what determines variations and fluctuations within it? This is a subject that, properly speaking, is beyond the purview of this book, but a few points need to be made here so that some of the empirical results of Chapters 7 and 8 can be properly interpreted. The standard neoclassical arguments in the literature of economics concerned with this topic revolve around "cost of time" and "income" effects. An extremely simplified version of the cost time hypothesis is as follows: It is supposed that couples treat children as a source of consumption satisfaction (this is a reasonable formulation once children no longer make important economic contributions to the household, i.e., once the economic costs of leverage over children exceed the benefits). Therefore if raising children is particularly time intensive relative to other consumption activities—and in particular if it requires significant time inputs on the part of the mother—it follows that factors that increase the value of a woman's time tend to depress levels of marital fertility. Thus if wages paid to women improve, we would expect, other things being equal, a fall in marital fertility according to the logic of this hypothesis.

Now consider the impact of the husband's wage in terms of the income effect. If his contributions to child rearing are not substantial in terms of time, then improvement in his wages should tend to constitute a pure income effect. As household income is enhanced, household consumption of all goods that have positive income elasticities of demand should increase. In particular, as income levels for a typical couple go up with a rise in real wages for the husband, we would expect marital fertility to increase in response to an outward shift in the demand for children occasioned by the improvement in the capacity to purchase goods and services. In sum, the cost-of-time effect should be associated with the wife's wages and the income effect with the husband's wages. These standard arguments of neoclassical economics developed principally by Becker (1976) do seem to make sense for a population that was originally patriarchal in nature (i.e., in which there was a sexual division of labor in the premodern period as assumed by the model of household behavior). Thus we would anticipate that one empirical sign of the ending of the premodern demographic regime in a population with a patriarchal stem family system is the appearance of statistically significant coefficients on male and female wages in regressions in marital fertility, which are consistent with the "cost-of-time" and "income" hypotheses. It is this deduction that will be applied in the empirical analysis of Chapters 7 and 8.

Now let us turn to the issue of nuptiality. In the discussion of the premodern demographic regime, a demographic adjustment model was developed that linked the age at marriage of females (and to a lesser extent the nuptiality of males) to infant mortality and natural fertility. As long as the patriarchal stem family system remains viable (in the sense that legal institutions and the social and economic environment have not undermined it), decisions about the nuptiality of unmarried persons rest largely with their parents (i.e., the patriarchs). The primary concern of the patriarch is the main line of family descent; the eventual living standards achieved by offspring who leave the house are decidedly less crucial. Thus daughters typically marry out of the descent line and leave the house; and the inferior status they enjoy among their siblings partly reflects this.

But as the institution of the patriarchal stem family system decays and the nuclear family gains prominence because of the erosion of the patriarch's position and the related change in the net economic benefits of his leverage over children), sons and daughters take an increasingly strong hand in arranging their own marriages. From the daughter's point of view, *her* future living standards and status within marriage are of paramount concern; in an environment in which she makes her own decisions about marriage, she will tend to hold out for a match that will guarantee her maximum status *within* her union and maximum *outward* status for the union itself (i.e., family position, which depends on family income, occupations of partners, etc.). Thus the critical considerations for a woman in an environment in which the patriarchal stem family system is crumbling are (a) how effective are birth control techniques (i.e., how sure can a wife be that she can efficiently enter and leave the labor market once she weds) and (b) what are the incomes and educational and occupational characteristics of prospective mates?

In short, relative male–female wage and occupational differentials and the degree of contraceptive efficiency will be crucial determinants of the ages of marriage for women, *once* the institution of the patriarchal stem family system has decayed sufficiently. In particular, as contraceptive efficiency improves, we would expect the female's age at marriage (and/or entry into extralegal regular cohabitation) to decline. Let us reiterate that these deductions hinge on the institutional environment in which couples are arriving at marital decisions.

We can now make some comparisons between Japan and Sweden on the basis of these points. As was argued earlier, and as Chapters 5 and 6 will show, the patriarchal stem family system decayed slowly in twentieth-century Japan, whereas it crumbled rapidly in Sweden. Through the mid-1950s in Japan, decisions about nuptiality of daughters rested largely in the hands of their parents; as long as a substantial segment of the population clung to the rules of the patriarchal stem family system and wished to perpetuate it through inheritance, the model of marriage involving the demographic adjustment mechanism continued to be valid. In Sweden, by contrast, the patriarchal stem family system waned early, during the late nineteenth and first quarter of the twentieth century; a model of nuptiality that revolves around wage differentials and contraceptive efficiency is relevant after 1930. This contrast will guide us in our later analysis of the evolution of marriage in Sweden during the period 1880–1960.

This completes a general characterization of the evolution of natality in societies having a patriarchal stem family system in premodern period.

2.7. Comparison with Other Theories

The argument and the associated mathematical models developed in the preceding analysis constitute the theoretical core of this volume. To properly appreciate the thesis, it would be useful to place it in the broader context of the literature that it contributes to and draws from. Two specialized fields of academic inquiry that are particularly relevant with respect to this broader picture are the economic analysis of the peasant household and the economic and sociological theories of fertility. It is impossible to give an adequate treatment of the literature devoted to these fields of inquiry here, but it is possible to suggest briefly what has already been accomplished and to highlight the salient differences between other approaches and the line of attack formulated in this book.

Let us first take up the literature dealing with the economics of the peasant household. It is generally agreed that the seminal piece in this area is the remarkable study by Chayanov (1966). (This work was originally published in Russian in the 1920s.) Chayanov defined the most important and lasting issues in this field as being the degree of interdependence between decisions about consumption and production within the peasant household; the degree to which household demographic composition (i.e., age, structure, and size) determines consumption and labor usage per person; and the degree to which a peasant economy functions differently from a capitalistic economy. Chayanov himself adapted marginalist principles involving subjective utility in attempting to demonstrate how maximization of household utility would lead to an equilibrium determined by the demand for leisure and material consumption secured largely at the expense of labor input. Sen (1966) and Nakajima (1969) have drawn from Chayanov's pioneering effort and have refined his basic insights into a more rigorous theory.

Economists working with a neoclassical perspective have attempted to explain the type of empirical evidence observed and cited by Chayanov and others—and explained by Chayanov in terms of his assumption of the peasant household's almost complete dependence on its own family labor supply—by the use of models that assumed that nonfamily labor is hired by the peasant household and that markets behave as one expects they would under typical capitalistic price-taking assumptions. Jorgenson and Lau (1969) and Lau and Mitchell (1970) pioneered the rigorous application of the linear logarithmic expenditure system. They have been followed in this direction by, among others, Yotopoulos and Lau (1974); Yotopoulos *et al.* (1976); Lau *et al.* (1978); Barnum and Squire (1979); Rosenzweig (1980); and Lau *et al.* (1981).

The approach taken in this volume is closer to that advanced by Chayanov than to that taken by the neoclassical school. It differs from both, however, in its explicit treatment of the institutional rules of the patriarchal stem family system, a treatment directly embedded into the formulation of the model of household behavior. It does follow Chayanov in the assumptions made about the dependence on household labor, but the model developed here emphasizes the adjustment of household demography to the needs of household economy, whereas Chayanov's thesis stresses the adjustment of household economy to the demography of the household.

Now let us consider the literature concerning the analysis of fertility and the fertility transition. Two major branches in this group of writings are one derivative of sociology and another stemming from economics. The sociological approach has mainly concerned itself with the supply of surviving children (i.e., infant mortality and natural fertility); the relationship of the institution of the family to demographic variables (e.g., in some approaches the institution of the household is taken to be a function of mortality); and the question of whether rationality governs decisions about natality before the fertility transition. Notestein (1945) is responsible for the classic thesis that it is mortality that determines natality over the long run and that fertility falls with a considerable lag after the death rate declines because rational behavior toward natality takes a long time to develop and diffuse itself throughout populations. Davis (1963), in his major critique of Notestein's approach and in his revision of the theory, argues that Notestein is correct in emphasizing mortality as the crucial determinant of fertility but incorrect in his supposition about rationality. Davis maintains that populations are always rational in their behavior with respect to fertility and that the lag Notestein emphasizes as an indicator of irrationality does not, in fact, occur. Friedlander (1969) has elaborated on Davis's approach considerably. More recently, Caldwell (1976, 1978, 1980) has taken the approaches of both Notestein and Davis to task. Caldwell agrees with Davis that households are always rational, but he rejects Davis's emphasis on mortality, arguing that social and cultural influences that determine whether net wealth flows from children to parents or from parents to children are crucial in explaining the transition. All three of these theories, however, grapple with the question of how the institutional rules governing household behavior interact with demographic variables.

The economic literature is different from this sociological literature in terms of its emphasis on a different set of themes. Economists tend to assume rational behavior at the outset and discuss this no further; to stress demand rather than supply factors (special weight is placed on the opportunity cost of a mother's time and the value of children as labor inputs in pinpointing determinants of demand); and to eschew detailed treatment of the institution of the household. The strictly neoclassical (Chicago–Columbia) approach pioneered by Becker (1976) is the most thoroughgoing in its emphasis on simple, constrained, utility maximization without regard for institutional considerations or for changes in attitudes. Becker has also pioneered work in the rigorous development of the household production function, which is used in showing how material and inputs are converted by the household into activities that are the source of utility for the household members. Easterlin (1978) (in addition, see Easterlin *et al.,* 1980 also relies on straightforward utility maximization and the idea of a household production function, but he integrates changing preferences and supply factors (natural fertility and infant mortality) systematically into his analysis. Leibenstein (1976) has developed a general model of human behavior that does not rely on utility maximization (he calls it a theory of selective rationality), and he has applied this to the problem of explaining fertility decline (see Leibenstein, 1975). Leibenstein also departs from standard neoclassical ideas by introducing principles involving social pressure and group identification into his analytical framework. Like Becker, however, Leibenstein emphasizes almost exclusively demand-side factors. In particular, Leibenstein emphasizes the value of children in providing labor services and security for the aged as he explains why the demand for children is especially strong in an agricultural setting. It should be stressed that these three economic approaches do share a concern for the factors determining demand for surviving children in terms of some weighing of costs of and benefits from children (whether this be understood in a utility maximizing framework or not) and a lack of interest in systematic treatment of household institutions. The main features of these three approaches and the approach used in this book are captured (for purposes of comparison) in a simple schematic presentation in Table 2.2.

However, economists have begun to give greater attention to institutions and other "sociological" concerns in this field than was true five years ago. Becker, for example, in his book (see Becker 1981) has come to conceptualize the household in agrarian society as an institution that helps protect its members against risk and uncertainty; in this context he also emphasizes its role in providing skills and certification of future work for the children. Lee (1980) and Willis (1980, 1981) have followed Samuelson (1958) in considering the household as an institution that facilitates the transfer of income from workers to nonworkers (either children or retired persons); this theme also treats the institution of the household in a functional sense (that is, in a manner close to that pioneered by the sociologists).

TABLE 2.2
A Comparison of Various Aspects of Selected Models of Fertility and Their Implications for the Analysis of the Fertility Transition of Populations

	Analysis of individual household			Analysis of fertility decline in aggregate populations			
Identification of model type	Decision-making process	Constraints	Objectives	Institutional rules	Technology	Factor endowments	Preferences
Chicago–Columbia	Maximization of household utility function (preference map) subject to constraints	(1) Budget constraint (wages, nonlabor income, prices of goods) (2) Household production function (technology)	Fixed and stable utility map	Assumed to depend on technology, factor endowments and preferences	Affects fertility through income (pure income and income elasticity of child quality effects) & price effects (cost of time)	Effects same as technology	Assumed fixed
University of Pennsylvania	Maximization of household utility function (preference map) subject to constraints	(1) Budget constraint (as above) (2) Household production function (3) Fertility production function (4) Infant mortality function	Variable; various specifications: (1) intrafamily (2) socialization	Exogenous. Not entered directly into model	Same as above. In addition, it assumes income effects fertility and incorporates production and infant mortality functions	Effects same as for technology	Variable, assumed to change

Leibenstein	Selective rationality. Utility maximization of individuals with constraint concern and pressure as arguments of utility function	(1) Pressure (2) Rules of family system (3) Income (approximately)	Utility depends on social status of household. Utility basis of consumption decision	Exogenous rules of family system directly entered into the model. Assumed to change systematically with income and occupational structure	Affects fertility through income effects mainly (decline in need for child labor and old age security)	Effects same as for technology	As occupational structure changes with rise in income, aggregate demand for social status expenditures rises
Mosk	Bargaining model of household decision involving costs and benefits of the patriarch's leverage over children	(1) Rules of family system (2) Income (3) Imperfections in labor and capital markets	Continuation of household line and maximization of income	Exogenous and entered into model (1) Rules of family system (2) Institutions of labor and capital markets both assumed to change systematically with income and occupational structure	(1) Affects fertility through income effects on costs and benefits of maintaining leverage over children (2) Technology also has additional impact on leverage	Affects fertility through income effects on costs and benefits of maintaining leverage over children	No systematic analysis undertaken

With this brief overview of the literature completed, it is now possible to see how the theory expounded here fits into this broad area of academic inquiry. As mentioned earlier, the approach used here goes further than that of other economists in directly integrating the institutional rules of the household into a theory of household behavior and fertility. In this sense it represents a step toward integrating sociological concerns with economic ones. It also emphasizes supply-side factors (e.g., natural fertility and mortality). On the other hand, the model is explicitly cast in terms of constrained maximization (although not in terms of utility maximization), and it does emphasize demand factors (especially the labor contributions from children). Of all the areas of academic inquiry just reviewed, it is closest in spirit to that economic literature that treats the household as an insurance institution and as a locus for the transfer of income from economically productive to economically inactive persons (e.g., children and retired people). Thus it would appear to match most closely the approaches taken by Lee (1980) and Willis (1980, 1981).

2.8. Conclusions

In this chapter a simple model of peasant household behavior in the context of a patriarchal stem family system was developed. We have shown how the essence of this model can be captured by a basic equation, which relates flow of births to future labor needs. We then proceeded to demonstrate how this model of the household can be utilized in formulating a stylized model of economic—demographic equilibrium for an aggregate population (the premodern demographic regime). Finally, we pinpointed the major forces associated with economic and social modernization that lead to the undermining of the premodern demographic regime.

The remainder of this book is devoted to testing the thesis empirically using data for Japan and Sweden. Part II explains why the particular choice of populations is apt (Chapter 3), and it advances documentation for the model of the peasant household for Japan and, to a lesser degree, Sweden (Chapter 4). The primary emphasis here and elsewhere is on Japan, but the Swedish material is essential in providing an appropriate comparative perspective.

Part III (Chapters 5 to 8) demonstrates that aggregate data for Japan and Sweden broadly supports the deductions of the theory of the household regarding fertility. These findings, taken in conjunction with the empirical material presented in Part II, constitute a thorough and systematic verification of the theory developed in this chapter.

Notes to Chapter 2

1. It is of course possible that some households might use the "terminating" instrument (i.e., practice some parity-specific control) if they were lucky and had many surviving sons in the early years of marriage. The existence of such stopping behavior in family reconstitution studies for Japan and other countries does not vitiate the argument that the population follows a natural fertility strategy as long as the incidence of such behavior is not typical, the proportion of total households behaving in this manner being relatively small.

2. Economic literature of the 1970s contains a number of articles that argue that "safety first" behavior characterized agricultural communities in a number of countries prior to the twentieth century. For example, with regard to the nineteenth-century American South, see Wright and Kunreuther (1975), and on preindustrial England, see McCloskey (1976).

3. Here the assumption is that the nonfamily worker is paid a regular wage. But it should be noted that other arrangements are possible, and have and do occur, in peasant agricultural villages. For example, one solution is division of the harvest among all workers, whether they be family members or not. The disadvantage of this method (and the reason why family members are preferable to nonfamily members even in an environment characterized by such labor market institutions) is that when the harvest is brought in, the nonfamily member is likely to steal what he or she can and, consequently, must be supervised. This tends to raise supervision costs. I am grateful to Pranab Bardhan for suggesting this point to me.

4. One way in which a household head could secure nonfamily labor for his land and still extract a surplus of the sort he obtains from family labor (i.e, pay less for the laborer's work than he would otherwise) is if he hired labor to rent the land out to and shared the output with the tenant according to some sharecropping arrangement. The problem encountered here is that the landlord encounters search costs, for he must screen prospective tenants to find those who are efficient in production. This is a serious economic incentive for preferring a family labor strategy, and it was commonly observed in prewar Japan, for example, that only farmers with fairly large landholdings leased out land to others in a systematic manner.

5. In Chapter 4 these figures are computed for Japanese farm households.

6. Mosk (1981b) also uses the results of simulations to establish that patriarchal stem family agricultural populations tend to move to equilibria in the absence of technological changes. At the equilibrium point the rate of growth for the population is, by definition, zero. Mosk (1981b) demonstrates that one secures equilibrium solutions with the parameters for natural fertility and mortality, which characterized premodern Japan and Sweden (i.e., the theoretical model developed here does not tend to produce collapse or extremely rapid growth for the population it is designed to characterize).

7. The previous section did not deal with artisans, officials, and merchants who, in agrarian peasant societies, may constitute up to around a fifth of the labor force. The model developed here, however, is applicable to merchants who pass a shop on to a son and also to artisans who own shops and lumpy capital equipment because both groups, like peasants, tend to rely on family labor prior to modernization. Moreover, as this section will argue, norms that bolster natural fertility generally keep the costs of parity-specific control extremely high when the vast majority of the population follows a natural fertility strategy; so the fertility transition tends to begin only when an important segment of the population (in an isolated subpopulation this need only be a substantial proportion of the subpopulation) attempts to abandon the natural fertility strategy.

8. For a general economic theory of signaling that treats the role of education as a screening mechanism, see Spence (1973).

9. Note that this argument concerns the costs and benefits of economic leverage. It is well to

keep this in mind because a change in the net benefits from leverage may occur—and as a result fertility may be affected—but the degree of leverage parents exercise over children may not change demonstrably, at least not in the medium term. I am grateful to Thomas C. Smith for pointing out that in Japan patriarchal leverage over sons remained high throughout the first half of the twentieth century despite a major shift in the costs of and benefits from that leverage. In the long run, however, the degree of economic leverage over children has demonstrably diminished in Japan, especially since the mid 1950s. It should be noted that this is partly due to institutional changes wrought by the American occupation authorities during the late 1940s and early 1950s and partly to the economically dependent changes in the costs of and benefits from children.

PART II

Japan and Sweden

CHAPTER 3

Japan and Sweden

3.1. Introduction

Part II of this book is devoted to accomplishing two main goals. The first goal is the setting of the stage for the empirical analysis of the volume. Specifically, it involves justification of the choice of countries on which the analysis is carried out. The principal focus in this volume is on Japan. To bring a comparative focus to bear on the study, Swedish materials are brought in as well. Why Sweden? In Chapter 3 this particular choice is explained. The second goal is to show that the model of household behavior, laid out in Chapter 2, is reasonable as a model (admittedly stylized and simplified) for understanding average Japanese and Swedish households and their evolution during the modern period (since the nineteenth century); this is accomplished in Chapter 4. Then, in Part III, the empirical study of natality in Japan and Sweden is considered to test the deductions concerning fertility arrived at from the model of the household developed in Chapter 2.

The purpose of Chapter 3 is to explain the choice of countries used in this study. At the outset, demographic criteria that both countries should meet are listed. The fertility transitions of the two nations should be sufficiently different so as to capture the range of diversity discussed in Chapter 1. That is, the interval of time between the beginning of the transition and the onset of economic and social modernization should differ substantially between the two countries; and their premodern demographic regimes should be different, so that the relative balance between nuptiality and marital fertility, and the trends in these two aspects of natality, would be dissimilar. Second, the demographic, economic, and social data for each country should be of sufficient quality, and available for each country over a duration of time that roughly encompasses its fertility transition, so that a serious statistical analysis of each nation's transition is possible. Third, each country should be relatively homogeneous in a linguistic and cultural sense, so that the national pattern does not emerge as the result of wholly different patterns obtaining for two or three subgroups of the nation; each country should enjoy substantial internal communication and intermarriage but be isolated from one another. For example, Belgium, analyzed by Lesthaeghe (1977), is a case of a linguistically divided nation with marked cultural segmentation between groups (Flanders and Wallonia). Fourth, the countries should both have begun their transitions in the prewar period, so that the international diffusion of contraceptives and family planning programs would not be a possible disturbing factor in the initiation of either country's transition. The preceding four points constitute the demographic conditions we desire in our choice of nations for study. The final point, involving other criteria, is that the broad features of economic development of the two countries should be roughly alike. It is desirable that both nations began to industrialize at about the same date, experienced relatively close structural transformations of income and labor force (i.e., the sectoral composition of production) at the same dates, and had approximately equal rates of growth in income per head.

The first point was touched on in the introductory chapter and will be pursued in more detail later in this chapter. As for the second issue, one should consult the appendixes, where the quantitative material and tapes that underlie this study are discussed. A large amount of quantitative material for the 46 prefectures of Japan, covering the years 1905–1970, has been assembled. This includes the demographic indices already discussed as well as figures on the structure of the labor force, educational attainment, tenancy status and density, and real wages and income. Many of these data are also available for the rural and urban sectors of each prefecture.[1] Moreover, for the period 1925–1938, a large file of variables has been assembled (including measures of demographic, economic, and social structure) for each of the approximately 600 individual cities (*shi*) and counties (*gun*) in Japan.[2] Finally, for the year 1929 a detailed set of measures of the economic and demographic structure of 219 Japanese peasant households has been secured that, as will be argued in Chapter 4, lends considerable support to the theoretical approach used here.[3] For Sweden, a tape has been prepared that includes figures for the demographic indices previously noted, the structure of the labor force, and real wages and income for the 24 counties of Sweden and Stockholm city over the period 1880–1960.[4] Moreover, many of these variables are also available on the tape for the rural and urban sectors of the counties. As suggested in Chapter 1 and as will be demonstrated more thoroughly later in this chapter and in Part III, the Swedish fertility transition commended in the late 1870s or early 1880s and was more or less complete by 1940, whereas the Japanese transition probably began in the period 1915–1920 at the earliest and was finished around 1960; thus the data sets are comprehensive and encompass the transitions for each country.[5] In sum, the two countries satisfy the second requirement. Moreover, both Japan and Sweden meet the third and fourth criteria because since they both began their transitions before 1940 and are culturally and linguistically homogeneous (with only minor exceptions in either case).

This brings us to the fifth and last criterion, which is the main subject of this chapter. Before embarking on the details of the argument, however, we wish to elaborate a bit on what can reasonably be expected. The goal is to suggest that the two nations experienced similar modern economic growth.[6] Similarity is a relative concept. The argument in this chapter is that, in relative terms, Swedish modern economic growth looks as much like, indeed is closer to, Japan's development than that of any other country that meets the first four criteria. Moreover, the similarities are not simply artificial. To make the case, attention will be restricted to developing quantitative data on the growth experience of these two countries, with occasional reference to other relevant countries. The reader should consult Kuznets (1966, 1971) for quantitative evidence for other nations that supports the claim for the relative superiority of Sweden as a country of comparison.[7]

We shall begin the set of systematic comparisons with income growth; then turn to the transformation of the structure of production, stressing the similarities. Next, we shall focus on developments within the agricultural and industrial sectors, stressing certain differences that will play a role in the theoretical argument concerning the timing of the fertility transition. After that, we shall turn to a comparison of trends in education and the general demographic and social structure (urbanization). Finally, we shall close with a comparison of the fertility transitions in Japan and Sweden. But prior to these matters, we wish to touch briefly on a few of the difficulties attendant on doing systematic comparative work using statistics of the sort carried out in this chapter and in Part III.

3.2. Some Methodological Problems in Comparative Quantitative Analysis

There are two basic problems involving systematic quantitative comparisons that are relevant to this study. The first is a general problem concerning definitions of variables; the second concerns age structure and specifically relates to the demographic variables examined in this work.

It may be the case that particular national statistics on, for example, income and labor force reflect the peculiarities of the statistical offices in a country; on that score, national statistics are difficult to compare with those produced in other countries. The very definition of employment, for instance, probably varies somewhat from nation to nation and, historically, from epoch to epoch. In this work, we have used standard official data available for Japan and Sweden and have adjusted these in some places to achieve consistency of comparison. Although we have certainly not been wholly successful in securing completely comparable measures for the two countries, the data sets worked with are reasonable for comparative purposes. Specific details may be found in Appendixes 3–6 and in the working papers cited there.

The second issue to be taken up concerns the possible distortions due to differing age structures. For example, consider the Hutterite index I_f. Although Coale, in formulating the definitions of the Hutterite indices, specifically attempted to purge them of any bias due to the age structure of the population for which the index is calculated, perusal of the formulas in Section 1.2 does suggest that there may be an index number problem associated with age structure. Because the Japanese and Swedish populations had very different age structures (partly stemming from emigration out of Sweden), there may be distortions that affect the empirical comparisons. Examination of specific cases, however, demonstrates that this is not really a problem. Consider I_f in 1930, for example. If we compute it for Sweden, we obtain .154. If we take the same total number of women in the age range 15–49 for Sweden in 1930 but divide them among the seven age classes 15–19, 20–24, . . . , 45–49 according to the proportions of women in those age classes for Japan in 1930, we can recalculate I_f as if the Japanese female age structure characterized Sweden. If we do so, we obtain a value of .153 instead of .154. It is clear from examples of this sort that potential distortions stemming from differences in age structure are not serious.

With this brief discussion of methodological problems complete, let us turn to a comparison of income (levels and growth) between Japan and Sweden.

3.3. Income

Modern economic growth, according to Kuznets (1966:1), who formulated the concept, is "a sustained increase in per capita or per worker product, most often accompanied by an increase in population and usually by sweeping structural changes." In this section, we shall demonstrate two points relevant to Kuznets' definition. First, both Japan and Sweden entered modern economic growth at about the same time and, relative to other countries that began economic development prior to World War II, started with fairly low per capita incomes. Second, both countries enjoyed brisk growth, outstripping the other nations that entered modern economic growth in the same broad historical epoch.

Much work has been done to measure accurately income in the nineteenth and twentieth centuries for presently developed countries. Yet, unfortunately, estimates for the period prior to 1900 are not precise; this is particularly the case if one wishes to compare two countries in the units of a common currency.[8] Kuznets (1971), using backward extrapolation of figures from a later period and using trends in growth, attempted to do this using 1965 United States dollars and arrived at the following estimates for Japan and Sweden at the approximate time they commenced modern economic growth: Japan in 1874 to 1879 had a per capita gross national product of about \$75 per head, and Sweden in 1861 to 1869 had a figure of about \$215 per head. As Kuznets readily admits, such estimates are only conjectural. Indeed, Ohkawa *et al.* (1979:8) suggest the Japanese figures may have been considerably higher than Kuznets's extrapolation predicts; but in any event, "Japan's initial per capita income was certainly lower than those of western nations . . ." [also see Ohkawa and Rosovsky (1973:5)]. In a comparative framework, Kuznets's figures suggest the following general points: First, both Japan and Sweden experienced a definite discontinuity in economic history, the onset of modern economic growth, at about the same date, circa 1870. Second, although initial Japanese income per head was probably below that of Sweden, Swedish income per capita was relatively low compared with most other European countries (or areas of European settlement) when they began modern development. Sandberg (1978:1) is categorical on this point, noting that "in 1850 Sweden was one of the very poorest countries in Europe. . . . " In short, Japan and Sweden were relatively similar in terms of income just before modern growth and began to spurt forward at about the same date.

Now let us turn to the process of growth. Consider the figures in Table 3.1. Two points emerge from these data. First, the rates of population growth across comparable time periods are roughly similar for the two nations. Second, real national output expanded rapidly within both countries, so that gross output per worker or per capita grew at a brisk pace in both cases. Indeed, of the nations that experienced sustained periods of economic development prior to World War I, Japan is regarded as having had the most rapid rate of growth in real income or output per head over the long period from its beginning of modern economic growth to 1970. Sweden is usually accorded second place, behind Japan, in this aspect. For example, Ohkawa *et al.* (1979) have written, "Sweden is the only western country whose

TABLE 3.1

Indices of Real Output, Population, Labor Force, Real Output per Capita, and Real Output per Worker: Quinquennial Averages for Selected Periods, 1886/90 = 100 and Annual Growth Rates, Japan and Sweden

	Indices (1886/90 = 100)					Growth rates (% per annum)					
Years	Domestic product	Population	Labor force	Domestic product per capita	Domestic product per worker	Periods	Domestic product	Population	Labor force	Domestic product per capita	Domestic product per worker
Sweden[a]											
1886/70	59.1[c]	87.9	89.8	67.3[c]	81.8[c]	1886/90 to 1936/40	3.0[c]	0.6	0.6	2.4[c]	2.4[c]
1886/90	100.0[c]	100.0	100.0	100.0[c]	100.0[c]						
1911/15	227.4[c]	118.5	137.6	191.8[c]	220.7[c]	1886/90 to 1951/55	3.3[c]	0.6	1.0	2.7[c]	—[e]
1936/40	429.3[c]	132.9	191.3	322.8[c]	318.8[c]						
1951/55	828.0[c]	151.2	—[e]	547.5[c]	—[e]	1936/40 to 1951/55	4.5[c]	0.9	—[e]	3.6[c]	—[e]
Japan[b]											
1886/90	100.0[d]	100.0	100.0	100.0[d]	100.0[d]	1886/90 to 1936/40	3.1[d]	1.2	0.7	1.9[d]	2.4[d]
1911/15	183.9[d]	131.5	114.4	140.4[d]	160.5[d]						
1936/40	460.0[d]	183.4	142.4	250.9[d]	323.1[d]	1953/55 to 1961/65[f]	11.3[d]	1.0	1.7	10.1[d]	9.4[d]

[a] Swedish figures given in terms of gross domestic product, are calculated from data in Johansson (1967: Table 56, pp. 152–153; Table 58, pp. 156–157; Table 60, pp. 160–161).

[b] Japanese figures, given in terms of net domestic product, except for growth rates for period 1953/55 to 1961/65 are from Ohkawa *et al.* (1979: Table A.9, pp. 271–272; Table A.53 pp. 392–393). Japanese growth rates for period 1953/55 to 1961/65 are from Ohkawa and Rosovsky (1973: Basic Statistical Table 4, pp. 284–285; Basic Statistical Table 15, pp. 310–311).

[c] 1913 prices.

[d] 1934–1936 prices.

[e] The dash indicates when data were not available.

[f] 1960 prices.

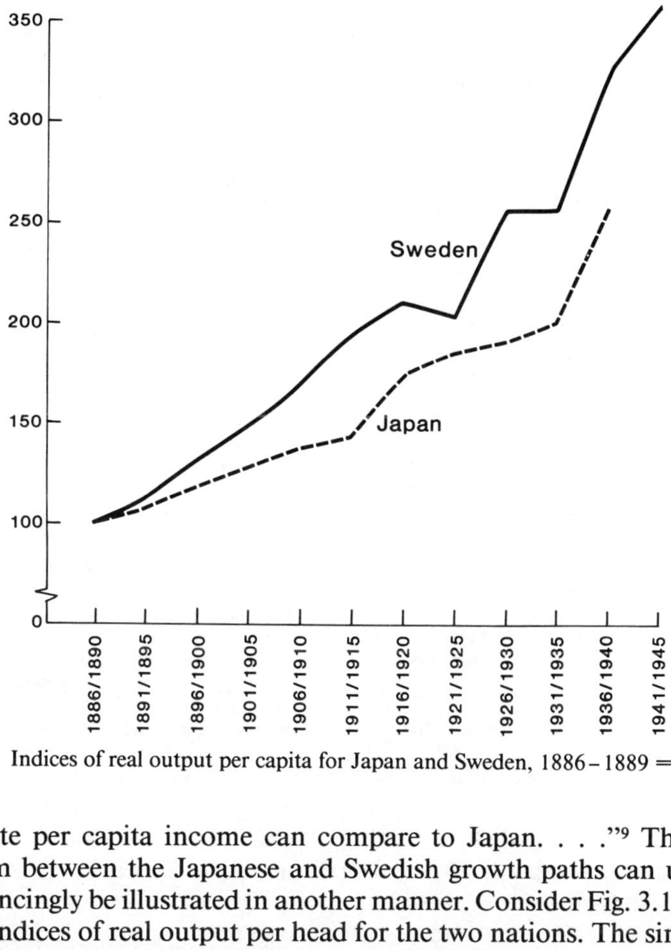

Fig. 3.1. Indices of real output per capita for Japan and Sweden, 1886–1889 = 100.

growth rate per capita income can compare to Japan. . . ."[9] The close parallelism between the Japanese and Swedish growth paths can usefully and convincingly be illustrated in another manner. Consider Fig. 3.1, which provides indices of real output per head for the two nations. The similarity in aggregate economic expansion is revealed by the tendency of the two countries to reach similar levels of increase in income per head at approximately the same times.

To summarize: Of the countries to which it is reasonable to compare the Japanese demographic experience, Sweden appears to be the most appropriate in terms of level and growth of income.

3.4. Structure

The parallelism in expansion of production for the two countries can also be gleaned from figures on the structure of the labor force and output. Recall

TABLE 3.2

Years (1)	Agriculture, forestry, fishing (2)	Manufacturing and mining (3)	Facilitating (4)	Construction (5)	Commerce and services (6)
	Percentage domestic product				
Sweden[a]					
1866/70	45.2	16.7	4.1	5.4	28.6
1886/90	36.8	16.3	7.0	9.1	30.8
1911/15	25.6	30.8	8.3	6.5	28.7
1936/40	14.0	39.1	9.9	7.4	29.6
1951/55	10.3	45.8	6.5	8.2	29.2
Japan[c]					
1886/90	43.5	13.6	2.5	3.8	36.5
1911/15	34.7	21.4	6.7	4.3	32.9
1936/40	18.6	36.3	8.0	7.9	29.3
1951/55	22.8	26.2	8.7	4.1	38.3
1966/70	9.5	31.3	8.1	7.3	45.1

[a] The Swedish figures are given in terms of the gross domestic product. The names of the sectoral categories used for Sweden are taken from the Japanese categories. The equivalent Swedish categories as given in the Swedish statistics are "Agriculture, Horticulture, Fisheries and Forestry," "Manufacturing Industry and Handicrafts," "Transport and Communications," "Building and Construction," and "Public Administration, Commerce, Hotels, and Restaurants, etc." The figures on Gross Domestic Product used here exclude "Services of Dwellings" and "Indirect Taxes and Customs Duties." Prior to 1910 the Swedish statistics on Employed Persons gives only the "Public Administration" category within "Commerce and Services." Gross Domestic Product is in current prices. Swedish figures are from Johansson (1967: Table 55, pp. 150–151 and Table 58, pp. 156–157).

[b] Note that "Transport and Communications" (facilitating) is not included as a separate category in the

that Kuznets emphasizes the transformation of economic structure in categorizing modern economic growth. Table 3.2 contains the relevant figures. As for the structure of output (columns 2–6, Table 3.2) and labor force (columns 7–11, Table 3.2), the comparisons are straightforward. The decline in dependence on primary production is evident for both cases. The increase in importance of manufacturing and mining is also a salient feature of both series. Moreover, these statements do not describe only the sequence of change, they also describe the composition of output and labor force at the same dates.

There are also somewhat weaker similarities revealed in the figures on differential productivity (differentials between the agricultural and manufacturing sectors). From the last two columns of Table 3.2, the relative average labor productivities of the two sectors can be compared. In general, the relative superiority of manufacturing over agriculture is more pronounced for Japan than for Sweden, but the differentials can be seen in both

Distribution of Domestic Product and Labor Force by Sectors, Japan and Sweden

<table>
<tr><th colspan="5">Percentage of employed labor force</th><th></th><th></th></tr>
<tr><th>Agriculture, forestry, fishing (7)</th><th>Manufacturing and mining (8)</th><th>Facilitating (9)</th><th>Construction (10)</th><th>Commerce and services (11)</th><th>Col. 2[b] ÷ Col. 7 (12)</th><th>Col. 3[b] ÷ Col. 8 (13)</th></tr>
<tr><td>81.0</td><td>13.3</td><td>1.5</td><td>—[e]</td><td>4.3</td><td>.56</td><td>1.26</td></tr>
<tr><td>74.2</td><td>17.6</td><td>3.0</td><td>—</td><td>5.1</td><td>.50</td><td>.93</td></tr>
<tr><td>48.8</td><td>26.8</td><td>4.7</td><td>—</td><td>19.7</td><td>.53</td><td>1.15</td></tr>
<tr><td>30.8</td><td>29.3</td><td>6.0</td><td>8.5</td><td>25.5</td><td>.46</td><td>1.33</td></tr>
<tr><td>—</td><td>—</td><td>—</td><td>—</td><td>—</td><td>—</td><td>—</td></tr>
<tr><td>70.0[d]</td><td colspan="4">30.0</td><td>.62</td><td>—</td></tr>
<tr><td>63.7</td><td>13.0</td><td>2.9</td><td>2.7</td><td>17.8</td><td>.55</td><td>1.65</td></tr>
<tr><td>44.1</td><td>20.4</td><td>4.4</td><td>3.0</td><td>28.0</td><td>.42</td><td>1.78</td></tr>
<tr><td>42.9</td><td>19.5</td><td>4.9</td><td>4.2</td><td>28.7</td><td>.53</td><td>1.34</td></tr>
<tr><td>20.2</td><td>26.5</td><td>6.7</td><td>7.3</td><td>39.3</td><td>.47</td><td>1.18</td></tr>
</table>

labor force breakdowns, which probably raises the percentage of labor force in "Manufacturing and Mining".

[c] The Japanese figures are given in terms of net domestic product. "Facilitating" sector is "Transportation, Communications and Public Utilities" in the product figures. In the labor force figures it is "Support and Utilities." There are a few missing categories in the labor force figures because the sum of employed persons in the categories given here is about 2% less than total employed persons. The income figures used here exclude "Imputed House Rent," and are in current prices. Japanese figures are from Ohkawa *et al.* (1979):Table A.54, pp. 392–395 and Tables A.10 and A.11, pp. 273–277.

[d] "Agriculture and Forestry" only.

[e] The dash indicates when data were not available.

cases. That Japan became involved as a belligerent in a number of major wars during this period, whereas Sweden did not, may partly explain this disparity concerning the relative superiority of manufacturing over agriculture. For example, Japan's shift toward heavy industry in the 1930s is related to the demand for war material. In short, if we examine the *broad* structural changes in labor input and output, the similarity already shown in terms of income per head is bolstered. However, as will now be shown, if we examine circumstances within the broad sectors, important differences emerge.

3.5. Agriculture

At the onset of modern growth, both Japan and Sweden were peasant societies, the vast majority of whose populations depended on agriculture for survival. The reliance on primary production prior to 1870 has already been demonstrated in Table 3.2. That the two agrarian sectors were composed primarily of peasants requires a brief discussion here before we proceed to an examination of factor proportions and social structure within the agricultural sectors of the two nations.

Prior to the Meiji Restoration in 1868, Japan had been a feudal society for nearly two and a half centuries, ruled by the Tokugawa shogunate that had established political control at the end of the sixteenth century. The Tokugawa regime pursued a policy of international isolation, so that the *daimyo,* the rulers of the feudal fiefdoms, the *han,* were prevented from establishing international alliances that could jeopardize the delicate balance of power maintaining internal peace. The populace of each *han* fell into various social classes. The former military class, the *samurai,* resided in the castle towns of the *han* and administered a realm that consisted primarily of peasants living in villages and merchants and craftsmen who gathered primarily in the urban centers. In theory, the peasants were not free to sell land, to migrate, or to grow crops other than those the *han* authorities permitted (this latter prohibition involved the fact that peasants paid their taxes in kind, primarily in rice). In practice, however, there was a market in land within the peasant villages, a fact attested by village documents on acquisition and sale of fields (Smith, 1966, 1977). When the Meiji oligarchs took power, these feudal regulations were abolished, the class designations were eliminated, and the peasants' freedom of movement, marketing of land, and choice of output to produce were guaranteed. In practice, however, these legal changes did not constitute the dramatic break one might have otherwise expected because, as noted, the Tokugawa peasant already operated in a relatively unfettered market environment despite the laws.

By the nineteenth century, the typical Japanese peasant family farmed a variety of small fields that it owned or rented (which were scattered throughout its village with perhaps a few located in a neighboring village), relinquishing a large proportion of its output for taxes in kind and providing a limited amount of corvee labor services to the fiefdom.[10] After the Meiji Restoration, tax payments were commuted to exactments of money, but the economic environment in which decisions about production and consumption were fashioned was probably affected in marginal ways only.

Prior to the late eighteenth century, Swedish society, similiar to much of Europe and to Tokugawa Japan, was divided into feudal classes, with the peasantry constituting the vast majority of the population. However, the political structure of the feudal regime was considerably different from that characterizing Japan. From the seventeenth century until the Parliamentary Reform of 1866, Sweden was controlled by a four-estate *Riksdag,* in which the peasantry was represented as one of the estates and played an important role in the determination of national policy (Sandberg, 1978:38). In the mid-sixteenth century, taxpaying peasants (freeholders of land who paid taxes directly to the state) owned approximately half the land, the rest being held by the Crown and tax-exempt nobles; but by 1700, the peasants' proportion had fallen to about one-third (Østerud, 1978:78–81). The peasantry, regardless of landowning status, was personally free, although there were labor codes that required men to secure legally sanctioned employment or be liable for compulsory military service (Montgomery, 1939:62–67).

In terms of organization of units of production, Swedish farming took two basic forms: peasant farms (either freely held or held in some form of tenancy) and estates (on which peasants often secured small holdings in exchange for their labor). Prior to the nineteenth century, the typical Swedish peasant farmed a portion of a hamlet's open fields; but between 1800 and 1830 there began a long process of enclosure of farmlands, with the state taking a fairly aggressive role in the transformation.[11] This occurred partly in response to the cries of reformers who looked to England, but it also stemmed from a sustained growth in population, which commenced around 1750. Enclosed lands were easier to subdivide, so peasant families who wished to provide lands for more than one male heir favored these reforms. The institutional reforms, in turn, helped promote improved systems of crop rotation and increased cultivation of fodder crops. After industrialization began in earnest in the 1870s, there were a number of other technological changes in Swedish farming which will be noted subsequently; but these appear to have involved market forces almost exclusively rather than changes in the institutional organization of peasant farming units.

In sum, both Japan and Sweden in the period just prior to modern economic growth were peasant economies. Despite institutional differences between the two nations and within each country over time, there is a similarity between the two settings—a point we shall return to in Chapter 4 in considerable detail when we discuss the family systems of peasant households in the two nations.

Having emphasized this basic likeness, attention should be called to those salient differences between Japanese and Swedish agricultural conditions in the period just prior to industrialization. For example, consider factor proportions and the types of crops produced. In Table 3.3, figures are provided on output per hectare, output per worker, and land area per worker in the two countries around 1870. The much greater output per worker in the Swedish case is to a large degree explicable in terms of the much larger Swedish ratio of land area per worker compared with that of Japan. Indeed, the assertion that income per capita in 1870 was lower in Japan than in Sweden is certainly a logical implication of these figures

TABLE 3.3

	Indices and ratios			
	1886/90 = 100			
Years	Output[b] (contribution to gross domestic product)	Arable land	Labor	Output per worker
Sweden				
1866/70	72.6	77.2	98.0	74.2
1886/90	100.0	100.0	100.0	100.0
1911/15	166.5	115.6	90.6	184.2
1936/40	171.3	116.6	79.6	215.8
1951/55	246.5	113.8	57.1	431.9
Japan				
1876/80	81.4	95.6	99.7	68.6
1886/90	100.0	100.0	100.0	100.0
1911/15	154.2	116.9	100.7	153.1
1936/40	208.0	125.6	86.1	241.5
1951/55	193.3	121.3	98.6	196.2
1966/70	353.9	120.8	65.2	543.1

[a] Swedish figures from Johansson (1967: Table 56, pp. 152–153 and Table 58, pp. 156–157); and Sweden. Statistiska Centralbyrån (1959: Table E6, pp. 38–39). Japanese figures from Hayami, Ruttan and Southworth (1979: Tables J-2 and J-4, p. 245) *WU* conversion ratios from Hayami and Ruttan (1971: Table 4.2, p. 73).

because both economies were primarily dependent on peasant agrarian production. These factor proportions are also reflected in the crops on which the peasant households in the two countries subsisted. The staple crop of Japan was rice, which can be produced by utilizing the land intensively. In contrast, in nineteenth-century Sweden the principal crops were grains—wheat, oats, and barley—with animals frequently grazed, a practice uncommon in densely populated Japan. That the Swedish peasant of the nineteenth century was relatively impoverished compared with the inhabitants of other European nations and countries of European settlement is due to geography; the Swedish climate is harsh and the soil is relatively poor. But given the factor proportions prevailing, we would still expect the Japanese peasant to have had a lower standard of living than the Swedish peasant.

The modernization of agricultural production in the two countries can be traced in Table 3.3. The implications of the initial balance of resources are extremely important for the fertility transition, as will be argued subse-

Agricultural Indices and Measures, Japan and Sweden[a]

Absolute measures			Growth rate (% per annum)			
	International (*WU*) units[c]					
Arable land per worker (hectares per worker)	Output per hectare	Output per worker	Periods	Arable land	Labor	Output per worker
2.36	0.95	2.24	1866/70 to 1936/40	0.6	−0.3	1.5
2.99	1.01	3.01				
3.82	1.45	5.55	1936/40 to 1951/55	−0.1	−2.2	4.7
4.39	1.48	6.50				
5.96	2.18	13.01	1866/70 to 1951/55	0.5	−0.7	2.1
.300	2.10	0.63	1876/80 to 1936/40	0.5	−0.4	2.1
.313	2.94	0.92				
.363	3.88	1.41	1936/40 to 1966/70	−0.1	−1.0	2.7
.456	4.87	2.22				
.385	4.69	1.81	1876/80 to 1966/70	0.2	−0.5	2.3
.580	8.61	4.99				

[b] Based on figures in 1913 prices for Sweden. Based on figures in 1934–1936 prices for Japan. These series are constructed by taking *WU* per hectare figures for each country (1955 for Sweden; 1965 for Japan) and adjusting these by an index of output per hectare (in constant prices) for each country.

[c] *WU* = wheat units (one wheat unit equals one ton of wheat)

quently. Hayami and Ruttan (1971) laid out the basic theoretical arguments concerning agricultural development that will be followed here. Briefly, their position is as follows. On the one hand, countries with a highly favorable man–land ratio (like the United States, Canada, and Australia) tend to have a relatively inelastic supply of labor, so the agricultural sector grows by substituting capital for labor; that is, mechanization plays a major role early on in the expansion of agricultural productivity. On the other hand, where the man–land ratio is highly unfavorable, such as in Japan, land is relatively scarce and labor abundant, so technological progress tends to be labor-using and capital is substituted for land. In such cases, fertilizer and new seed varieties play a major role; that is, biological and chemical technical progress occurs, which preserves the labor-intensive nature of farming, and capital is invested to permit more intensive farming of each acre of land. Countries like Sweden, Belgium, and Denmark, which are between these two extremes, experience agricultural modernization by

TABLE 3.4A

Size Distributions of Agricultural Holdings, Japan and Sweden

	Land ownership (%)		Tenancy status of farm households (%)		
Year	% of farm land leased	% of arable land leased	Owner	Part-owner part-tenant	Tenant
Sweden					
1927	23.9	25.5	—	—	—
1937	25.4	26.5	—	—	—
1951	21.5	25.9	—	—	—
Japan					
1920	—	—	30.7	40.9	28.4
1935	—	—	31.0	42.0	27.0
1941	—	—	31.2	40.7	27.7
1950	—	—	61.8	32.5	5.0

moving along a middle path, with biological and chemical progress as well as mechanization playing important roles.

Some details from the history of agricultural development in Japan and Sweden may be helpful in illustrating this argument. Let us first consider Japan. A number of studies have carefully delineated the path of productivity growth in Japan; they find acceleration in the growth rate of output from about 1900 until around World War I, followed by a period of stagnation between the wars, and finally a rapid spurt after World War II.[12] The first period was characterized by a rapidly increasing demand for fertilizer, which was met by a dramatic increase in supply, occasioning a falling price of fertilizer. In turn, the decline in fertilizer costs induced farmers and government experimental stations to develop high-yielding, fertilizer-responsive crop varieties. A plateau was reached around World War I because diffusion of the best practice techniques of early Meiji agriculture (through pure-line selection of existing seed varieties) had been completed. The next big step involved the application of Mendelian principles of cross-breeding, a task achieved in the 1930s. But the shortage of fertilizer occasioned by the war prevented farmers from effectively exploiting these new varieties. After the war the constraint on fertilizer availability vanished, and this undoubtedly accounts for much of the early postwar spurt. With the rapid growth of manufacturing in Japan after 1955, labor has become a scarce factor (this is particularly the case since the middle 1960s), and mechanization has quickly proceeded Tsuchiya, 1976:179). The first wave of mechanization occurred between 1955 and 1965, when power tillers played the crucial role. The second phase, from 1965 to the present, primarily involves rice trans-

TABLE 3.4B

Social Structure of Agricultural Population, Japan and Sweden[a]

Year	Entrepreneurs	Working members of families of entrepreneurs	Crofter class	Statare	Day laborers, etc.	Farm servants and other laborers living in	Others
Distribution of productive agricultural population for Sweden							
1880	20.3	21.8	10.4	3.2	19.4	24.4	0.5
1910	26.8	26.3	8.3	3.5	22.7	10.8	1.6
1930	29.3	27.3	2.3	4.5	23.8	9.7	3.1
	0–5 *tan*	5 *tan* to 1 *chō*[b]	1 *chō* to 2 *chō*	2 *chō* to 3 *chō*	3 *chō* to 5 *chō*	5 *chō* & over	
Distribution of farm households by amount of land farmed for Japan							
1920	35.3	33.4	20.7	6.2	2.8	1.7	
1941	33.3	30.0	26.7	6.1	2.2	1.3	
1946	39.2	31.3	23.5	3.7	1.4	0.8	
1954	39.8	32.5	22.1	3.4	1.5	0.8	

[a] For Sweden, land ownership figures from Sweden. Statistiska Centralbyrån (1959), *Historical Statistics, II (1955)*; distribution of agricultural population from Thomas (1941: Table 18, p. 97). For Japan, figures for 1920 and 1935 from Bank of Japan (1938, pp. 122–123); figures for 1941, 1946, 1950 and 1954 from Dore (1959: Table 9, p. 176 and Table 10, p. 181).

[b] One *chō* = one hectare approximately; 10 *tan* = 1 *chō*.

planters and combines. In sum, Japanese agricultural productivity growth follows the path predicted by the theoretical arguments advanced by Hayami and Ruttan.

In the Swedish case, mechanization came much earlier, but biological and chemical innovations were also crucial from the onset of rapid productivity growth. Before World War I, and especially after the appearance of American grain in European markets at the end of the 1870s, crop rotation was improved; systematic subsoil drainage was adopted; and sugar, beets, and turnips became common crops. These changes served as the basis for the dramatic concentration on animal husbandry [this latter specialization was almost surely a response to the movement in relative prices of grain and animal products after American grain exports swamped Europe, see Heckscher (1954:257)]. The development of animal husbandry, especially of the dairy industry, encouraged early mechanization. An outstanding example of this is the cream separator, which Swedish inventors developed. Mechanization is also indicated by the utilization of tractors; a survey conducted in 1927 testified to the widespread adoption of tractors in the first quarter of the twentieth century (Thomas, 1941:75). Thus Swedish technological progress in farming reflects the factor proportions with which Sweden commenced modern growth.

In addition to the differences in the balance between population and cultivatable land, the social structure of Swedish peasant agriculture, especially in land ownership, was unlike that prevailing in Japan. Tables 3.4A and B help us to appreciate this point. As already emphasized, in preindustrial Japan there were no manorial estates. Tenancy, however, was of considerable importance throughout the period 1870–1945, until the postwar land reform that was encouraged by the American authorities (a comparison of the 1941 and 1950 figures on land ownership succinctly captures the impact of the reform).[13] As previously indicated, land was exchanged during the Tokugawa period despite legal prohibition. Thus tenancy also developed, although, until 1880 and the Matsukata deflation, only about one-third of the land was not directly owned by the cultivator. As a result of the Matsukata deflation, which hit small cultivators the hardest, the proportion of arable land under tenancy rose gradually until, by 1930, it amounted to almost one-half of all land. As will be demonstrated in Chapter 4, the distinctions among owner–cultivators, part-owners, and tenants were essential to the concept of status differences in the Japanese village. A similar cleavage is indicated by the figures in Tables 3.4A and B on farm land cultivated by the household.

As one can gather from the figures in Tables 3.4A and B, in Sweden tenancy was considerably less prevalent than in Japan. But status differences associated with land were nevertheless of great importance among Swedish peasants, as the figures on productive agricultural population suggest. Because sustained population growth occurred in Sweden between 1750 and 1850, sons of land-owning farmers found it increasingly difficult to acquire their own property. Before, such individuals had taken positions as farm servants for a time, carefully husbanding and building their capital until they could acquire land. If this proved impossible, negotiation of a long-term contract as a crofter (*torpore*) or a short-term lease of land as a cottager were less desirable alternatives (Montgomery, 1939:69; Thomas, 1941:53–54). The period of population expansion saw the gradual proletarianization of the agricultural population, with increasing numbers of males becoming crofters or leasors of cottages. Finally, many landlords and estate owners experimented with another system of securing labor for their land because the increase in population and the institutional reorganization of agriculture in emulation of England encouraged innovations. They hired laborers on annual contracts and paid them wages in kind (the *stat,* i.e., food and housing).[14] Such workers were known as *statare.* The importance of crofters, *statare,* and other more casual laborers in 1880 is indicated by the figures in Tables 3.4A and B. In sum, the Swedish peasantry like the Japanese was sharply differentiated into social classes according to land ownership.

The differences between the two cases are twofold. First, the institutional arrangements were considerably different, with contracted labor playing a greater role in the Swedish case (crofters, *statare,* and day laborers) and tenancy taking a much more prevalent position in Japan. Second, modern economic growth in Sweden between 1880 and 1930 witnessed a decline in the proportions of people occupying inferior statuses, whereas an increase in those groups accompanied Japanese development during the same epoch. (Swedish emigration, to be noted in the following text, accounts for some of this latter difference.)

Let us summarize what we have learned about agriculture in the two countries. First, both nations were populated primarily by peasants prior to industrialization. Among the peasantry, major status distinctions associated with land tenure were apparent in both cases. But the institutions and forms these social differences took were somewhat different in the two countries, as were their ebb and flow over time. Finally, initial factor proportions were very dissimilar in the two nations; this played a major role in shaping the types of technological progress taking place in the two settings.

3.6. Industry

We have already suggested how initial resource endowments and factor proportions can be important in shaping economic modernization. What is

TABLE 3.5

Composition of Manufacturing Output by Type of Subsector, Japan and Sweden (%)

Years	Food products	Textiles, clothing, leather, hair, and rubber products	Wood products	Chemicals	Stone, clay, and glass	Mining and metals	Pulp, paper, and printing	Electricity, gas, and water works
Sweden[a]								
1866/70	34.7	13.2	19.0	4.7	1.3	24.7	2.0	0.3
1886/90	33.6	14.1	18.3	5.7	2.6	22.2	3.7	0.5
1911/15	29.4	16.5	10.5	4.2	4.2	24.7	9.0	1.6
1936/40	22.8	15.5	7.2	4.3	3.3	32.6	10.4	3.7
1951/55	17.2	12.5	7.6	6.2	3.2	37.2	12.6	3.5

Years	Food products	Textiles	Lumber and wood products	Chemicals	Stone, clay, and glass	Iron and steel, nonferrous metals, and machinery	Printing and publishing	Others
Japan[b]								
1886/90	36.0	35.3	3.0	13.1	1.8	5.3	0.4	5.3
1911/15	31.1	33.2	2.7	11.6	2.5	13.5	1.4	4.1
1936/40	13.2	21.3	3.5	16.2	2.3	38.3	1.8	3.5
1952/55	19.6	17.3	4.7	18.3	3.4	31.7	3.3	1.7
1966/70	12.5	8.4	4.8	15.9	3.6	48.4	3.0	3.3

[a] Percentages of Gross Output in "Manufacturing and Mining" (current prices). Swedish figures are from Johansson (1967: Table 6, pp. 48–67).

[b] Percentages of Total "Manufacturing" Production (current prices). Japanese figures are from Ohkawa *et al.* (1979: Table A.19, pp. 298–301).

true for agriculture is also true for the industrial sector, where geography and resources have been crucial elements in determining Swedish and Japanese development. Table 3.5 provides us with the relevant information.

In comparing these two sets of figures concerning changes in the structure of industrial output, two points spring immediately to our attention. First, if we think about broad types of industries, then we see substantial similarities. For example, let us divide the industries into three groups: food processing and related industries; textile production (light manufacturing); and chemicals, metals, and machinery (heavy manufacturing). In terms of these categories there are clear parallels. For example, food-processing industries initially constituted about 35% of output in both cases, and their proportion steadily fell, reaching approximately 20% around 1950. Second, heavy industry grew dramatically in both countries, especially metals and machinery. There are also marked dissimilarities. Initially, textiles played a major role in Japanese manufacturing (constituting a major demand for unskilled and semiskilled youthful female employees); but this was never a major sector in Sweden. Rather, wood and paper products acted as a critical industrial block in the Swedish case, a notable contrast to Japan.

The reasons for these differences lie almost certainly in geography and natural resources. Historically, nineteenth-century Sweden lay on the periphery of the industrial heartland of Western Europe, which was concentrated in England, France, Belgium, and parts of Germany. Sweden played a prominent role in supplying raw materials to these countries, especially timber and iron ore from the central and northern districts. Because of its mines and abundant forests, on the one hand, Sweden retained a comparative advantage in these products after industrialization began; thus growth was initially built around a few crucial export sectors. Textiles, on the other hand, was not an especially attractive industry, in light of the domination of European textile markets by England and France.

Japan, in contrast, was isolated geographically from Europe and located in an area having virtually no modern industrial regions at the end of the nineteenth century. This meant that the low-income Japanese domestic market had to play a more major role with respect to demand than did the Swedish domestic market in the Swedish case (and in any event the closest foreign markets in Asia were all low-income agricultural nations). Thus the Japanese manufacturing industry initially specialized in cheap textiles for which the demand, even in a low-income setting, was buoyant and unlikely to fall off rapidly. Moreover, Japan was not especially abundant in mineral ores, coal excepted. For example, in 1931 coal production constituted over 60% of the value of all minerals mined [see Mosk (1981d) for a discussion of Japanese mining]. Thus Japanese manufacturing initially centered around food processing industries and textiles; the great surge in heavy industry was delayed until fairly late, the 1930s, and even then was partially related to Japanese military advances on the Chinese continent.

In sum, despite broad structural parallels between the two economies over the period 1880–1960, a brief scrutiny of circumstances within the major sectors of employment and production—agriculture and manufacturing—reveals important differences. These differences, as will be argued subsequently, had a considerable impact on the timing of the fertility transitions in the two nations.

3.7. Urbanization

Urbanization is commonly thought to accompany modern economic growth. Among other reasons for this assumption, it is argued that industrial production in a technologically sophisticated economy receives substantial economies of scale from centralization of labor force. That economic development was indeed accompanied by urbanization is suggested by the second and third columns of Table 3.6, which provide a capsule summary of the growth of the urban and rural sectors of Japan and Sweden.[15] The areas designated as rural actually lost population in absolute terms, whereas the urban districts increased by multiples of about six during the time periods compared here. The urbanization proportions given at the center of the table also suggest similarities. If we are to believe the early pre-1920 estimates for Japan, they suggest that the urban population around 1880 constituted about 10% of the total national population, a figure comparable to that indicated for Sweden at about the same time.[16] Similarly, by 1960 both countries had over 50% of their populations living in cities. In short, indicators of levels and trends in urbanization and the relative expansion or decrease of total numbers of people residing in rural and urban districts are roughly equal in the two nations over the time period 1880–1965.

What does differ between these two countries is the sex ratio. In the Japanese series, females remain in surplus in the rural areas at all dates, whereas they are initially in deficit in the prewar urban areas. In contrast, the figures for Sweden show that the initial surplus of females in the rural areas gives way to a deficit in the period after 1930, whereas females always remain in surplus in the urban districts. At least two reasons can be adduced for these discrepancies, both of which suggest important differences in the growth experience of the two countries. During the nineteenth and early twentieth centuries, geography and international patterns of migration established in the original settlement of America were such that Swedish emigration to the United States was considerable. Thus the heavily female sex ratios in *both* the urban and rural sectors of Sweden up to world War I

TABLE 3.6

Indices and Rates of Growth of Urban and Rural Population, Urbanization (%), and Sex Ratios, Japan and Sweden[a]

	Indices and ratios								Growth rates (% per annum)			
			Females/1,000 Males				% in locales with 10,000 or more people[b]	% in locales with 50,000 or more people[b]				
Years	Rural population	Urban population	Rural population	Urban population	Total population	Urbanization (%)			Period	Rural population	Urban population	Total population
Sweden[c]												
1876/80	100.0	100.0	1042	1189	1057	14.8	N.A.	N.A.	1876/80 to 1936/40	0.1	2.1	0.6
1886/90	101.3	129.1	1037	1186	1062	18.1	N.A.	N.A.				
1911/15	108.1	222.8	1006	1163	1045	26.4	N.A.	N.A.	1936/40 to 1961/64	−0.4	2.3	0.8
1936/40	105.0	341.6	950	1154	1019	36.1	N.A.	N.A.				
1951/55	96.5	522.2	939	1085	1007	48.5	N.A.	N.A.	1876/80 to 1961/64	−0.1	2.1	0.6
1961/64	94.5	596.4	937	1069	1004	52.3	N.A.	N.A.				
Japan[d]												
1888	—	—	—	—	—	—	12.9	7.4				
1903	—	—	—	—	—	—	20.7	11.4	1920 to 1935	0.0	5.5	1.4
1918	—	—	—	—	—	—	31.9	16.5				
1920	100.0	100.0	1013	920	—	18.0	—	—	1935 to 1965	−1.3	3.7	1.2
1935	100.5	223.7	1016	947	—	32.9	—	—				
1955	85.0	498.1	1041	1033	—	56.3	—	—	1920 to 1965	−0.8	4.3	1.3
1965	68.4	662.8	1068	1025	—	68.1	—	—				

[a] Swedish figures are from Sweden. Statistiska Centralbyrån (1969, Table 4:46–48), *Historical statistics of Sweden, part 1 population.* Japanese figures are from Nihon. Naikaku Tōkeikyoku (various years) *Kokusei chōsa hōkoku* for various years, and Japan. Prime Minister's statistical Bureau (various years) *Report of the population census* for various years. The dash indicates that data were not available.

[b] Percent urbanization for legal (*honseki*) population. The *honseki* population of a district is all persons who are listed in a *koseki* (family registration book) kept by a government office of the district. N.A. indicates not applicable.

[c] For rural and urban populations the index is 1876/80 = 100.

[d] For rural and urban populations the index is 1920 = 100.

reflect the tendency of Swedish males to leave their country of birth for North America. After World War I, the Swedish economy was strong enough to hold its population better (and the United States began to impose restrictions on immigration). Thus female deficits in the rural zones, where labor demand (timber, mining, etc.) tends to run in favor of men, are complemented by an excess of females in the cities, where white-collar work and light industrial opportunities abound. (Given a roughly equal balance of sexes for the national population, we would expect this complement of the ratios.)

By comparison, the opportunities for Japanese prewar emigration were not nearly as good as those for the Swedes, the colonies of Taiwan, Korea, and Manchuria (Manchuko) being the major locales for settlement outside Japan. Thus Japanese national sex ratios prior to the onset of World War II tend to be fairly normal, and the rural excess of females, occasioned perhaps by the concentration of much light manufacturing in the rural zones, is matched by an excess of males in the cities. However, because of losses of men sustained during World War II, the Japanese sex ratios show an excess of females in both urban and rural areas after 1945.

In short, setting aside the contrast in sex ratios, the parallelism in urbanization between the two countries is compelling. However, the contrast in sex ratios is something that must be taken into account in the demographic analysis of Part III. In Chapters 5–8, a proxy for the sex ratio will be introduced to deal with its possible influence (especially on nuptiality).

3.8. Education

The next topic of comparison is education, and some basic points can be made succinctly. Both Sweden and Japan had highly developed educational systems at the outset of modern economic growth, and these enjoyed sustained and rapid expansion with industrialization. In comparative terms, however, it is probably safe to say that Swedish schools were more universally attended during the nineteenth and early twentieth centuries than were Japanese. The relatively early development of education in these two countries (which stands in stark contrast to Great Britain, whose educational system expanded around 1870, after a century of modern economic growth) is undoubtedly attributable primarily to religious and political factors; the cultural and linguistic homogeneity of the two nations played an additional part.[17]

Let us begin our discussion with a few quantitative indicators. In Table 3.7, figures concerning educational attainment for Sweden are provided, at various dates, and for Japan, for a number of cohorts (the cohorts fell into the age classes given in the table headings on October 1, 1970). The term "have not graduated from a school," used in connection with the Japanese data, refers to failure to graduate from a prewar primary school. As the reader can quickly gather from these figures, attendance in primary schools was virtually universal in Sweden by 1880, and graduation from a primary school in Japan was virtually universal by 1905 or so. Given that these two countries were relatively poor and backward compared with other western nations in the last quarter of the nineteenth century, what explains the early acceptance of schooling in these nations?

To understand the early Meiji educational system, it is first necessary to sketch in the background of Tokugawa schooling. Tokugawa schools fell into two broad classes: those designed to train the sons of *samurai* in the Chinese classics and in the management of institutions run by fief (*han*) administrations; and those that trained the children of merchants and farmers, the *terakoya* schools (other more minor categories of schools also existed). Between the mid-eighteenth and mid-nineteenth centuries, the number of feudal fiefdoms not having domain schools to educate their *samurai* fell sharply [see Dore (1965) and Passin (1965)]. In these schools, the sons of upper-class *samurai* studied the Chinese classics and learned Confucian philosophy and ethics; the sons of lower-class *samurai* often learned the more practical subjects of arithmetic and the like. The point is that the fiefdoms came to feel that they needed a literate bureaucracy to manage their affairs, and the domain schools filled this need. The status of a fief was partly a function of the education it provided its *samurai.* The privately run *terakoya* schools were another matter altogether. In these schools, which were especially prevalent in the cities, teaching was oriented toward learning to read and write the Japanese language and to perform arithmetical computations. It is estimated that between 1803 and 1867 over 9000 *terakoya* schools were established. In sum, during the later Tokugawa period, as the peace brought by the feudal regime permitted the *samurai* to turn away from purely military pursuits, Confucian-inspired education spread among the upper strata of society. Undoubtedly partly through emulation, the other feudal classes, especially merchants, also began trying to educate their children on a wide scale; the emphasis on the type of education they sought probably reflected status differences and economic needs of the various groups.

Thus when the Meiji government set up the new Department of Education (*Mombushō*) in 1871, it already had a tradition of learning to fall back on—and, equally important, a stock of domain and *terakoya* instructors from whom it could recruit teachers. Initially, primary schooling was declared compulsory for all children, but in 1879 the Meiji government rejected its first Education Code of 1872 but later reinstituted it on several occasions, so that the early Meiji period did not witness the smooth implementation of a school system. It is usually recognized that by 1908 compul-

TABLE 3.7

Measures of Educational Attainment, Japan and Sweden[a]

Year(s)	Percentage of persons aged 7–14 receiving or not receiving schooling					
	Receiving schooling			Not receiving schooling		
	Primary[b]	Secondary	Other	Left school	Not yet begun school	Other
Sweden						
Country						
1871/1875	83.6	4.2	9.8	—	—	—
1891/1895	84.7	3.7	4.0	4.3	—	3.3
1911/1915	86.7	4.2	0.9	5.8	—	2.4
1915/1919	74.7	3.9	0.5	8.1	11.8	1.0
1920	74.4	4.6	0.5	7.1	12.5	0.9
1935	83.5	3.8	0.7	0.1	11.6	0.3
1959	82.0	5.5	0.9	0.0	11.4	0.2
Rural						
1891/1895	86.5	1.2	4.6	4.2	—	3.3
1911/1914	88.7	1.3	1.1	6.3	—	2.6

1916/1919	76.6	1.1	0.5	9.0	11.9	0.9	
1920	76.8	1.3	0.4	7.9	12.8	0.8	
1959	83.9	4.2	0.4	0.0	11.3	0.1	
Urban							
1891/1895	75.1	15.6	1.2	4.5	—	3.6	
1911/1914	80.0	14.2	0.5	3.7	—	1.7	
1916/1919	68.2	12.4	0.7	5.5	12.1	1.1	
1920	67.6	13.9	0.6	5.0	11.6	1.2	
1959	80.0	6.8	1.4	0.0	11.5	0.3	
	Percentage of males and females at various ages who have not graduated from a school (1970)						
Sex	55–59	60–64	65–69	70–74	75–79	80–84	85–over
Japan							
Male	0.4	0.7	0.9	1.4	2.3	4.5	10.7
Female	0.8	1.5	2.6	4.6	9.0	18.9	34.1

[a] Swedish figures are from Sweden. Statistiska Centralbyrån (1974: *Pupils in Compulsory Schools in Sweden 1847–1962* Tables 1.4, p. 52 and 1.6, p. 54). Japanese figures are from Nihon. Sōrifu Tōkeikyoku (1973: *1970 Population Census of Japan. Vol. 5. Part 1* Table 6, pp. 73–82).

[b] Includes continuation course attendance after 1920.

sory education (in a primary school) had become a reality throughout Japan (Shimahara, 1979). The Japanese government's insistence on this program was probably due as much to military and political needs (i.e., the need to provide a literate, disciplined populace that was sufficiently imbued with the values of the Meiji regime to be extremely loyal to it) as to any economic advantages that might accrue to it. Moreover, the regime's willingness to educate the entire populace probably stemmed from its lack of fear that any serious internal threats to its power would arise from the diffusion of popular education among the common people (Dore, 1965).

The prewar system of Japanese education consisted of 6 years of required elementary schooling. After that, students could elect to continue their schooling in academically oriented middle schools, which were segregated by sex, or in a wide variety of specialized technical schools, including institutions that specialized in agricultural or commercial affairs. In the postwar reforms inspired by the American occupation authorities, this system was considerably revamped. Education was made compulsory for 6 years of elementary and 3 years of junior high school. Students now typically enter 3-year high schools, which are not compulsory, following graduation from junior high school.

To summarize, Japanese education in the Tokugawa period developed extensively among the *samurai* because the country enjoyed internal peace and because the feudal elite was strongly influenced by Confucian values. The other classes emulated them, and by the time the Meiji Restoration occurred, a tradition of education had firmly taken root. The Meiji oligarchs found education to be a useful means of building a strong military and a cooperative populace (by making indoctrination in the political values of the Meiji government part and parcel of education), so they expanded its scope with considerable vigor. By the 1930s, Japan had a well developed system of schools and illiteracy was almost unknown. Building on this, the postwar Japanese government expanded the system further to make compulsory education cover middle school.

The modern Swedish system of compulsory education, like the Japanese, rests on a vigorous tradition stretching back before the nineteenth century —in the Swedish case, to the reformation statutes of the 1530s (Dixion, 1965:69). After the Lutheran religion had taken hold in Scandinavia, Luther's plea that children be taught to read so that they could read the Bible on their own encouraged the spread of education. Latin schools, the precursors of the *gymnasium,* were set up, and the children of the elite were educated in these institutions at the expense of their parents. For the mass of the peasantry, financial circumstances precluded sending their offspring to such schools, and in any event the liberal education secured there was of little use to their children, but the clergy encouraged teaching in the home in lieu of formal schooling. Interest in universal education continued among the peasantry, however, and as economic circumstances began to improve in the first half of the nineteenth century, the *Riksdag* finally passed a bill, in 1842, requiring the local parishes to provide compulsory education for children aged 7 to 13. Thus the public elementary school (*folkskola*), designed to educate both boys and girls in reading, writing, and arithmetic, was created in the mid-nineteenth century. On paper at least, all children were required to attend these schools; however, in the countryside, where transportation was poor, population densities low, and children a useful source of family labor, attendance was spotty until later in the nineteenth century (cf. the rural and urban figures for Sweden in Table 3.7). An important feature of Swedish educational history is that in the early stages, when basic literacy was spreading, education was promoted on a family basis; that is, all family members, regardless of age, were taught to read.

Later reforms of the Swedish system, as of the Japanese, increased the duration of compulsory education and widened the options for pursuing different programs, both academic and technical. Major reforms occurred in 1904, 1927, 1946, and the early 1960s. In 1904, the *realskola* was created to serve as a middle school, following the elementary school, and to prepare the student for entry into the upper secondary school, the *gymnasium* [see King (1978:17) and Orring (1969:13–14)]. In 1927 the *realskola* was transformed to make it more flexible in meeting the needs of children from the rural areas, and in the early 1930s experiments were started with practical junior secondary schools (*pratisk realskola*). The postwar reforms were aimed at lengthening the period during which all students received a formal academic training; the school commission report of 1946 recommended 9 years of compulsory schooling; differentiation into practical and academic courses would not occur until the final year. The reforms of the 1960s were also aimed at this problem of when to differentiate into separate courses.[18]

In sum, by the early postwar period both Japan and Sweden had managed to create school systems that provided for 9 years of compulsory education, covering approximately the ages 7 to 16. The parallels between both the early and continued development of the educational systems of the two countries are impressive. Indeed, the educational data reviewed here support (as do the figures on income and structure of production) the choice of Sweden and Japan for comparative analysis.

3.9. The Fertility Transition

The final issue considered in this chapter concerns comparisons of premodern fertility levels and fertility transitions between Japan and Sweden. We already touched on aspects of this in the discussion of fertility transitions in

TABLE 3.8

Characteristics of Natality, Sweden and Japan—Selected Dates[a]

Approximate date	Nuptiality: Males, % single 25–29	Nuptiality: Males, % single 45–49	Nuptiality: Females, % single 20–24	Nuptiality: Females, % single 45–49	I_m	I_m^*	Age gap at marriage at age of wife 20	Age gap at marriage at age of wife 25	Marital fertility I_g	Illegitimacy I_h	Illegitimacy rate
Sweden											
1800	49.6	6.9	77.6	11.7	.46	.49	—[b]	—	.68	.03	—
1880	59.6	10.9	82.3	19.8	.41	.46	.9	1.7	.70	.05	10.2
1900	60.6	13.5	80.4	19.4	.41	.45	.8	1.9	.65	.04	12.7
1930	66.9	16.6	80.4	22.9	.42	.45	.9	2.5	.30	.04	13.9
1950	48.6	16.2	59.7	18.5	.63	.60	.8	2.3	.27	.05	10.2
1960	40.4	14.5	56.0	11.1	.63	.64	—	—	.24	.05	12.8
Japan											
1920	25.8	2.3	31.4	1.9	.70	.73	3.0	4.3	.59	.05	8.2
1925	25.0	1.9	29.6	1.8	.70	.75	2.5	4.1	.55	.05	7.3
1930	28.8	1.8	37.7	1.6	.68	.73	2.7	4.1	.53	.05	6.5
1935	34.9	1.8	44.9	1.5	.66	.70	2.4	4.1	.52	—	5.7
1950	34.5	1.5	55.3	1.5	.59	.64	.9	3.2	.51	—	2.5
1955	41.1	1.3	66.5	1.7	.57	.61	.8	2.4	.35	—	1.7
1960	46.2	1.3	68.4	1.9	.58	.61	.8	2.4	.29	—	1.2

[a] Mosk (1979d) and Sweden Statistika centralbyrån, *Historisk statistik för Sverige* (1969).
[b] The dash indicates that the figures were not estimated.

Europe and Asia, so the broad contrasts should already be apparent to the reader. Here we would like to present more details about fertility levels and trends in the two nations and to couch this discussion in slightly more technical terms than was done in Chapter 1. A general understanding of this technical material is essential to the subsequent analysis of fertility in Part III (Chapters 5–8), so its introduction here serves two purposes: it assists us in describing the fertility transitions in the two populations under study, and it deals with methodological issues we must consider before we can delve into the detailed analysis of natality that Chapters 5–8 contain.

In light of the contrasts between European and Asian transitions pointed out in Chapter 1, it is clearly useful to split the discussion into details concerning nuptiality and details concerning marital fertility. Concerning nuptiality, the first (left-hand) nine columns of Table 3.8 provide us with our focus. We have already mentioned the Hutterite indices I_m and I_m^*, the proportions of single men and women, and the age gap at marriage, respectively, in Chapter 1, so we need not go into a discussion of these terms here. However, one other index of nuptiality that, like the others in Table 3.8, can be computed from census data alone should be mentioned here. This is the singulate mean age at marriage, which is calculated by the formula given in note.[19] Intuitively, it can be thought of as a measure of the average number of years a person spends in single (i.e., never married) status. This index will be used extensively in Part III.

Now let us turn to the substantive issues highlighted in Table 3.8. First, note the sharp contrast in nuptiality patterns between the two countries before their transitions got underway (i.e., Sweden around 1880 compared with Japan around 1920). In Sweden, marriage for *both* males and females was late, age gaps at marriage were small, and proportions of those still unmarried by age 50 were high. In Japan, marriage for males came relatively late (although, as can be seen from the proportions of those single for the age group 25–29, Japanese men married considerably earlier in 1920 than did Swedish males in the nineteenth century), but women married considerably earlier than did men (and, consequently, Japanese women in 1920 married much earlier than did Swedish women in the nineteenth century). The age gaps at marriage for Japanese couples in 1920 were far larger than those for Swedish couples in 1880, and Japanese proportions of those still single at age 50 were exceedingly small around the beginning of the fertility transition. Thus the contrast in the conditions characterizing nuptiality just before the fertility transitions in Japan and Sweden is both sharp and substantial in magnitude. It most certainly captures the range of diversity in Eurasian fertility transitions highlighted in Chapter 1.

Now consider the evolution of nuptiality as the transition proceeded in the two populations. Note the pronounced convergence to a common pattern in 1960.[20] By 1960, marriage ages were at moderate levels, age gaps at marriage were small, and proportions of those permanently single were relatively low in both populations. In effect, the nuptiality trends in the two countries converged from opposite directions. The notion of convergence has already been hinted at in the graphical material discussed in Chapter 1 (Figs. 1.1 and 1.2), and it is highlighted most simply in a comparison of levels and movements in the hutterite index of marriage I_m, which is detailed in Table 3.8.

Now let us turn to the other main component of natality, marital fertility, commencing our discussion with the data in the last three columns of Table 3.8. The last two columns at the far right of the table give measures of illegitimacy, the Hutterite index I_h and the proportion of all births that are illegitimate. These figures substantiate the claim that we can restrict our study to nuptiality and marital fertility in analyzing the transitions of these two populations. The Hutterite index of marital fertility dropped in Sweden from 1880 to 1930, when it reached very low levels. In Japan, this decline commenced around 1920 and was largely complete by 1960. The question of the timing of the fertility transitions in Japan and Sweden is taken up in considerably greater detail in Chapters 5–8.

Looking at fertility transitions in terms of I_g is useful, but there are problems with relying on I_g alone. Levels of I_g may reflect deliberate control of reproduction, but they may also reflect constraints on natural fertility (e.g., limitations on the fecundability, or reproductive capacity, of married couples). Ideally, we would want an index that separates the degree of regulation of fertility from total marital fertility, purging our measure of variations due to factors like reproductive capacity. In Chapter 1, we mentioned the concepts of natural fertility and parity-specific control. By working with these concepts scholars at the Office of Population Research at Princeton University have attempted to produce more precise and sensitive measures of fertility control than I_g; these are the Coale–Trussell indices of natural fertility and parity-specific control.

The Coale–Trussell Indices of Marital Fertility

The Coale–Trussell indices of natural fertility and parity-specific control were developed by Coale (1971) and Coale and Trussell (1974, 1978).[21] Whenever age-specific marital fertility rates are known, we can estimate these indices. An index of the overall level of marital fertility M is usually interpreted as a proxy for natural fertility; a set of age-specific indicators $m(a)$ (and their mean value m), which numerically describe the deviation of the curve of age-specific fertility away from natural (unregulated) fertility, serves as a measure of parity-specific control.[22] In populations with little parity-specific control (m $\cong$ 0) or when parity-specific control is just beginning to characterize natality, the values of m (and $m(a)$) are less than .2; as the transition takes place, they approach or exceed one.

The utility of the Coale–Trussell formulation is considerable. There is no doubt that movement in m gives an extremely useful characterization of the fertility transition, and analysis of its value and trend provides a fruitful approach to delineating and understanding the fertility transition. Because modern reproductive behavior is characterized by complete cessation of reproduction after a certain number of children are born, a value of m near 0 suggests that modern deliberate family limitation is not being practiced on a significant scale within that population.[23] Other approaches typically involve determination of the level of marital fertility or, even more crudely (because of nuptiality), of the crude birth rate. But changes in the level of natural fertility of a population (and hence its reproductive capacity) can affect its value of marital fertility even when modern parity-specific control is absent.

As Coale and Trussell probably originally intended when developing their indices, the Coale–Trussell formulation is supposed to yield a complete decomposition of fertility into two "orthogonal" components: one measuring the level of marital fertility that would obtain among married women if they did not control their reproduction (M) and the other capturing the extent to which they do (or do not) control or regulate their reproduction (m). This interpretation is far too simple, as will be shown subsequently at considerable length. Rather, the distinction in reproductive behavior involves contrasting reproductive behavior designed to maximize the total number of surviving children out of a given number of births (i.e., control related to the survivorship ratio) with that designed to control the total number of surviving children a couple has. It is, of course, likely that a third type of reproductive behavior—no control whatsoever—also exists. Indeed, within any given population, all three types of behavior may be observed. The argument here is that much of what we observe in (at least some) fertility transitions is a movement from the type of behavior that attempts to maximize survivorship rates to a behavior that tries to limit the total number of surviving children.

The problem of interpreting M and m arises at this point. Both M and m may well involve control; as couples in a population begin to control their total surviving family sizes, they may use methods of reducing M (which they originally employed for controlling the survivorship rate) as well as increasing m to obtain this goal. That is, they may continue to rely on their traditional methods of control, although the aim and purpose that underlie their adoption of these methods are now shifting and changing. As a result, a fertility transition may be characterized by a simultaneous reduction in M

TABLE 3.9

Values of the Coale–Trussell Indices of Natural Fertility (*M*), Parity-Specific Control (*m*), and the Mean Square Error (*MSE*) of the Regression, for Selected Countries at Selected Dates[a]

Country and date	*M*	*m*	*MSE*
Sweden			
1871/1880	.92	−.01	.009
1901/1910	.90	.23	.004
1911/1920	.77	.32	.006
1930	.66	.79	.024
1949	.60	1.06	.012
1957	.64	1.47	.022
1967	.62	1.60	.006
Portugal			
1930	.73	.18	.020
1940	.64	.31	.006
1950	.64	.39	.009
1960	.72	.69	.006
1968	.61	.69	.029
Hungary			
1948/1949[b]	.60	1.08	.003
1956[c]	.48	1.95	.005
1968[b]	.56	2.03	.002
Japan			
1925	.72	.19	.001
1930	.72	.29	.001
1950	.92	1.02	.029
1955	.88	1.07	.027
1960[c]	.89	2.21	.018
1965[c]	1.03	2.56	.045
1970[c]	1.07	2.71	.069
Korea			
1960[c]	.98	.29	.006
1966[c]	.90	.53	.004
1970[c]	.91	.82	.002
Taiwan			
1963	.91	.47	.015
1968	.97	1.10	.039
Sri Lanka			
1963	.94	.64	.012
1970	.94	.76	.006

[a] Swedish and Hungarian (1956) figures from United Nations Department of Economic and

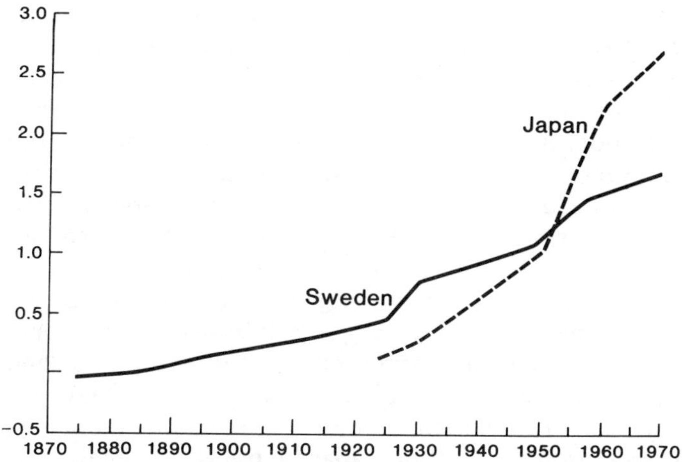

Fig. 3.2. Values of the Coale–Trussell index of parity-specific control m for Japan and Sweden.

and increase in m; the new kind of control (designed to limit family size) may, initially at least, show up in both parameters.

This does not mean m is not a useful index. Indeed, the point is that it is very useful, if interpreted with proper care. To see how it can capture the timing and progress of fertility transitions, let us consider Table 3.9, which shows, for a variety of countries, that parity-specific control is initially absent and then increases substantially.[24] Moreover, the transitions, once begun, seem to be irreversible. Graphically, this process is captured in Fig. 3.2, which displays the paths taken by the fertility transitions of Japan and Sweden. The steady upward climb of m serves as a concise indicator of the fertility transitions in these two nations. Note also that the Japanese transition is far more rapid than the Swedish; the slope of the curve for m in Japan is much steeper than for Sweden.

As suggested in Chapter 1, it has frequently been observed that the fertility transition accompanies economic and social modernization. (It should be noted that "modernization," as a term, is ambiguous and difficult to define.

Social Affairs (1958). Hungarian figures for 1948–1949 and 1968 from Berent (1970). Portuguese figures from Livi-Bacci (1971). Japanese figures from Nihon. Koseishō. Jinkō Mondai Kenkyūjo (1966,1967), adjusted by myself for malregistration and illegitimacy; and from Kobayashi and Tsubouchi (1979). Taiwanese figures from United Nations. Statistical Office of the United Nations (1968). Figures for Sri Lanka from Fernando (1972). Figures for Korea from Mosk (1979c).

[b] Based on figures for four age groups (excluding age groups 40–44 and 45–49).

[c] Based on figures for five age groups (excluding age group 45–49).

As used in this chapter and the following chapters, it refers to modern economic growth *and* to improvements in the educational attainment of national populations.) From the perspective of pure logic, a rigorous statement of that principle in terms of the Coale–Trussell parameters is that the fertility transition in terms of *m* occurs if and only if modernization takes place. However, this statement is too sweeping. Even if we restrict our attention to transitions that commenced before World War II and the introduction of birth control programs in the less developed nations, this statement can be shown to be an exaggeration. In some cases, the transition commences before industrialization (e.g., in France and Hungary during the first half of the nineteenth century), and in others, only after economic development has taken place for several generations (e.g., England's transition began in earnest only after 1870). Indeed, as we have shown, the Japanese and Swedish economies modernized at about the same time, but (as can be seen from Fig. 3.2) the Japanese transition began long after the Swedish.

Nevertheless, there is a broad and compelling association between the standard of living and the modern control of natality, as measured in terms of *m*. We demonstrate this point, somewhat crudely because income per head is admittedly only a rough index of welfare, with Table 3.10, which provides average values of *m* for countries grouped by per capita income and region, circa 1965.[25] An unmistakable pattern emerges from the data. For nations in which the standard of living is high ($1000 or more), parity-specific control is substantial. In the moderate income ranges ($500–1000), the mean value of *m* significantly exceeds zero but is not nearly as great as in the more developed regions. Finally, for the group of less-developed countries with per capita incomes below $500 per annum, there is little evidence of parity-specific control.

In any event, describing the fertility transitions of Japan and Sweden in terms of the index *m* is clearly useful for comparing both the general characteristics and the timing and speed of the transitions. What we have learned is that the Swedish transition began almost a half-century earlier than the Japanese, that it was slower than the Japanese, and that the general pattern of an upward trend in *m* was common to both transitions. The contrast in timing and pace echoes the contrasts in the nuptiality trends. However, the one common feature, namely, the movement of *m* from levels near zero to levels around one or above, is also notable. That is to say, the Swedish and Japanese transitions share one common feature (which all fertility transitions have in evidence), the irreversible fall in I_g or, equivalently, the irreversible increase in *m*; the remaining aspects of the transitions (those involving nuptiality, for instance) show stark and striking differences between the two populations. It is precisely the sharpness of these differences, to reiterate preceding points, that serves as one of the basic motiva-

TABLE 3.10

Average Values[a] of the Coale–Trussell Index of Natural Fertility (M), the Index of Parity-Specific Control m, and the Mean Square Error (MSE) of the Regression, for Countries Grouped by Per-Capita Income Y/P for Circa 1965: Market Economies Only[b]

Region and Income Group	Number of countries	M	m	MSE
Y/P < $500	5	.70	.12	.110
Africa	1	.64	−.19	.130
America	3	.79	.24	.124
Asia	1	.52	.10	.045
$500 ≤ Y/P < $1000	9	.84	.52	.017
America	5	.90	.37	.022
Asia	1	.66	.58	.036
Europe	3	.81	.76	.003
$1000 ≤ Y/P < $1500	2	.97	1.16	.031
Europe	2	.97	1.16	.031
$1500 ≤ Y/P	15	.74	1.43	.010
America	3	.73	1.20	.002
Asia	1	1.07	2.71	.069
Europe	9	.67	1.37	.008
Oceania	2	.91	1.37	.004

[a] Calculated by taking simple means of the values of M, m, and the MSE for the individual nations within each group.

[b] United Nations. Statistical Office of the United Nations (1965).

tions for the choice of these two populations for systematic comparative analysis.

3.10. Conclusions

In this chapter, we have provided a variety of evidence that supports the choice of Japan and Sweden for the purposes of this study. Using several indicators that scholars utilize in quantitatively measuring modern economic growth, it has been shown that, of the countries meeting the conditions for a demographic comparison, Sweden and Japan are the most logical choices for study. It is, of course, no accident that Sweden and Japan look quite similar in terms of all the general indicators of economic growth, such as income per head, structure of total output and labor force, and urbanization. As Kuznets (1966, 1971) went to great lengths to demonstrate, modern economic growth is a process through which technological changes raise productivity and reshape the structure of production at the *same* time. Thus demonstrating that income per capita grew in a similar fasion in the two settings implies the other broad similarities pointed to here. At the same time, we have pinpointed important differences in economic conditions; these should be kept in mind as we proceed to a detailed discussion of the forces underlying the fertility transitions in the two countries.

What is perhaps most compelling, however, is the similarity in the developments of the educational systems in the two countries. Because education is so loosely tied to economic development in a historical sense, at first glance this finding appears very striking. On reflection, however, it does not appear strange. Recall that, of the countries that began modern economic growth prior to the twentieth century, Japan and Sweden were relatively late developers that experienced especially rapid growth. It is likely that part of the reason for their success lies in the early development of education, which permitted their populations to borrow effectively technology from the leading countries and to adapt quickly to change in international markets. Thus we should view all of the factors we have drawn attention to as constituting portions of a simultaneous evolution in economic and social affairs. The burden of this chapter was to show that, if we are carefully and seriously to confront the problems outlined in the introductory chapter, undertaking a comparative study of Japan and Sweden will be the most illuminating approach.

Notes to Chapter 3

1. See Appendix 3 and Mosk *et al.* (1980) for a discussion of the data set. The names and geographical locations of the prefectures appear in Chapters 5 and 7.
2. See Appendix 4 and Mosk and Faris (1979) for a discussion of this data tape.
3. See Appendix 5 and Mosk and Stoft (1979) for a discussion of this data tape.
4. See Appendix 6 and Mosk *et al.* (1980) for a discussion of this data tape.
5. The dating of the beginning of the Japanese transition is discussed in Chapters 5 and 7.
6. Kuznets (1966) is responsible for developing the concept of modern economic growth and utilizing the various quantitative measures to capture it numerically.
7. Kuznets (1966, 1971) provides historical data for the United Kingdom, France, Norway, the United States, Canada, Belgium, the Netherlands, Germany, Italy, Australia, Switzerland, and Russia in addition to Japan and Sweden. The United States, Canada, Russia, and Switzerland fail to meet the homogeneity test. France fails to have an adequate statistical record of the transition. The United Kingdom and Germany began to industrialize substantially before Japan. Australia was a country of tremendous population inflow, a complicating factor because the fertility of immigrants may reflect the conditions of the mother country to a large extent.
8. For Sweden, there are four major series of real income estimates that cover the period after 1870; they differ partly in the periods covered by the figures, the scope and comprehensiveness of the definitions of income, and the price deflation procedures that were utilized in making the estimates. There is the early series covering the period 1860–1930 appearing in

Lindahl *et al.* (1937) and the series developed by Åberg (1969), Johansson (1967), and Krantz and Nilsson (1975). In Table 2.1, we utilize the Johansson estimates because they cover the time period of interest and appear to have been very carefully done. For Japan, there is the widely accepted series that was developed by the scholars at Hitotsubashi University in Tokyo during the 1950s, 1960s, and 1970s. Early estimates from this project were reported in Ohkawa *et al.* (1957) and were later substantially revised and published as Volume 1 of the LTES (Estimates of Long-Term Economic Statistics of Japan) in Ohkawa *et al.* (1974). These latter estimates form the basis for the figures utilized by Ohkawa and Rosovsky (1973). Finally, further modifications were made on the series and the results were published by Ohkawa *et al.* (1979). Whenever possible we use the final, and apparently most definitive, estimates from this massive research project.

9. Ohkawa *et al.* (1979:51). Because of the changes in the Japanese currency system after World War II and the dramatic postwar changes in economic structure and production facilities after the devastation of the war, it is not common for scholars to calculate indices of real output for the postwar period with prewar output figures as the base.

10. The typical family also engaged in some forms of communal village labor. These are described in Chapter 4.

11. Montgomery (1939:50–58). The subject of enclosure of Swedish farmland is controversial. See Sivesand (1979) for a treatment of the issue that stresses the long, drawn-out nature of the process. I am grateful to John Rogers for this reference.

12. See, for example, Hayami *et al.* (1975) and Hayami *et al.* (1979) for details and references to other works. It should be noted that these works rely on the Hitotsubashi (LTES) statistics for agricultural production. Nakamura (1966) launched a trenchant criticism of the official government statistics on agriculture prior to World War I from which the scholars who worked up the LTES series obtained their primary source material. Nakamura proposes a new series, for the years 1874–1920, that he has constructed under a variety of assumptions. He arrives at much higher initial levels of output (circa 1875) and consequently at considerably lower growth rates for agricultural output and productivity. The authors of the LTES series took into account some of Nakamura's points in revising their series, however, and the consensus among scholars who work with these data seems to favor the latest reworked LTES series. For a rebuttal of some of Nakamura's arguments, see, among others, Hayami and Yamada (1970).

13. For details concerning prewar tenancy, see Waswo (1977) and Dore (1959). Also see Dore (1959) for an account of the land reform program.

14. On the *statare* system, see Eriksson and Rogers (1978:18).

15. Discussions and measures of urbanization are plagued at the outset by the very definitions of "urban" and "rural," which are legal, administrative concepts and do not necessarily correspond closely to "concentrated" versus "unconcentrated" population districts. For example, in some cases cities do not incorporate their suburbs, which remain rural by definition, whereas in other cases they legally incorporate agricultural hinterland, which, as a result, becomes urban. In Japan during the mid-1950s, it was common for cities to incorporate a good deal of the surrounding rural territory into their boundaries, producing an artificially rapid "urbanization" when measured statistically. Before the war this was not such a problem because cities usually did not grow in this manner. Rather, when villages became large, reaching about 30,000 in population, they were administratively transformed into cities. In Japan, each prefecture (*ken*) is divided into the urban (*shi*) sector and the rural (*gun*) sector. The urban sector consists of all the cities (*shi*) in the prefecture, and the rural sector consists of all the counties (*gun*) in the prefecture. In Sweden, each county (*län*), except Stockholm city, which is also a county, is divided into the urban (*städer*) sector and the rural (*landsbygd*) sector; the total of individual city (*stad*) populations in a county constitutes the population of its urban sector.

16. For a discussion of Japanese population statistics prior to 1920 and their deficiencies, see Chapter 5 and Appendix 3.

17. For a discussion of why some countries that experienced early industrialization developed educational facilities rather late, see Cipolla (1969).

18. Husén (1962:17). In Chapter 4 the issue of differentiation in Swedish schooling is discussed from another angle.

19. The singulate mean age at marriage (*SMAM*), which is calculated on this data set, referred to in the text, from figures on percentage of single adults in quinquennial age classes, is

$$SMAM = \frac{[\Sigma_{i=1}^{10} S_i] - 10S_{10}}{1 - S_{10}} \times 5$$

where S_i is the percentage of those single in age group i (a decimal number less than or equal to 1), and $i = 1$ stands for ages 0–4, $i = 2$ for ages 5–9, etc.

20. Trends in Swedish nuptiality after 1960 have vitiated this similarity, however, because it has become considerably more common for Swedish women to remain unmarried now than in the 1950s. Indeed, the entire concept of nuptiality has undergone a dramatic transformation in Sweden and a number of other countries with low fertility since 1960. For the purposes of the analysis in this book, however, we wish to focus solely on the premodern and transitional periods. As will be argued in Chapter 4, it is possible to utilize a single model of the household to analyze fertility just before and during the Swedish transition. But once the transition moves toward completion, the model itself loses cogency; in an environment in which parity-specific control is widely diffused, the considerations and constraints that the model used here pinpoints cease to be of great importance.

21. See the discussion in Chapter 1. In computing the index of national fertility M and the indices of parity-specific control (the age-specific values $M(a)$ and their average value m), the computer program developed by Coale and Trussell (1978) was utilized. For a defense of the robustness of the Coale–Trussell indices and a comparison with other methodologies for measuring natural fertility, see Trussell (1979).

22. The idea is that, in parity-specific populations, women in the older reproductive ages have relatively low marital fertility in comparison with the rates of reproduction of the women in the younger reproductive ages 15–19 and 20–24. Because reproductive capacity diminishes with age in a natural fertility population, the critical factor is the *degree* to which the reproduction of older women is diminished.

23. Here we mean deliberate family limitation in the sense of Henry's definition, as discussed in Chapter 1.

24. The mean square error (*MSE*) of the regression used to simultaneously approximate M, $m(a)$, and m is a measure of the goodness of fit of the Coale–Trussell indices. Coale and Trussell (1978) suggest that a mean square error of .01 is fairly poor and about .005 is better, but not especially good. Note the fall in the index of natural fertility M for the European countries (which probably represents the practice of deliberately spacing out births across a longer duration). This means, as argued in the text, that M is really a precise indicator of natural fertility only before the transition begins and that some control of overall surviving family size may appear in M and not be exclusively captured by the m index.

For several of the nations presented in Table 3.9, data were unavailable for some phases of the transition. The index m cannot be calculated for Japan prior to 1925 because age-specific marital fertility rates are unavailable before then.

25. Income figures are in 1970 U.S. dollars.

CHAPTER 4

Leverage and Life Cycle

4.1. Introduction

Is the model of household behavior set forth in Chapter 2 a reasonable stylization of household behavior in Japan and Sweden? Are the concepts of patriarchal leverage, the extraction of labor services, and the life cycle adjustment of work effort and capacity reasonable for these two populations? Does descriptive evidence suggest that the behavioral mechanisms and the institutional rules emphasized here are reasonable in the stylization underling the model? Is there evidence supporting the interpretation of education given to it in Chapter 2? These are the concerns of this chapter. And because the theoretical model revolves around the dependence of household age structure on the economic constraints of production facing the household, the term "life cycle model" as a shorthand phrase is used to capture this concept in the discussion that follows.

The chapter is organized as follows. In Section 4.2 qualitative evidence on the operation of the peasant household in rural Japan is discussed. This is followed by the quantitative discussion of Japanese peasant families in Section 4.3—a discussion that centers around data on Japanese farm families in 1929. Then in the next two sections examination of the Japanese case is concluded by looking at education and the labor market (Section 4.4) and some institutional aspects of marriage (Section 4.5). Sections 4.6 and 4.7 consider, respectively, the institution of the Swedish family and the relationship of education to the labor market in Sweden.

4.2. Labor and Life Cycle in the Japanese Village

In this section we shall be concerned with providing evidence about the operation of the stem family system among Japanese peasants.[1] Here attention will be restricted to a discussion of qualitative material; in the next section statistical evidence in support of the approach used here will be offered. Six main points will be made in this section. We shall first, establish that the Japanese peasantry have pursued a patriarchal stem family system in the nineteenth and twentieth centuries; second, show that this system can be traced back to the eighteenth century; third, demonstrate how the demographic life cycle strategy (which relies on generating family labor for farming) operated in the typical Japanese village prior to the 1960s; fourth, indicate how the rising standard of living of the peasantry in the prewar period led to the gradual growth of labor markets and the substitution of hired hands for family labor; fifth, make note of the slow growth in capital markets prior to the Second World War; and, finally, show how the rapid industrial development of the 1960s and 1970s has completely undermined the operation of the patriarchal stem family system.

There are a substantial number of studies of Japanese villages. Most of these were written during the period after World War II, though some date back to the interwar era.[2] Despite the changes wrought by the occupation of Japan and by the postwar reforms (especially the Land Reform), village studies from the 1950s appear to be in close agreement with those conducted before the war, at least in terms of the variables and patterns we are interested in (except for tenancy status). The dramatic changes associated with mechanization of agriculture and the brisk drawing out of labor from the countryside mainly occurred after the middle 1950s.[3] Thus citations are restricted to descriptions of circumstances that obtained in the interwar period, the late 1940s, and the 1950s. During this period, the village (*mura*) was the lowest level of national governmental administration. Below the administrative entity called the *mura,* however, was the *buraku* (hamlet). Most of the village studies are actually accounts of life in *buraku* because this was the major social unit of village life for individual farming households during our period of analysis.

All authorities indicate that the *ie,* the household, was (and is) the principal unit of social and economic organization in rural Japan.[4] The economic basis of the household is its property (land, residence, material means of production, the graveyard where the ancestors are buried, family shrines and altars, etc.). This economic realization of the *ie* is handed down from father to son. The *ie* continues through time, the heir serving as a means of transmission (see Shimpo, 1976:xiii). The rules governing the heir are straightforward: the head of the house must always be "the son"; and there should be only one "son," not two or more sons jointly occupying the headship. In a typical succession the eldest son inherits; the parents remain with him, along with his wife and children, composing the *ie*. The brothers and sisters leave the *ie* to marry into other *ie* or establish their own *ie*. Two qualifications should be noted here (see Nakane, 1967:4–5). The first is that although the "headship" itself is indivisible, the property may be divided. Tokugawa law discouraged the division of the land, and Meiji law even more stringently restricted division of land (but not necessarily other real property). However in the early twentieth century in certain regions of Japan where densities of population were still relatively low (mainly Hokkaidō and Tōhoku, in the northeast), second and third sons occasionally received small plots of land as part of their inheritance. In such a case the bulk of the land passed to the heir receiving the headship (the main branch, the *honke*) and the other sons established branch families (*bunke*). Second, although the Meiji Civil Codes encouraged primogeniture, in some cases second or third sons secured the headship, rather than the eldest son. Typically, however, the eldest son was groomed for the headship from an early age on. He was usually treated as a superior to his siblings from infancy, receiving larger and better shares of food, a seat at the table closer to the patriarch, and more deferential address in conversation than his brothers and sisters.

Something must be said at this point concerning the practice of adoption as a means of securing the "son" if a biological son is unavailable. A man can be "adopted" into another *ie* in one of two ways. (1) He can enter the other house as the husband of their daughter, in which case he takes on her name. This is called *nyūfu ko'nin.* (2) He can legally be adopted as the son of the couple in the *ie*, and then later marry either their daughter (if they have an unmarried daughter) or, if not, then a woman from another house. This is called *muko yoshi ko'nin.* The possibility of being adopted in this fashion is obviously in part a function of the mortality and fertility of the rural population. If natural fertility is relatively low, as it was in Tokugawa and early Meiji Japan, and mortality relatively high, the number of couples failing to have a biological heir will be numerous enough to absorb most of the sons of other families who do not inherit their own parents' land. As mortality declines and natural fertility increases, the situation clearly changes. One indication of this—testified to in the accounts of the village studies and in aggregate statistics—is that the proportion of males marrying in either *nyūfu ko'nin* or *muko yoshi ko'nin* unions has been declining over time.[5] The reader can see this in Table 4.1, which gives the proportions of marriage in these categories in the prefectures of Japan for the years 1920 and 1935. The table also shows the relative insignificance of these deviant forms of nuptiality in all of Japan during the period of the fertility transition.

TABLE 4.1

Percentages of All Marriages in 1920 and 1935 That Are *nyūfu ko'nin* or *muko yoshi ko'nin* in the Prefectures of Japan[a]

Prefecture	Percentage that are *nyūfu ko'nin* 1920	1935	Percentage that are *muko yoshi ko'nin* 1920	1935
Hokkaidō	1.9	1.3	5.2	3.9
Aomori	1.9	1.6	9.3	7.9
Iwate	2.1	1.8	10.0	8.5
Miyagi	2.3	2.1	9.9	8.9
Akita	2.5	2.3	11.0	8.5
Yamagata	2.8	2.2	7.5	6.0
Fukushima	2.2	1.9	8.9	6.9
Ibaraki	3.0	2.8	9.0	8.0
Tochigi	2.5	1.8	7.5	6.1
Gumma	3.0	2.0	6.4	6.3
Saitama	2.7	2.3	6.1	5.8
Chiba	3.7	3.4	8.2	7.6
Tokyo	3.2	2.4	3.8	4.1
Kanagawa	3.1	2.5	5.2	4.7
Niigata	3.8	3.3	7.3	6.2
Toyama	2.8	2.2	4.0	3.6
Ishikawa	3.5	2.9	3.9	3.9
Fukui	3.6	2.8	5.0	5.0
Yamanashi	3.9	2.5	6.4	5.3
Nagano	3.2	2.8	6.1	5.7
Gifu	3.2	2.6	5.0	4.6
Shizuoka	3.0	2.5	8.1	5.8
Aichi	2.8	2.3	4.3	4.4
Mie	3.1	2.5	6.0	5.6
Shiga	3.8	3.5	3.0	3.7
Kyōto	3.6	3.2	5.5	5.7
Ōsaka	3.1	2.6	4.4	4.5
Hyōgo	3.1	2.8	5.1	4.6
Nara	3.2	2.5	5.4	4.9
Wakayama	2.9	2.3	4.3	4.7
Tottori	3.3	2.8	8.9	7.2
Shimane	4.3	3.5	5.6	5.6
Okayama	3.1	2.7	6.6	6.4
Hiroshima	2.3	2.3	4.4	4.1
Yamaguchi	3.5	3.4	5.1	4.6
Tokushima	4.1	3.6	6.4	5.7
Kagawa	3.0	2.9	5.1	6.0
Ehime	2.8	2.2	4.4	3.4
Kōchi	2.4	2.1	3.6	3.4
Fukuoka	1.7	2.1	3.3	3.0

TABLE 4.1 (Cont.)

	Percentage that are *nyūfu ko'nin*		Percentage that are *muko yoshi ko'nin*	
Prefecture	1920	1935	1920	1935
Saga	2.3	1.7	3.4	2.6
Nagasaki	2.4	1.8	3.8	3.5
Kumamoto	2.2	1.9	3.0	2.9
Ōita	2.8	2.5	5.2	5.0
Miyazaki	2.4	2.1	3.8	2.8
Kagoshima	1.3	1.3	1.9	1.6

[a] *Sources:* See Chapter 5 and Appendix A.3.

The reader should note that the possibility of in-adoption, however, does not invalidate the model in which the patriarch strives to have sons who will mature before he reaches a certain age. There are two main reasons why this is so. (1) If the son is raised by the patriarch himself, he learns farm-specific tasks from a young age and, consequently, does not need to be taught about these special features of the family farm when the patriarch begins his retirement from active work. (2) In-adoption often creates tension within the village. The reason lies in the fact—to be mentioned in the following text—that many village activities are communal. Male household heads play the dominant role in organizing and managing these activities. Males born and raised in the village have a clear sense of the village traditions, personalities of their neighbors, etc. that outsiders do not. Moreover, the in-adopted son is often viewed as an inferior within his family of adoption (particularly if he marries one of the family's daughters as part of the in-adoption arrangement). Thus his position as household head and authority is compromised.[6]

What about the female side of the marriage market? We have argued that a dowry eventually comes to characterize marriages, as natural fertility rises, infant mortality falls and the demand for young brides falls off. Ariga (1968), the expert on the financial arrangements surrounding marriages in the prewar period, discusses regional patterns of gift-giving at marriage (*yuinō*). He argues that although the gifts exchanged are often of little value, in some locales they are of considerable importance, and the bride's family ends up giving more to the groom and his family than the groom's family gives to the bride's family. Thus the practice of *yuinō* is consistent with the preceding interpretation of dowry, for it appears to be similar to a dowry system and, at the same time, there is evidence that it was not of great importance in many districts before the war. Ariga (1968) also suggests it was more commonly practiced in cities, where women wed later and incomes were higher than in most villages. The implication is that the *yuinō* system spread as marriage ages for women rose and incomes improved.

The preceding discussion supports my contention that a patriarchal stem family system has been characteristic of Japan since the late nineteenth century. But has this always been the case historically? T. C. Smith (1966), basing his analysis on a considerable body of literature produced by Japanese historians, argues that the stem family system emerged in the late seventeenth and eighteenth centuries as population growth and technological changes gradually encouraged a stem family system to develop out of an earlier extended joint family system. In the joint family system, the sons farmed the land as a collectivity, working along with servants and *nago* (the latter obtaining a separate dwelling and land in exchange for their labor services). Population densities were still fairly low, and the landholdings of such extended families were often quite extensive. But human numbers increased in the seventeenth century (see Chapter 5), increasing population densities. And a certain type of technological change occurred (perhaps itself resulting from the increase in density): the introduction of new seed varieties, organic fertilizers, more systematic planting techniques, irrigation systems, and the like. These new techniques encouraged more overall labor intensity in production and especially more skill and diligence in planting because all of the changes involved increasing the utilization rate of land but few involved the substitution of capital (e.g., machines) for labor. It is quite plausible that the secular increase in population during the seventeenth century eventually induced this form of labor-utilizing, land-saving transformation of techniques because an increasing scarcity of land (and its rising relative value as compared with labor) would tend to encourage farmers to seek more efficient methods of extracting output from each acre of soil. Because labor was falling in value relative to land, the incentive would presumably be to substitute labor for land and to augment land through an improvement in quality (e.g., fertilizers and irrigation).[7] In any event the new techniques rendered the large joint families inefficient because the supervision and management required for each acre with the new methods came to exceed that available in the extended joint household, with its collateral relatives, *nago,* and servants. More profitable was the division and leasing out of land to stem families. So gradually the sons divided the land (by late Tokugawa this process had been completed) into units of a size that, on the average, a stem family could most efficiently farm, and tenancy replaced the *nago* system. In short, by the nineteenth century the stem family system, in which peasant households farmed land almost exclusively with family labor, came to characterize rural Japan.

It should be noted, in passing, that the existence of gradual productivity gains during the Tokugawa period is consistent not only with a falling or unchanging average level of income (because productivity per land unit may have increased, but productivity per worker may not have increased) but also with a dramatic flourishing of agricultural productivity after the Meiji Restoration. The institutions of feudalism—the stifling of geographical mobility and the exclusiveness of the *han,* the feudal fiefdoms—discouraged the diffusion of best practice techniques throughout the nation. Thus regional variations in techniques, seed varieties, and the like were probably extremely marked at the close of the Tokugawa period. The abolition of the fiefdoms, and the encouragement of interregional migration and dissemination of knowledge of agricultural technology, quickly led to productivity increases in the less developed regions. Moreover, the Meiji government encouraged farmers to learn from the West and to adopt suitable American and European innovations, including chemical fertilizers and the like. Thus the hypothesis that early Tokugawa population growth encouraged the gradual development of labor-using, land-saving agricultural methods is consistent with the picture of the development of agricultural productivity after 1870 described in Chapter 3.

Now let us turn to the utilization of family labor within the farm household. Here we wish to concentrate on family labor alone, postponing the discussion of the gradual development of a market for hired labor during the twentieth century.

The members of the *ie* perform economic activities according to their age, sex, and heirarchical relationship to the household head. Children begin to learn simple tasks at an early age and soon become involved in serious labor, particularly during the periods of peak labor demand.[8] The following remark is typical: "The *buraku* farmer does not regard his children as mere domestic laborers of course, but in the tight schedule of the annual cycle of work a sizable labor force of healthy children is a decided advantage to any household." (Cornell, 1956:152). But although children play an important role in the labor force, "most hard work is performed by men between the ages of eighteen to forty, termed collectively *seinen* (commonly translated as 'young men'). Men from forty to sixty, while doing plenty of work, act as advisers to the *seinen*" (Embree, 1939:87). Here we get to the crux of the life cycle: the gradual retirement of the parents as they reach their middle forties and can hand over the most onerous work to their children. That this is related to their state of health is attested to by study after study. The following characterization typifies the situation: "Older men and women appear to have aged quickly after entering their forties, partly because their unrelieved, physical labor with its special features such as tramping knee-deep in water throughout a wintry day bends their backs and knots their hands in arthritis . . ." (Beardsley *et al.,* 1959:337). Finally, when individuals reach their sixty-first birthday, they hold a party celebrating their entry into the oldest age group, where they "escape to the relative leisure and prestige of old age."[9] In these descriptions of the age groupings and their economic differentiation, we witness the operation of the life cycle considerations we have pinpointed, morbidity intertwining with skill formation and knowledge.

By the interwar period, the sole reliance on family labor was definitely giving way to the employment of labor, and improvements in income and wealth within the village appear to account for this. For, as we shall show, it was the wealthier households who hired labor and the poorer who supplied it. But before considering hired labor *per se,* we must briefly make note of labor exchange in the village. Most Japanese peasants participated in some form of "team" labor pooling during the spring transplanting season (and less frequently at harvest and other times of the year). Because it might be argued that the existence of labor pooling among all households tends to mitigate seriously the needs for a demographic life cycle strategy among low or moderate income families, it is necessary to review the evidence on labor exchange to demonstrate that this objection is not a serious one.

Family members are not the sole source of labor utilized by the household. In the Japanese village, there are groupings of households among which there are exchanges of labor (and, sometimes, material goods and money). Three forms of alliance are observed: *dōzoku, oyako-kankei,* and *kumi.*[10] *Dōzoku* are groups of households in which branch households (*bunke*) cluster about a main household (*honke*). Often the branch families are related through kinship, though this is not always the case. *Oyako-kankei* involves a master–client relationship. The *oyabun* is in heirarchically superior position vis-à-vis the *kobun* client household. Finally, the most common group in the Japanese village is the local corporate group, the *kumi.* Usually the *kumi* consists of a neighborhood grouping of households who engage in various forms of exchange and mutual aid. All three forms of corporate relationships just outlined can involve credit, mutual participation in rituals, and exchange of labor. This is especially the case with the *kumi,* in which labor exchange is common.

Labor exchange between households in the Japanese village is usually known as *yui, i,* or *kattari,* depending on the locality. It customarily takes place during the periods of peak labor demand, especially during the time of spring rice transplanting. Tasks must be completed in an extremely brief period, and no single household can manage all of the requisite operations.[11] The exchanges are exact: for instance, if household A receives two days' work from a man of family B, it later gets the equivalent back (the equivalent could be three woman-days, or one horse for two days, depending on the particular circumstances of the locale and families). It should be emphasized that the existence of communal labor does not undermine the need of households to raise children to meet labor needs, precisely because labor exchanges are exact and must be repaid at approximately the same time of the year (e.g., exchanges in rice transplanting). Other types of *kumi* exchange involve managing the village's irrigation system, mending roads and bridges, house building, and the like. These practices do not diminish reliance of the household on its own labor (which, in fact, must be available for exchange); but rather the villagers secure economies of scale by combining their efforts. In the case of tasks where such clear efficiency gains are realized, the practice of labor pooling or exchange is common in the Japanese village.

Whereas the development of practices of labor exchange did not weaken the basis for a life cycle demographic strategy, the expansion of labor markets in the village certainly did erode the reliance on such a strategy, at least for the higher income groups within the village. Embree (1939:137–138) notes that hired labor only became significant during the 1920s and 1930s in Suye, the village he studied, and he indicates that it took three forms: (1) temporary employment of villagers hired directly by the farmer, (2) payment of a fee to a contractor who then hires laborers himself, (3) employment of domestic servants on long-term contracts. Embree observes that only landowners with abundant fields hire temporary labor or contract out their work and that this supplements the family labor force but does not substitute for it. He also notes that only a small upper class of farmers can afford servants and that this labor comes mainly from the lower and landless classes, as do the temporary workers (Embree [1939:159–160]). In short, observations from the 1930s suggest that the hiring of workers was relatively recent and that only the wealthier farmers could rely on that market to any significant degree.

Embree's work also documents the fifth point, concerning the gradual development of capital markets in the prewar Japanese village. He describes in some detail the rise of the system of cooperative credit clubs, the *kō* (Embree [1939:138–153]): "More money is tied up in *kō* than in banks, village credit association, and postal savings put together. Money *kō* did not exist in the old days" (Embree, 1939:146). As he shows, membership in a *kō* permits one to lend and borrow, and thus the *kō* serves as a capital market for the villagers. But he also shows that the magnitude of "loans" in a *kō* was quite limited in the 1930s, as was membership itself. Generally *kō* that extended credit to any major degree were limited to the more prosperous villagers, those who had assets extensive enough to offer security in event of default. Thus the expansion of the *kō* system was mainly a response to prosperity.

The final point in this section is that the disintegration of the patriarchal stem family system in rural Japan since the 1960s, as people have left the village for the cities and industrial work, even in rural areas, has expanded. Three points most succinctly capture the process: the difficulty of finding or keeping an heir for the farm; the tendency of farming to become a mere part-time supplement to industrial work, even among former full-time farmers; and the erosion of patriarch's position vis-à-vis his son or sons because of technological changes.

Studies by Dore (1978) and R. J. Smith (1978) capture this process extremely well. Both note that because nonagricultural employment in the late 1960s and the 1970s offered higher wages and less strenuous working conditions than farming, many sons of farmers abandoned agriculture altogether. Moreover, even if a son could be cajoled to stay on, finding a bride for him was even more difficult: "The problem of getting a son to be a farmer is as nothing compared with the problem of getting a girl to be the bride of a farming son . . . by the sixties . . . a salary-man husband came to seem like every girl's birthright" (Dore, 1978:151).

Thus the bargaining position of the patriarch has been tremendously reduced by industrialization. Second, many farmers now work in factories, turning the management of the property over to their wives and putting in labor for farming only on weekends. R. J. Smith (1978) shows how this has seriously eroded the cooperative work team and management of village affairs and the family's commitment to staying on the land altogether. However, the relative position of the wife is enhanced. Finally, with wholesale mechanization and the substitution of capital for labor in the 1960s and 1970s, sons have acquired a considerable advantage over their fathers in many areas. For the young are far better educated and can more quickly learn how to utilize the new equipment and techniques. The economic rationale of patriarchal control partly rested on the empirical nature of farming techniques, long experience on the land being an essential prerequisite for sound management. Modern economic growth has almost completely eroded this economic basis for the patriarchy. In short, the patriarchal system has rather thoroughly given way even in agricultural areas. A farmer's remark to R. J. Smith captures this neatly: ". . . in the old days parents demanded of their children what was in the parents' best interests. All that talk about filial piety was just a cover. I think its best to let one's children develop as best suits their talents" (Smith, 1978:107).

In sum, the qualitative evidence concerning Japanese village life assembled here provides useful documentation concerning the operation of the patriarchal stem family system in rural Japan. We shall now proceed to bolster these findings with some results from the quantitative analysis of Japanese farm family budget data for the interwar period.

4.3. The Life Cycle: Japanese Farm Households in 1929

In this section we utilize a comprehensive set of data for 219 Japanese farm households in 1929 to document further the assertions regarding peasant households. The figures were secured from the Ministry of Agriculture and Forestry's survey of the economy of agricultural households in 1929.[12] During the interwar period the Ministry of Agriculture and Forestry published annual surveys of farm household data, but the detail of the information surveyed and size of the sample varied greatly from year to year. The figures available for 1929 are especially comprehensive, and the sample size is adequate for statistical analysis. Although the figures for the 1930s are also detailed, the data for a number of those years reflects the semiwartime conditions characterizing Japan after the invasion of China. (For example, as already noted in Chapter 3, fertilizer was in relatively short supply in the late 1930s, and household composition was markedly affected by the needs of the troops.) In short, the choice of the 1929 survey is a good one for attempting to capture the economics and demography of the peasant life cycle before the war.

The variables that the life-cycle model of the peasant household focuses on are household composition and density on the land, consumption, labor, and income. To measure aspects of the first category, the following measures are used: total household members (*HHM*), total children (*HHMC*), percentage of the household members who are adults (*PHMAD*), cultivable land area (*CL*), worker units per cultivable land unit (*W/CL*), cultivable land area owned (*CLO*), and cultivable land area rented (*CLR*).[13] The consumption variables are total consumer units (*C*), total consumption per consumer unit (*TC/C*), primary consumption per consumer unit (*TPC/C*), and the percentage of total consumption that is primary consumption (*TPC/TC*).[14] The labor variables are total worker units (*W*), hours worked per worker unit (*WH/W*), the ratio of hours worked by nonhousehold members to hours worked by household members (100 *WHNH/WH*), and the percentage of all workers in (nonagricultural) side work (*PSWT*).[15] Finally, the income variables are total net income *Y*, net agricultural income *AY*, side financial income *SY*, income per worker *Y/W*, and income per household member *Y/HHM*.[16] As the reader can see, the list of variables available completely covers those used in developing the theoretical model, with the exception of work hours of the husband (*WHH*) and work hours of the wife (*WHW*). So we are afforded a detailed quantitative glimpse of the life cycle of the Japanese peasant household.

With this data we wish to establish four points. First, the patriarch secured an economic rent from his position, that is, he could utilize family labor at a

TABLE 4.2

C/W Group	Number of families	Household composition: Household members HHM	Children HHMC	Percentage adults PHMAD	Consumption: Consumer units C	Consumption per consumer unit TC/C
$C/W < 1.1$	33	5.3	.6	90	4.4	267
		(1.7)	(.6)	(10)	(1.3)	(107)
$1.1 \le C/W < 1.2$	42	7.1	2.0	73	5.2	230
		(1.9)	(.8)	(7)	(1.5)	(69)
$1.2 \le C/W < 1.3$	44	7.9	2.9	64	5.5	208
		(2.0)	(.8)	(5)	(1.5)	(67)
$1.3 \le C/W < 1.4$	38	8.1	3.5	56	5.3	204
		(1.7)	(.8)	(5)	(1.3)	(57)
$1.4 \le C/W < 1.6$	43	7.7	3.8	49	4.9	212
		(2.1)	(.8)	(5)	(1.4)	(94)
$1.6 \le C/W$	19	7.5	4.5	39	4.5	187
		(1.6)	(1.1)	(5)	(1.1)	(61)
All families	219	7.3	2.8	63	5.0	219
		(2.1)	(1.5)	(16)	(1.4)	(81)

[a] Classified by the consumer–worker (*C/W*) ratio standard deviation is in parenthesis below the mean of the variable.

unit cost to himself below what he would have to pay for hired labor. Second, the life cycle of the household is of considerable quantitative significance in explaining variations in the consumption, income, and intensity of work experienced by household members of farm households. Third, reliance on family labor was a function of income and assets (wealth). And, fourth, the bargaining position of patriarchs probably varied with their social status (a point we shall make note of a bit later), so that the ability to retain the labor of sons varies somewhat from social class to social class.

The first point can be dealt with quickly. The average hourly wage paid out in 1929 for the sample of farm households was .0989 yen. The average *total* family consumption per hour worked by family members was .0895 yen. The cost of retaining a family worker (his or her consumption) must be considerably less than .0895 yen because this includes the total consumption of *all* nonworkers and workers per hour worked. And even this total falls below the hourly wage of .0989 yen. Thus the patriarch was clearly earning a substantial rent, as measured by the 1929 data, in the sense that the opportunity cost of employing family members as workers was considerably less than the cost of hiring that labor in the market. The precise measurement of this rent is obviously difficult to make, but the point remains that a disparity between the two costs existed. However, a qualification to this

Mean of Variables for the Farm Family Budget Data[a]

Consumption		Labor			Income	
Primary consumption per consumer unit TPC/C	Percent of consumption that is primary $100TPC/TC$	Hours worked per worker unit WH/W	Percent of hours worked by nonhousehold members per household member hours worked $100WHNH/WH$	Worker units W	Income per worker Y/W	Income per household member Y/HHM
150	60	3020	3.2	4.2	286	230
(39)	(15)	(988)	(8.0)	(1.2)	(133)	(109)
137	62	3092	7.1	4.5	293	185
(37)	(12)	(1127)	(11.1)	(1.2)	(103)	(66)
125	62	2947	6.3	4.4	275	155
(33)	(11)	(642)	(10.0)	(1.2)	(132)	(79)
132	67	3177	7.2	4.0	294	144
(32)	(13)	(977)	(14.7)	(1.0)	(111)	(56)
130	66	3369	11.3	2.3	358	153
(30)	(14)	(922)	(15.1)	(1.0)	(156)	(72)
123	70	3650	5.1	2.6	344	119
(23)	(15)	(1043)	(5.7)	(.7)	(126)	(44)
133	64	3170	7.0	4.0	306	167
(34)	(13)	(959)	(11.9)	(1.2)	(131)	(81)

argument should be noted here. Usually outside labor is brought in to work for the family when demand for labor is especially strong (in the season of peak labor demand), and thus wages may be especially high (relative to a yearly average wage for such hired labor). As a consequence, it is not at all clear exactly how much rent patriarchs were actually securing in 1929. Indeed we would not expect them to be earning large rents by 1929 in any event because by that date much modernization had already occurred in labor markets in Japan.

The second point concerns verifying that the position of the household in the life cycle was important in determining various aspects of household economy, including consumption per consumer and average hours worked (and, consequently, income) per worker. To do this I wish to explore several cross classifications of the households, utilizing proxies—the number of workers W and the consumer–worker ratio C/W—as (albeit imperfect) measures for the position of a household in the life cycle. It is unfortunate, in regard to this discussion, that the Japanese farm family data does not provide the age of the patriarch (household head) directly. It should be emphasized that C and W are calculated by weighting the age groups, separately for each sex, by a set of age–sex-specific weights (see notes 14 and 15 for details).

TABLE 4.3

		Household composition land and density				Consumption	
W Group	Number of families	Household members *HHM*	Percentage (%) adults *PHMAD*	Cultivable land area *CL*	Workers per cultivable land unit *W/CL*	Consumer units *C*	Consumption per consumer unit *TC/C*
$W < 2$	13	4.9	46	142	.015	2.9	257
		(1.4)	(19)	(56)	(.007)	(.6)	(148)
$2 \leq W < 3$	42	5.6	58	132	.023	3.7	231
		(1.5)	(19)	(48)	(.009)	(.7)	(77)
$3 \leq W < 4$	62	6.9	62	170	.023	4.6	214
		(1.6)	(16)	(61)	(.009)	(.6)	(62)
$4 \leq W < 5$	50	7.8	68	172	.028	5.5	217
		(1.6)	(15)	(46)	(.009)	(.7)	(97)
$5 \leq W < 6$	36	9.0	68	209	.030	6.5	216
		(1.3)	(75)	(99)	(.013)	(.6)	(66)
$6 \leq W$	16	10.1	75	243	.033	7.7	193
		(1.4)	(11)	(120)	(.016)	(.7)	(52)

[a] Classified by worker units (*W*) standard deviation is in parenthesis below the mean of the variable.

What we do here with these data is to scratch merely the surface to make some elementary points of direct empirical relevance to the theory of the peasant household. We would like to commence the discussion of the findings with an analysis of the relationship between the consumer–worker ratio (*C/W*) and the other variables. Table 4.2 provides us with our focus. Four points emerge from considerations of this table. First, *C/W* clearly depends on household composition. When *C/W* is very low, there are on the average few children; when *C/W* is large, the mean number of children is sizeable. This is also apparent in the percentages of household members who are adults. Second, consumption per consumer unit reflects the changing pressure of consumers on workers. The range between averages for consumption per consumer unit for the two extreme *C/W* groups is very large. Third, the pressure of consumers on workers is revealed in the amount of effort the workers must exert in working (i.e., the number of hours they work). And fourth, the figures on income per worker and income per household member show a sharp division between households with little pressure of consumers on workers and those with great pressure. For instance, when *C/W* is small, on the one hand, workers are not compelled to exert great effort because consumption pressures are not especially demanding and average *Y/W* is relatively low. On the other hand, income per household member is sizeable, reflecting the high proportion of workers in

Means of Variables for the Farm Family Budget Data[a]

Consumption		Labor			Income	
Primary consumption per consumer unit TPC/C	Percent of consumption that is primary $100TPC/TC$	Hours worked per worker unit WH/W	Percent of hours worked by nonhousehold members per hours worked by household member $100WHNH/WH$	Percent of hours worked that is side work $PSWT$	Income per worker Y/W	Income per household member Y/HHM
157	70	3954	12.8	5.7	419	172
(42)	(18)	(897)	(15.9)	(4.3)	(151)	(86)
141	64	3653	9.1	8.4	366	186
(32)	(13)	(1017)	(14.0)	(10.1)	(151)	(104)
137	66	3387	7.4	6.0	302	162
(35)	(12)	(1016)	(12.9)	(6.9)	(95)	(62)
128	64	2832	4.4	5.6	273	163
(31)	(15)	(674)	(9.2)	(5.8)	(125)	(89)
126	60	2655	6.9	6.9	288	169
(35)	(13)	(625)	(11.0)	(7.3)	(132)	(74)
112	60	2636	3.7	8.7	212	140
(26)	(11)	(773)	(4.1)	(13.0)	(65)	(50)

the household. The opposite situation obtains in the case where C/W is comparatively large.

In Table 4.3 the life cycle in terms of the total number of worker units is explored. Two new points can be treated usefully with the figures given here. First, the effort exerted per worker is a function of the number of workers. Indeed the range of values spanned by hours worked per worker unit, as we contrast households with large and small numbers of workers, is considerable (over 1300 hours on an annual basis). Second, households with substantial numbers of workers are less dependent on communal and/or hired labor to meet labor needs. Because the proportion of labor input that is communal labor is probably almost a constant for most households in a given village regardless of the number of workers (because exchanges are exact and suppliers and demanders of communal labor must have similar needs), it stands to reason that much of the variation in the variable $WHNH/WH$ must be due to the hiring of labor from outside the family. On the one hand, for a household whose income is relatively small and risks in production are substantial, the need to rely on the outside labor market is clearly undesirable, and, therefore, strategies of avoiding this dependence (e.g., the life-cycle strategy we discuss) are attractive as a result.

On the other hand, for households with substantial assets (i.e., the ones cultivating relatively large farms), hiring labor is an efficient strategy for

TABLE 4.4

CL Group	Number of families	Household composition and density: Household members *HHM*	Household composition and density: Workers per unit of cultivable land *W/CL*	Consumption: Consumer units *C*	Consumption: Consumption per consumer unit *TC/C*	Consumption: Percent of consumption that is primary 100*TPC/TC*
$C/W < 1.2$						
$CL < 160$	32	5.4	.033	4.2	250	61
		(1.8)	(.010)	(1.3)	(88)	(12)
$160 \leq CL < 220$	27	6.8	.025	5.2	249	63
		(1.4)	(.006)	(1.2)	(109)	(14)
$220 \leq CL$	16	7.4	.018	5.6	234	58
		(2.5)	(.006)	(1.6)	(49)	(14)
$1.2 \leq C/W < 1.4$						
$CL < 160$	44	7.4	.034	5.1	195	64
		(2.0)	(.012)	(1.5)	(60)	(12)
$160 \leq Cl < 220$	17	8.4	.023	5.6	206	66
		(1.2)	(.005)	(.9)	(54)	(9)
$220 \leq CL$	21	8.9	.017	6.1	228	63
		(1.6)	(.005)	(1.4)	(70)	(13)
$1.4 \leq C/W$						
$CL < 160$	34	7.3	.025	4.5	193	67
		(1.7)	(.011)	(1.1)	(64)	(13)
$160 \leq CL < 220$	22	7.9	.018	5.0	204	69
		(1.8)	(.004)	(1.2)	(106)	(16)
$220 < CL$	6	8.3	.013	5.3	265	62
		(3.3)	(.006)	(2.1)	(104)	(14)

[a] Cross classified by the consumer–worker ratio (*C/W*) and cultivable land area (*CL*) standard deviation is in parenthesis below the mean of the variable.

reducing the labor input of family members, in effect, buying leisure. When income is substantial and risk of economic collapse unlikely, this is one principal "luxury" a family expends its income on (at the same time reducing its need to rely on a demographic life-cycle strategy). One means of exploring this issue is to cross classify the households into farm size groups. Let us explore variations with respect to farm size. The relevant cross tabulations appear in Table 4.4. These figures show three things. First, farm households with relatively large amounts of land are better able to retain workers than those with small amounts of land (a point we shall return to subsequently). The ratio of workers to land area is less on large farms than on small farms. Second, income (especially agricultural income) and consumption reflect the amount of land the household cultivates. The households with larger farms enjoy both greater absolute incomes and higher

Means of Variables for the Farm Family Budget Data[a]

Labor				Income		
Worker units W	Hours worked per worker WH/W	Percent of hours worked by nonhousehold members per hours worked by household members $100WHNH/WH$	Percent of hours worked that is side work $PSWT$	Income per worker Y/W	Side financial income SFY	Agricultural income AY
3.9	3338	3.4	6.5	301	70	788
(1.1)	(1235)	(5.7)	(4.3)	(138)	(169)	(331)
4.6	3006	5.2	5.0	307	97	1028
(1.0)	(974)	(9.7)	(4.7)	(109)	(273)	(350)
5.1	2599	9.6	3.0	239	128	938
(1.4)	(604)	(15.4)	(4.6)	(58)	(210)	(374)
4.0	3174	3.5	8.4	276	55	712
(1.2)	(930)	(6.4)	(11.4)	(129)	(75)	(310)
4.3	2849	6.6	7.7	256	86	751
(.7)	(632)	(8.7)	(7.2)	(93)	(184)	(263)
4.7	2966	13.6	6.2	322	156	1079
(1.1)	(656)	(19.8)	(7.5)	(123)	(222)	(426)
2.9	3476	6.5	7.2	329	87	639
(.8)	(815)	(9.3)	(8.2)	(130)	(272)	(266)
3.3	3577	8.6	6.4	366	33	872
(.9)	(1221)	(12.5)	(9.1)	(166)	(47)	(369)
3.5	2882	28.5	7.6	450	144	1153
(1.5)	(398)	(20.1)	(9.0)	(132)	(169)	(576)

income per worker and consumption per consumer unit (there is a single exception to this proposition in the class of households with $C/W < 1.2$). Third, workers in households with relatively abundant amounts of land exert themselves less (enjoy more leisure) than do the households with moderate or very small amounts of land. These points testify to the critical importance of holding onto land—a concern the model builds into Eq. 2.3 using the assumption that households pursue a strategy of keeping total work capacity above a minimum, so the total household labor controlled by the patriarch will be sufficient to farm the land that the patriarch controls.

Table 4.5 permits us to explore the implications of the balance of workers and land by focusing on the ratio of workers to cultivable land units. Because density of workers reflects both the life cycle and the land controlled by the household (as well as other factors), this table usefully summarizes

TABLE 4.5

Means of Variables for the Farm Family Budget Data[a]

W/CL group	Number of families	Household composition and land: Household members HHM	Household composition and land: Cultivable land area CL	Consumption: Consumption per consumer unit TC/C	Consumption: Primary consumption per consumer unit TPC/C	Labor: Worker units W	Labor: Hours worked per worker unit WH/W	Labor: Percent of hours worked by nonhousehold members per hours worked by household members $100WHNH/WH$	Labor: Percent of hours worked that is side work $PSWT$	Income: Income per worker Y/W	Income: Percent income that is agricultural PAY
$W/CL < .015$	24	6.8	291	264	156	3.4	3329	20.2	3.5	371	78
		(2.5)	(108)	(110)	(38)	(1.5)	(1094)	(22.6)	(3.5)	(171)	(11)
$.015 \leq W/CL < .02$	51	7.1	198	213	135	3.5	3296	9.3	6.3	328	78
		(1.6)	(61)	(68)	(33)	(1.1)	(905)	(12.2)	(7.8)	(112)	(11)
$.02 \leq W/CL < .025$	48	7.3	169	233	135	3.8	3243	5.6	6.5	326	73
		(2.3)	(42)	(94)	(32)	(.9)	(970)	(9.5)	(8.2)	(134)	(16)
$.025 \leq W/CL < .03$	39	7.4	155	215	129	4.3	3203	3.9	6.7	280	73
		(2.1)	(46)	(67)	(31)	(1.3)	(983)	(5.1)	(6.6)	(111)	(14)
$.03 \leq W/CL < .035$	26	7.0	133	214	136	4.3	2896	3.3	7.3	284	70
		(2.1)	(35)	(74)	(36)	(1.2)	(796)	(3.3)	(5.2)	(102)	(13)
$.035 \leq W/CL < .04$	8	8.0	113	201	124	4.2	3299	2.2	5.0	314	67
		(1.5)	(23)	(69)	(25)	(.8)	(1460)	(2.3)	(4.6)	(214)	(19)
$.04 \leq W/CL$	23	8.4	102	177	108	4.9	2779	2.2	11.3	210	67
		(1.8)	(27)	(54)	(28)	(1.2)	(767)	(3.1)	(13.3)	(76)	(16)

[a] Classified by worker–land ratio (W/CL) standard deviation is in parenthesis below the mean of the variable.

what we have learned from the other material. The declining average product per worker as the *W/CL* ratio (ratio of workers to cultivate land) increases and emerges as the most salient point here. Also instructive, however, are the figures on composition of total income and effort. A larger number of workers per land unit increases the pressure on the patriarch to direct his coresident family members into work on other farms or into nonagricultural employments, either by working as temporary farm or factory workers or by producing nonagricultural goods for the market. This is reflected in the *PSWT* and *PAY* variables (dependence on side work and agricultural income, respectively), which clearly display the variation in dependence on agricultural output with the life cycle.

We have attempted to summarize the findings from these data in a simple manner. Correlation coefficients for all the variables previously discussed are provided in Table 4.6. The connections between the variables most closely associated with the life cycle (the indicators of household composition like *HHMC* and *PHMAD*) and the total number of workers and consumers can be gleaned clearly, albeit crudely, from these figures. Equally instructive are the interrelationships between the several different measures of consumption and income. The reader should make special note of the variable *WHNH/WH* that measures the relative dependence on nonfamily labor. It is positively correlated with the average family income, farm size, and the burden of consumers to workers (*C/W*), as we have argued.

The raw farm family data for 1929 are so arranged that they allow us to explore more fully two points that bear on other parts of the model, especially the question of the bargaining position of the patriarch, the fourth major issue we wish to take up using these data. The first point involves the question of landowning status (i.e., tenancy). The second is the regional distribution of the farm household variables. The latter is of some relevance to the analysis in Chapters 5 and 7, which involves regional variations in natality and other factors.

Let us first consider tenancy. As we shall suggest in the following text, the status of the household head was important in determining his ability to place second and third sons in industrial jobs and as in-adopted sons on other farms. On the one hand, in an environment in which education was not a screening device for jobs, a head with low social status enjoyed less leverage in placing offspring than a socially prominent head. Thus tenants generally had weaker bargaining positions vis-à-vis their children than did owners, and, consequently, they tended to experience greater difficulty in retaining their offspring as workers. As the rural market for servants expanded, the tendency for tenants to lose workers earlier was probably accentuated. On the other hand, as we shall suggest, education became a more important screening device for high status jobs in cities than for

TABLE 4.6

Variable	Household composition, land and density					Consumption		
	Household members *HHM*	Children *HHMC*	Percentage adults *PHMAD*	Cultivable land area *CL*	Worker per cultivable land unit *W/CL*	Consumer units *C*	Consumption per consumer unit *TC/C*	Primary consumption per consumer unit *TPC/C*
HHM	—							
HHMC	.74[a]							
PHMAD	−.30[a]	−.85[a]						
CL	.35[a]	.13[b]	.05					
W/CL	.20[a]	−.08	.24[a]	−.59[a]				
C	.50[a]	.43[a]	−.01	.39[a]	.33[a]			
TC/C	−.31[a]	−.30[a]	.25[a]	.12[b]	−.24[a]	−.27[a]		
TPC/C	−.40[a]	−.30[a]	.20[a]	.10[c]	−.33[a]	−.39[a]	.70[a]	
TPC/TC	−.00	.14[b]	−.20[a]	−.09	−.02	−.06	−.66[a]	−.02
W	−.40[a]	−.03	.38[a]	.39[a]	.40[a]	.90[a]	−.13[b]	−.28[a]
WH/W	−.28[a]	−.01	−.20[a]	−.20[a]	−.17[a]	−.38[a]	.08	.15[b]
WHNH/WH	−.05[a]	.08	−.14[b]	.30[a]	−.35[a]	−.11[b]	.36[a]	.38[a]
PSWT	.01	.02	−.00	−.19[a]	.04	.04	−.08	−.11[c]
Y/W	−.25[a]	−.02	−.14[b]	.02	−.33[a]	−.31[a]	.62[a]	.55[a]
Y/HHM	−.43[a]	−.49[a]	.45[a]	.02	−.14[b]	−.28[a]	.71[a]	.60[a]
PAY	.01	.07	−.08	.20[a]	−.28[a]	−.05	−.17[a]	.02
C/W	.26[a]	.75[a]	−.89[a]	−.10[c]	−.23[a]	−.02	−.25[a]	−.19[a]

[a] Significant at the 1% level.
[b] Significant at the 5% level.
[c] Significant at the 10% level.

positions of moderate status. This would tend to encourage sons in the *highest* status families to seek a more advanced education than the sons of moderate status families were receiving, and it would weaken the bargaining position of the patriarch in the highest status families. (But the sons would tend to stay as residents on the farm while they were students and presumably provide some work inputs during that period.) Moreover, the real opportunity cost to the wealthy patriarch (in terms of foregone opportunities and risk of maintaining the farm) of relinquishing his sons and hiring paid workers would presumably be less than that of the patriarch of a lower status family. Thus patriarchs in the middle status categories would probably find their bargaining position eroded most slowly.

The data on farm households are grouped into three classes of approximately equal size: owners, part-owners, and tenants. Means for a number of the variables we are interested in are provided in Tables 4.7.A and 4.7.B and

Correlation Matrix for Selected Variables for the Farm Family Budget Data (219 Families)

Consumption	Labor				Income			
Percentage consumption that is primary *TPC/TC*	Worker units *W*	Hours worked per worker unit *WH/W*	Percent of hours worked by nonhousehold members per hours worked by household members 100*WHNH/WH*	Percent of hours worked that is side work *PSWT*	Income per worker *Y/W*	Income per household member *Y/HHM*	Percent income that is agricultural *PAY*	Consumer–worker ratio *C/W*
−.16[a]								
.05	−.44[a]							
−.14[b]	−.15[a]	−.12[b]						
−.04	.01	.02	−.05					
−.30[a]	−.35[a]	.23[a]	.35[a]	−.05				
−.40[a]	−.10[c]	.08	.20[a]	−.03	.79[a]			
.25[a]	−.07	.06	.01	−.51[a]	−.11[c]	−.16[a]		
.24[a]	−.43[a]	.20[a]	.09[c]	−.03	.16[a]	−.37[a]	.05	—

classified into the three tenancy groups. In addition, we test (using an *F* test) whether the differences between the groups are large as compared with the intragroup differences among the households (i.e., the differences within each group). The significance level tells us whether the *intergroup* differences are significant; a small value (say, of less than .05) indicates that the intergroup differences *are* substantial, that is, the tenancy status of a household is important in explaining variation in the particular characteristics under consideration. Tables 4.7.A and 4.7.B clearly show that many variables—income, household composition, the number of workers, and consumption—*do* vary significantly among the three tenancy groups. Landowners have a greater capacity to retain adult workers (note that the number of *children* does not vary much between the groups) and enjoy higher income, consumption, and leisure, than do tenants or part-tenants.

A similar analysis for the cultural regions of Japan (Hokkaidō is excluded

TABLE 4.7.A

Means of Household Structure, Land, and Income Variables for the Farm Family Budget Data Classified by Tenancy Status

Variables	Tenancy status: Owners	Part-owners	Tenants	Significance[a]
Number of families	88	73	58	—
Household members *HHM*	7.7	7.1	6.9	.04
Adult household members *HHMAD*	4.8	4.3	4.3	.02
Children *HHMC*	2.9	2.8	2.7	.59
Cultivable land owned: area *CLO*	168	86	10	.00
Cultivable land rented: area *CLR*	8	89	155	.00
Cultivable land area *CL*	177	175	165	.65
Percent cultivable land owned 100*CLO/CL*	95.2	48.8	6.5	.00
Agricultural income *AY*	986	817	623	.00
Side financial income *SFY*	151	58	18	.00
Income *Y*	1366	1110	874	.00
Income per household member *Y/HHM*	189	166	135	.00
Income per hour worked *Y/WH*	.119	.099	.079	.00

[a] The significance level tests whether, of the variation of the variables across the 219 families, the variation within tenancy groups is "small" compared to the variation between the groups (i.e., whether the groups tend to be relatively homogenous). The statistical test is by analysis of variance, and the significance level measures the degree to which this "homogeneity" hypothesis is supported.

here) is pursued in Table 4.8. The regions, which are listed in Appendix 1, run geographically from the northeast (Tōhoku) to the southwest (Kyūshū). Each region has slightly different climatic and geologic conditions from the others, and they are usually considered to enjoy some unique cultural features (such as varieties of dialect, special craft products, etc.).[17] Here again we utilize an *F*-test to reveal whether the differences are significant (in the case of all variables given in the table except income per hour worked, the intergroup differences *are* significant). Of special interest are the number of children, consumption, hours worked, and income per worker, which all show significant regional variation.[18] Noteworthy are the low numbers of children recorded for the Kinki and Chugoku regions and their correspondingly high incomes and consumption per head. This suggests that by 1929 at least parts of the life-cycle strategy had ceased to operate in those regions. As we shall see, these two regions were leaders in the fertility transition. It should also be noted that income per hour worked (*Y/WH*) does not show a particularly significant regional variation. This suggests that *hourly* returns

TABLE 4.7.B

Means of Labor and Consumption Variables for the Farm Family Budget Data Classified by Tenancy Status

Variables	Tenancy status			
	Owners	Part-owners	Tenants	Significance[a]
Worker units W	4.2	3.8	3.8	.02
Income per worker Y/W	338	309	252	.00
Agricultural income per worker AY/W	244	231	180	.00
Hours worked per worker unit WH/W	2900	3268	3319	.07
Worker units per cultivable land unit W/CL	.027	.024	.026	.31
Consumer units C	5.4	4.8	4.8	.01
Consumer–worker ratio C/W	1.3	1.3	1.3	.80
Consumption per consumer unit TC/C	243	210	194	.00
Consumption per household member TC/HHM	172	147	135	.00
Percentage of consumption that is primary $100TPC/TC$	59.8	65.8	68.1	.00

[a] The significance level tests whether, of the variation of the variables across the 219 families, the variation within tenancy groups is "small" compared to the variation between the groups (i.e., whether the groups tend to be relatively homogenous). The statistical test is by analysis of variance, and the significance level measures the degree to which this "homogeneity" hypothesis is supported.

to labor were approximately equal across the districts of Japan by the late 1920s.

By way of closing this section, it will be useful to systematically elaborate my remarks about the interaction of household structure and economic and social variables that are independent of the life cycle, so that the reader can see the full context in which the life-cycle model operates. The idea, to repeat, is that a life-cycle strategy is important for the continuation of the family line and the provision of labor, but that it is gradually eroded by modern economic growth and the associated social changes. As an illustration of this gradual breakdown of the life-cycle strategy in response to modernization, let us return to the issue of outmigration. We have argued that the ability to retain children as they mature depends on the asset position, status, and surrounding economic environment of the individual household. Where opportunities within the household enterprise are relatively good (for instance, the land can be partially divided) or the *local* labor market offers remunerative employment so that the children can reside at home and work in a nearby plant (this argument would apply mainly to

TABLE 4.8

Region	Number of families	Household composition, land, and density				Consumption	
		Household members *HHM*	Children *HHMC*	Cultivable land area *CL*	Worker units per land area *W/CL*	Consumer units *C*	Consumption per consumer unit *TC/C*
Tōhoku	31	8.4	3.2	219	.022	5.7	198
Kantō	33	8.2	3.1	230	.023	5.7	219
Hokuriku	22	6.6	2.6	160	.022	4.4	197
Tosan	19	7.1	3.1	148	.027	4.8	228
Tokai	20	7.5	3.2	180	.022	4.9	200
Kinki	24	5.8	1.6	141	.029	4.3	300
Chūgoku	18	6.9	2.3	146	.028	4.9	222
Shikoku	21	7.2	2.9	117	.034	5.0	200
Kyūshū	31	7.4	3.0	167	.026	5.0	212
Significance[a]	—	.00	.00	.00	.00	.00	.00

[a] Classified by the Regions of Japan. The significance level tests whether, of the variation of the variables across the 219 families, the variation within tenancy groups is "small" compared with the variation between the groups (i.e., whether the groups tend to be relatively homogeneous). The statistical test is by analysis of variance, and the significance level measures the degree to which this "homogeneity" hypothesis is supported.

females because the patriarch retains his leverage over them longer—his ability to arrange marriages not being eroded as rapidly as his ability to secure jobs for sons), households may be able to retain workers (and keep the *C/W* ratio from rising so rapidly) as the headship of the house passes from one generation to the next. Areal (county, *gun*) data are used in Table 4.9 to show this. The figures are for those *gun* that most heavily depend on agriculture during the late 1920s. The female employment ratio (E_f) measures job opportunities for women outside agriculture; the percentage of women in domestic service (*PDSFO*) measures local job opportunities for females, income per head, and the extent to which higher-income families have substituted hired labor for family labor; and the percentage cultivable land in mulberry product (*PCHM*) captures the degree to which the labor-intensive industry of raising cocoons for silk production (largely an industry utilizing female child labor) characterizes the agricultural district.[19] These variables represent forces holding persons to the household. Tenancy (1 minus the value of *PCHO*) and density represent forces associated with relatively youthful emigration from the family residence. As the reader can see from Table 4.9, the probable inference is that the status of households; local employment opportunities, especially for women; income (and presumably the delaying of emigration for the purposes of education); and

Means of Variables for the Farm Family Budget Data[a]

Consumption	Labor				Income	
Percentage of consumption that is primary 100*TPC/TC*	Worker units *W*	Hours worked per worker *WH/W*	Hours worked by nonhousehold members *WHNH*	Percentage of hours worked by nonhousehold members of hours worked by household members 100*WHNH/WH*	Income per worker *Y/W*	Income per hour worked *Y/WH*
70.6	4.5	2686	1638	14.6	265	.103
63.3	4.5	2988	708	6.1	266	.092
67.2	3.5	3050	190	2.1	273	.093
61.8	3.6	3226	464	5.7	369	.119
64.3	3.7	4277	320	2.1	340	.092
57.6	3.8	3207	793	7.4	386	.127
62.8	4.0	3213	515	4.6	296	.097
68.1	3.7	3178	500	4.5	306	.100
59.7	3.8	3123	900	10.8	293	.098
.01	.01	.01	.00	.00	.00	.13

density (the inverse of the opportunity to secure land), have all conditioned the retention of family members as they mature, in the manner suggested by the preceding arguments.

In short, by the interwar period modern labor markets and improvements in the standard of living were already having a marked impact on the household structure of patriarchal stem farm families and the pure economic basis of the demographic life cycle strategy was gradually being eroded. Nevertheless, the analysis of the farm family budget data from 1929 suggests that, although the life cycle strategy was undoubtedly gradually giving ground in some villages, it was still flourishing in most locales, though modernization was presumably being felt in all quarters to some extent. That the life-cycle strategy continued to hold sway in the rural areas of Japan as late as the 1950s has already been suggested by the village studies noted previously. The following citation, drawn from a report on a survey of villages in 1950 prepared by Professor Tadashi Fukutake and his colleagues for the Population Problems Research Council, Mainichi Newspapers Company (1952:52–53), summarizes the argument neatly:

> It may be seen from the above survey that the traditional family institution in Japan is fairly closely related to various aspects of the rural population. Under the Japanese system of primogeniture, importance is attached to the succession of the family from

TABLE 4.9

Regressions for Net Outmigration from *Gun* (Counties) in Which Percentage Labor Force in Primary Industry Is Greater than or Equal to 60%, 1925–1930

			Independent variables					
Dependent variable	Number of observations	Constant	Percentage cultivated land that is owned *PCHO*	Female employment ratio E_f	Percentage occupied females in domestic service *PDSFO*	Persons 15–49 per cultivable land unit *D*	Percentage cultivable land in mulberry production *PCHM*	R^2
Net outmigration with natural rate of increase based on 1925 data alone (NOMA)	418	25.0[a]	−28.5[a]	−99.4[a]	−55.6	6.0[a]	10.3[b]	.41
Net outmigration with natural rate of increase based on 1925 data alone (NOMA)	418	22.2[a]	−26.1[a]	−100.4[a]	n.e.[d]	5.9[a]	11.6[a]	.40
Net outmigration with natural rate of increase based on average of 1925 and 1930 figures (NOMB)	418	24.7[a]	−27.6[a]	−100.6[a]	−59.0[c]	5.9[a]	11.6[a]	.40
Net outmigration with natural rate of increase based on average of 1925 and 1930 figures (NOMB)	418	21.7[a]	−25.1[a]	−101.7[a]	n.e.	5.9[a]	13.0[a]	.40

[a] Significant at 1% level (two-tailed test).
[b] Significant at 5% level (two-tailed test).
[c] Significant at 10% level (two-tailed test).
[d] n.e. = Not entered into the regression as an independent variable.

> generation to generation rather than to the happiness of each member of the family . . . the desire to secure the heir brings about relatively early marriage which in turn results in many births . . . the low technological level of agriculture, together with paddy cultivation, is responsible for the fact that although there is abundant labor on a yearly basis, there is such labor shortage at the peak of labor demand that any helping hand is very much appreciated . . . child labor is not regarded as useless because it can help the primitive agricultural operation in many ways and therefore farmers do not worry about the large number of children. . . .

This quotation touches on most of the major facets of the argument developed here.

4.4. Education and the Labor Market in Japan

Because the theory of the fertility transition puts a great weight on education, and because it gives a manifold interpretation to the ramifications of education (e.g., bargaining position in the family, job screening, and productivity), it is useful to note briefly some evidence that supports the interpretations we give. We shall commence the discussion with the problem of the patriarch's ability to place children in jobs; then turn to the relationship between job screening and educational attainment of applicants in large firms; and conclude with the possible influence of child labor laws on the breakdown of the patriarchal stem family system.

Vogel (1967:95) provides an excellent discussion of the patriarch's role in placing his children in jobs prior to the late 1950s:

> In Japan placing a child in the city meant finding him a job in a good organization. The success of the placement depended in large part on the contacts which the rural family was able to command . . . tenant farmers, for example, were frequently dependent on their landlords for assistance . . . an employer expected to give a young man on-the-job training and so did not look for specific ability but rather sought a young man who had good general intelligence, reliable character, and most important, a special connection with his friends or relatives so he could be assured of the employee's willingness to work long hours without high wages.

And he goes on to say (Vogel, 1967:97): "Second and third sons who had no hope of sharing in the family inheritance could not find a desirable position in the city without their family's assistance." This system, as he points out, gradually gave way to the criterion of educational attainment (Vogel, 1967:96–97):

> Within the last generation the importance of universalistic criteria for hiring and promoting has increased drastically as a result of the increased size of business organizations . . . [that] must rely on such universalistic criteria as educational achievement, school, or university attended . . . entrance examinations. . . .

And he concludes by pointing out that parents since the 1960s now rely on the educational system, and their own related experiences concerning tutors and the like, to place their offspring in jobs. That this has effectively eliminated the opportunity to extract significant labor services from children will be evident from the discussion immediately following, concerning the competitiveness of Japanese education and the extreme demands it makes on pupils.

To motivate this discussion we can begin with the recent period. One of the most striking developments in Japanese education during the 1970s has been the expansion of the *juku,* the afterschool tutoring academies, in which students cram information to surpass their peers in the entrance examinations to higher schools.[20] Indeed many Japanese children now attend *juku* on weekdays after public school, on Saturdays and Sundays, and during the entire summer recess to eke out top scores on the junior high, high school, and college entrance examinations. The logic of this brutal competition is simple: to get into a good university (like Tokyo National or Ōsaka National) requires getting into a good high school; to qualify for a good high school requires excellent performance on the high school entrance examinations, and so forth. Indeed this is often dubbed the "examination hell" of Japanese schooling. Why do the Japanese put such an inordinate emphasis on education—to the degree that at present many children sacrifice the opportunity to play sports to attend *juku* and study until midnight or even later?

The answer is that education has become crucial both for job placement in the modern sector and for productivity in agriculture. Vogel (1963:41) writes about large firms as follows:

> Because the firm commits itself to a young man for life and because business in contemporary Japan is highly competitive, the firm must be careful to select men of unusual promise and ability . . . because there is such wide agreement in Japanese society as to which universities are most desirable, firms consider the university attended as important or even more important than their own examinations for selecting [professional employees]. . . .

The logic of the situation is simple. Firms seek some indicator of ability and a sign of diligence on the part of their recruits. Because of the ruthless competition to enter the best universities, the choicest firms (and most prestigious government ministries) tend to limit their offers to those graduating from the most selective and famous universities. Moreover, there are definite real returns to education in the form of productivity gains. This point can be seen most directly in the case of agriculture, where two points immediately emerge: the returns to education for individual farmers, and the returns to public expenditure on agricultural research and extension. Hayami *et al.* (1975:101) have studied this question at great length and they conclude:

> For the whole period of analysis from 1880 to 1965 . . . the rate of output growth is almost completely explained by changes in the four conventional inputs, in education, and in research and extension. . . . [The] three major sources for the whole period are: (a). changes in weights for input aggregation from factor shares to production elasticities; (b). the contribution of rural education; and (c). the contribution of agricultural research and extension. . . .

The expansion of technical institutes and vocational schools for farmers and workers in response to the demand for this specialized training is a clear sign of the purely economic returns to investment in this type of education. And as noted several times previously, the expansion of education has weakened the patriarch's position, both in his control over job placement and in the productivity advantage his many years of experience gives him vis-à-vis his children.

An interesting and related issue concerns the possible role of child labor laws in effecting some of the changes associated with education. Four reasons suggest, however, that such legislation was not of great moment in contrast to the expansion of the school system. First, labor legislation directly affecting child labor was restricted to only certain branches of modern industry and did not have a direct impact on family enterprises whose labor force consisted mainly of members, such as peasant farms and shops in cities. Second, the major piece of legislation, the Factory Law of 1911, was passed relatively late; although it prohibited employment of children under the age of twelve, according to the education laws such children were supposed to already be attending a public school, so the articles of the Factory Law added little extra, at least in principle. Third, the decline of child labor was as much due to technological changes in factory production as to legislation. And finally, the law was extremely difficult to enforce in practice because many inspectors would have been needed to impose the law.

This completes the discussion of Japanese education and its relation to the job market. The remaining issues that must be discussed regarding the assumptions of the model for Japan concern the status of women and the arrangement of marriages.

4.5. Marriage and the Status of Women in Japan

In discussing this issue we must be clear about one point at the outset: although the status of Japanese women has been transformed partly because of institutional changes due to American Occupational (SCAP) policies, the improvement of women's social status (and the associated decline of the patriarchal system) began before the war and was associated, mainly, with education and the evolution of the labor market.

However, it must be acknowledged that the occupation reforms of the civil code were very thoroughgoing and striking. The household (*ie*) system had been carefully delineated in the Meiji Civil Code and it specifically limited the rights of women regarding inheritance, the control of property, and the initiation of divorce. In general, the concept of the woman's role in the *ie* system, as codified by the Meiji lawmakers, was service to the *ie* in which she was a member (her own family of birth before marriage and her husband's *ie* after marriage). The occupation reforms abolished the Meiji Civil Code and established a new one, in which husband and wife were legal equals within marriage and need not have their parents' consent to wed or divorce. Moreover, schooling was declared coeducational, and women secured the right to vote. However, as important as the legal changes may have been, the literature on the status of Japanese women gives far greater weight to the economic and social aspects of education in the enhancement of their position in Japan.

That women were narrowing the gap between themselves and men, regarding schooling, even before the war is suggested by a number of statistics. Consider the accompanying tabulation showing the percentages of students receiving a middle school education (which was not compulsory before the war) who are boys or girls (Koyama, 1961:23).

1873	Boys (%)	Girls (%)	Total (%)
1873	98	2	100
1890	82	18	100
1910	74	26	100
1920	63	37	100
1930	57	43	100
1940	55	45	100

The closing of the gap has also been captured by figures on the sex differential of newspaper reading: the early Meiji cohorts had a large gap in this statistic between males and females, a gap that was closed considerably for the cohorts born and reared in the late 1920s and 1930s (Koyama, 1961:23–25). In short, even under the Meiji code, the position of women appears to have been improving.

There is no doubt that educational achievement strengthened the status of women in at least two areas. First, as noted previously in this section, the job placement of children depends on their academic achievement, and well-educated women are at an advantage in helping to propel their offspring forward in the school system. Second—and this is mainly a postwar phenomenon—education has improved the market skills of women, especially unmarried women, although there has been a pronounced trend toward the employment of married females in industrial firms and government. By enhancing the importance of women both in home activities (rearing children who will be high achievers) and in the marketplace, education has played an important role in breaking down the stem family system in which males dominate decision making. This is especially true in urban areas since the mid-1950s and early 1960s.

Because a prospective bridegroom now places more emphasis on the education of his bride-to-be and less emphasis on her family connections (because if her academic abilities are greater, his children may more readily perform in school and her potential for earning income in employment will be greater), the leverage the patriarch has in using his role of arranging the marriages of his daughters to extract income and labor services has been severely diminished. A few figures on marriages by type illustrate this point. In 1956 the Prime Minister's Office asked, "In regard to the choice of a spouse, which of the two is preferred—choice made by parents or by oneself" (Koyama, 1961:41). The percentage preferring parental arrangement, by sex and age category, is as follows:

males, 60+	49%
males, 40–49	24%
males, 20–29	9%
females, 60+	41%
females, 40–49	35%
females, 20–29	16%

(It should be noted, however, that these data are hardly conclusive on this point because they may reflect the age of the respondents, that is, they may be a life-cycle effect.)

This transformation is also seen in the decline of *miai* marriages as a proportion of all marriages. A *miai* marriage is often one in which the parents select a spouse for the child and employ a go-between to arrange the introduction (*miai,* literally, means "seeing each other").[21] By contrast a love marriage is one in which the partners to the marriage usually meet completely independently of parental involvement. The proportions of *miai* marriage (as opposed to love marriage) in 1955 for large cities and farming districts were as follows (Koyama, 1961:43):

large cities	73%
small cities	86%

Over time the proportion of *miai* marriages has declined considerably everywhere in Japan since the mid-1950s.

This completes the discussion of the appropriateness of the assumptions insofar as Japan is concerned. In this chapter (and also in Chapter 3), we have shown that the patriarchal stem family system, with household production, characterized Japan from the eighteenth century on, and that the absence of any sustained population increase from about 1700 to 1850 permitted this sytem to perpetuate itself with a relatively equal distribution of assets (landholdings) and income. After the Meiji Restoration, population began to grow (see Chapters 3, 5, and 7), but the simultaneous development of industry opened up job opportunities. Sons who were not expected to inherit land sought positions in this expanding modern sector, and initially they depended on their fathers for placement through family connections. The patriarchal stem family system thus perpetuated itself without disruption because all sons eventually managed to locate income-generating positions. But modernization, and especially education and the adjustment of labor markets to the diffusion of education, undermined the economic and social basis of the patriarchal stem family system in Japan. This completes our discussion of the Japanese evidence supporting the thesis concerning the Japanese family and household production. Now let us turn to the Swedish case.

4.6. The Stem Family System in Premodern Sweden

The goal in this section is to show that the assumptions concerning the stem family system, family labor, and the existence of a market for hired labor are reasonable for the premodern Swedish peasantry. We begin by discussing some literature concerning the stem family system of Western Europe as a whole, and then proceed to consider the issues for Sweden.

In thinking about the family systems of Western Europe from the Middle Ages to the nineteenth century, one can certainly find considerable variation in specific practices governing inheritance and the like. But if one takes a broad comparative view, contrasting the family systems of regions like traditional Africa, say, with those of premodern Europe, the structural similarities between the family systems of the Western European countries immediately become evident. Goody (1976:10) is struck by the relative uniformity of stem family systems throughout Europe, noting that they were all characterized by some form of dowry:

> If one looks in a broad comparative way at systems of agricultural production, one of the significant features of European societies, as indeed of the major states of Asia, is the fact that the property from some kind of conjugal estate devolves on both men and women, either by inheritance or by some form of pre-mortem endowment.
> . . . One implication is that even when a certain type of property is restricted to males, women are nevertheless seen as the residual heirs, in preference to more distant males.

Shorter (1975) has also looked at evidence concerning family systems throughout premodern Europe. He describes the stem family as commonplace throughout Western and Central Europe, and he argues, as we have for Japan, that the lineage of the family was of paramount importance in the behavior of premodern European peasants: ". . . popular marriage in former centuries was usually affectionless, held together by considerations of property and lineage. . . ."[22] Therefore, on a general level of discussion, it is safe to characterize the Western European premodern family pattern as a stem family system.

Moreover, for Sweden and other parts of Scandinavia there are more specific descriptions of the premodern family, all of which point to the stem family system. For instance, Thomas (1941) notes that the land usually passed from father to (eldest) son and that the land was typically left undivided, so the siblings of the heir had to leave the holdings: "When the farmer became old, or upon his death, his real property usually passed to one son, who bound himself to compensate the other children for their inheritance rights."[23] As for the woman's side of the marriage market, we have the unusually detailed descriptions of neighboring Norway for the early nineteenth century drawn from the publications of the Norwegian social philosopher Eilert Sundt:

> a young boy . . . marries a girl about his own age or a little older who has been so long in service and used her pay so well that she, in addition to good wearing apparel and bed linen, owns two pots, a baking pan, and a couple of candlesticks and perhaps at most a cow running with her master's herd.[24]

In short, men postponed marriage until an opportunity to acquire a farm or holding (croft, cottage, or *statare* position) became available. And women tended to work and save their earnings in order to build dowries that would make them attractive on the marriage market. Where the son inherited his father's farm, a stem family situation was realized, with the son residing with his wife and children and one or both of his parents before they died.

That children played an important role in premodern Swedish peasant farming is suggested by a number of authorities. For instance, Montgomery (1939:219) suggests that children of 5 to 6 years in age worked as late as 1837. Moreover, the *statare* system was considered advantageous to estate owners because the *statare* brought with him a family labor force (wives and children), unlike the unmarried male domestic servant. Finally, the connection between natural fertility and the peasant life-cycle considerations involving labor and old-age security has been remarked on by Swedish authorities. For example, Winberg (1978:181) wrote:

> In modern industrial society, the family is not a unit of production, but the woman tries to enter production as quickly as possible after the birth of children. In agricultural society, where the family to a great extent constitutes a unit of production, there

> are few rational motives for such a 'modern' form of birth control. Having children of different ages could be just as convenient as they could perform different tasks on the farm. To give birth to children at a relatively late age could also be an advantage as there would then be children at home during the parents' old age.

This quotation clearly reflects life-cycle considerations for the premodern Swedish peasantry.

The final issue to be considered concerns the existence of a market for paid labor in rural Sweden prior to modern economic growth, a factor that, according to the model, reflects the standard of living and income distribution and that may reduce the proportion of the populace that needs to rely solely on a demographic life-cycle strategy (the distribution of wealth and income being an important factor in determining this proportion). A quote from Eriksson and Rogers (1978:63) addresses this issue neatly. They are describing unmarried servants (*pigor, drängar*):

> This group included farmhands and servant girls who were employed to do a variety of menial tasks, from working in the fields to working in the kitchen. They were employed mainly by persons of standing and peasants although crofters, artisans and others might also employ them. They were contracted on a yearly basis and economic differences within the group were small (with the exception that farmhands received more pay than servant girls). . . . The group consisted mainly of the youth of an area who were engaged in this work only on a temporary basis. It was a normal part of many people's occupational careers. From the time they left home to the time they married, they worked as servants with only a small portion of them remaining in this position throughout their lives.

The Japanese data already cited suggests that a similar system developed in the rural villages of Japan as the standard of living rose, although the simultaneous expansion of industrial employment and productivity improvements in agriculture worked to slow its development there. In any event, the Swedish evidence on servants is consistent with the other evidence concerning the standard of living and natural fertility.

To summarize the argument concerning the premodern family system in Sweden, it is useful to return to the discussion of the slow transformation of Swedish rural social structure as the population grew between 1750 and 1850 (see Chapter 3). Two points can easily be grasped from this. First, the peasantry tended to cling to the stem family system, and the population increase generated downward mobility for the sons of peasants and crofters who could not inherit. It should be emphasized, however, that the downward mobility that occurred did strain the operation of the stem family system in Sweden and that some subpopulations began to abandon the stem family institutions as the century of sustained population increase continued. Second, landowners developed the *statare* system (partly in response to the expansion of population) as a means of securing a portion of the rents that accrued to patriarchs because the latter controlled, to a degree, the labor of their children and spouses. The landlords preferred the *statare* system over the hiring of unmarried males and females for that reason. In short, the institutional developments characteristic of the Swedish rural sector prior to 1870 support the general interpretation we have given to the patriarchal stem family system under conditions of household production.

4.7. Education, Status, and the Labor Market: Differentiation in the Swedish School System

Because most of the arguments concerning Swedish education center around the separate development of various facets of schooling (i.e., technical training, division into separate male and female systems, etc.), it is useful to commence this section with a discussion of the postwar debate over differentiation in the public schools. The issue of differentiation (i.e., tracking of students into vocational and academic courses) became controversial in Sweden soon after the Second World War (see Husén, 1962). In 1946 the Swedish recommended the introduction of compulsory nine-year schooling, which was to be undifferentiated until the ninth year. Torsten Husén was a principal advocate of the undifferentiated program, arguing that differentiation perpetuated class divisions and wasted potential talent of the lower classes who were not encouraged to develop their abilities and academic proclivities. During the 1960s, Sweden in fact carried out a radical reform of the school system, in response to reports of ad hoc committees that were appointed to analyze specific problems.

Differentiation had two major social aspects associated with it: the economic return to schooling and the dividing up of the student population according to sex. The advocates of the policy of abolishing differentiation were concerned with the perpetuation of class divisions—the children of the professional classes becoming professionals and the children of workers becoming workers. Their concentration on educational reform as a means of attacking social differentiation reveals that education did and continues to serve both as a means of screening persons for positions and as a source of productivity gain. Before the war, the professional and wealthy classes typically sent their children to the universities, whereas children of the working class were encouraged to select commercial and technical gymnasia, where they could learn a trade. By the same token, the differentiation of education that this implied served a practical economic function. The children of farmers and workers were expected to acquire a practical knowledge that would lead to a high economic payoff in terms of productivity. Graduation from the universities, by contrast, served as a job-screening function, as it does in Japan. Thus the differentiation of Swedish education before 1960 reflects the manifold aspects of education emphasized in the model.

Finally, differentiation in education by sex was common before 1950. It has been noted that the design of the Swedish school system in the first half of the twentieth century resulted in a girl's education being more expensive than a boy's. Moreover, the differentiation encouraged women to specialize in the arts instead of in the vocational and professional areas. Indeed, the emancipation of women in Sweden has been associated with three main changes: the family legislation of 1845 and 1858, which gave women the right to inherit land and unmarried women mobility and choice of employment in the labor market (later legislation also permitted unmarried women to select their own spouses without securing the permission of their fathers); the abolition (1846–1864) of the guild system, which had excluded most women from entry into craft employ; and the breaking down of sexual differentiation in the public schools, a process that permitted women more readily to acquire remunerative skills or graduation from a university as a means of passing job-screening hurdles (Qvist, 1977:180).

The last issue concerning education involves the question of whether or not labor legislation had an important impact on the process of the fertility transition, independent of education. As with the Japanese case, we argue it did not. Here only two points need be made. First, the major early legislation came in the 1870s and 1880s, long after the education law of 1842, and the laws were generally considered ineffective because inspection was grossly inadequate. Second, when the statutes finally were rendered relatively effective in 1900 and 1912, the group excluded was children under 13 years of age; these boys and girls, in principle, were required to attend a public school [see Olsson (1980) for a study of child labor in Sweden during the last two centuries].

In short, the material on Swedish education, which we have briefly reviewed in this section, supports the multifaceted interpretation of the expansion of the Swedish school system.

4.8. Conclusions

In this chapter we have concentrated on laying out empirical evidence for Japan and Sweden that directly bears on the operation of the household in these nations and, in particular, on the concepts of leverage and life cycle that underlie the model of household behavior. In Part III of this volume we turn to the empirical evidence concerning Japanese and Swedish natality. The model of the household is used as a theoretical basis for a theory of the evolution of natality; we must now examine the empirical evidence on natality to see if the theoretical approach regarding fertility is consistent with that data.

Notes to Chapter 4

1. It should be emphasized that the model is for a "typical" family and may not describe all subpopulations of the national populations we are concerned with. For instance, Thomas C. Smith in private correspondence has pointed out that there were a substantial number of slum dwellers (*hijin*) in the towns and cities of Japan, before and especially after the Meiji Restoration. Apparently, few of these families were stem families. The model of the premodern demographic regime does not deal with nuclear families per se, but the existence of such a subpopulation does not necessarily question the universal validity of the discussion we gave concerning the costs of and benefits for economic leverage over children for all subpopulations. One must be careful about drawing this conclusion. For example, as long as the subpopulations in question are relatively small within their geographical areas of location, their nuptiality patterns are likely to reflect that of their surrounding milieu because many of the brides and grooms within these subpopulations are likely to marry persons outside the subpopulations, reducing any variability attributable to the particular circumstances of such groups. I am grateful to Thomas Smith for pointing these matters out to me.

2. Writings in Japanese that Westerners would recognize as anthropological studies of villages fit almost exclusively into the period after World War II.

3. For the tremendous impact of these transformations on the institutions and behavior described in this section, see, among others, R. J. Smith (1978), Dore (1978), and Shimpo (1976).

4. For instance, Nakane (1967) wrote, "The primary unit of social organization in Japan is the household. In an agrarian community a household has a particularly important function as a distinct body for economic management." The *ie* as a legal concept was a product of the Meiji period, and the legal rules concerning its definition and operation were codified in the civil code of 1896. After the American occupation began, a new civil code was promulgated in 1947 and, theoretically, this did away with the laws that bolstered the prewar *ie*, including the practice of passing land from the father to one son (usually the eldest). But in practice these codes did not abolish the old system (see Nakane, 1972) and the Meiji and Tokugawa rules of succession continued, the other siblings "voluntarily" relinquished their claims to the land. However, as industrialization has drained the countryside over the last fifteen years, many sons who could inherit the family estate have opted for urban work and have given up their claim on the land, and the *ie* as an economic unit, an idealized stem family, has gradually died out in Japan. This is especially true of urban areas. It should be noted, on the one hand, that this disintegration of the *ie* in the rural areas refers to the period after 1960, and, consequently, to a period after fertility had reached low levels. On the other hand, the *ie* had probably lost a good deal of its meaning in cities even prior to World War II. See, for instance, Nakane (1972) and the subsequent discussion in the text.

5. In the late 1960s and 1970s, the possibility of becoming an in-adopted son had increased for males in the countryside because many sons who stand to inherit the family estate prefer to take up employment in industrial or professional occupations. This phenomenon, however, is limited mainly to the period after 1965. For a map of Japan showing the location of the prefectures, see Appendix 1.

6. For a discussion of village tensions that are created when many of the "sons" of village households are not biological, see Smith (1978).

7. It should be emphasized that T. C. Smith himself gives a very different interpretation to this phenomenon. It should also be noted that the interpretation we use suggests that the *average* standard of living (per capita income) may actually have fallen during the seventeenth and eighteenth centuries, despite the technological changes that did occur. This may well have happened because the increase in numbers would, in and of itself, tend to depress income per head. As land productivity rose, the gains would go into increases in rents; thus the tenants might suffer a decline in income no matter what. And if the productivity gains on a per capita basis were not sufficient to counteract the decline in output per worker due to the previous population increase (and this is an open question), the standard of living may actually have fallen for most landowners as well. See Chapter 5.

8. This is especially true at spring transplanting time in rice-growing villages. Thus Embree (1939:133), observing a village in the 1930s, wrote: "rice-transplanting is one of the biggest events of the year . . . at this time the whole *mura* is busy at the same labor so that a *buraku* looks like a deserted village, with a few babies and ancient crones here and there in a vacant lot." School children were given special leave to be at home, bending their backs working with their parents in the rice fields.

9. Beardsley *et al.* (1959:64) note that as improvements in public health and medicine have enhanced life expectancies, the vigor of persons in their middle age and old age has improved, gradually transforming the meaning of the traditional age classifications.

10. For an extensive discussion of these concepts, see Nakane (1967:82–85).

11. However, in the village of Niiike studied by Beardsley *et al.* (1959), the spring transplanting was almost exclusively performed by the individual households working separately.

12. See Appendix 5 for some of the details. Mosk and Stoft (1979) provide comprehensive discussion of the data tape on which the calculations in this section are based, as well as a precise examination of the meaning of the Japanese terms underlying the categories used in the analysis here.

13. In what follows we use the terms family or house (*ie*) and household (*kazoku*) interchangeably. Technically, the two concepts are different because, for example, domestic servants could be household members (i.e., residents of the family estate) but not necessarily members of the family. The data analyzed here are technically for farm families (*nōka*) but in fact concern farm households (i.e., residents). The age categories available in the raw data are 1–7 years; 8–14 years; 15–25 years; 26–40 years; 41–60 years; and 61 years and over. We define an adult as a person 15 years or older and a child as 14 years or younger. The calculation of worker units (W) is explained below. Land area is measured in *tan se bu* where 1 *tan* = 10 *se* = .245 acres and 30 *bu* = 1 *se*.

14. Consumption figures are in yen.

In calculating C, we weighted the age groups, separately for each sex, by the following weights:

	1–7	8–14	15–25	26–40	41–60	61+
Males	.4	.6	1.0	1.0	1.0	.8
Females	.2	.4	.8	.8	.8	.7

Then we summed the age-weighted males and females.

15. In calculating W, we weighted the age groups, separately for each sex, by the following weights:

	1–7	8–14	15–25	26–40	41–60	61+
Males	0	0	1.0	1.0	1.0	.8
Females	0	0	.8	.8	.8	.7

Then we summed the age-weighted males and females. Hours are hours worked per year. It should be noted that the labor weights differ from those used as examples in Chapter 2, Section 2.3. A more reasonable set of weights than those just shown would have the male labor weight dropping off below 1.0 for the age group 41–60. Adjustment of these weights and recalculation of the empirical results shown in the tables that follow would involve considerable cost, and the results are unlikely to be very sensitive to this adjustment, so we do not do so here.

16. The income figures are in yen. The income figures used here are all net of intermediate production costs (i.e., the cost of intermediate inputs like fertilizer and rent have been subtracted from the gross income measures so the income figures implicitly represent payments to the factors of production, capital, and labor actually *owned* by the family).

17. We were able to ascertain the region that each household is in because the original tables contain the name of the village (*mura*), county (*gun*), and prefecture that each household is in; and the regions are defined in terms of the prefectures they include (see Chapter 5). For a list of the households and their associated prefectures and regions, see Mosk and Stoft (1979).

18. The regional variation in the dependence on nonhousehold labor is also interesting, particularly because it suggests that regional factors like the timing of the harvest and the changeability of the climate may influence the degree to which households must rely on paid labor or labor exchange. These figures suggest that considerable caution must be exercised in drawing inferences from a particular village study because the region it lies in may be relatively atypical as compared with the national average. In the case of dependence on outside labor, the Tōhoku and Kyūshū regions stand out as unusual.

19. See Appendix 4 for a discussion of the data tape for the *gun*. In Chapters 5 and 7 we discuss the reasons for using these variables as proxies for job opportunities and income. E_f is defined as E_f = women employed outside primary industry/women 20–44.

20. On the *juku* see Rohlen (1980). On the general competitiveness of Japanese schooling and one interpretation (largely different from the one presented here of its relationship to postwar Japanese fertility, see Yamamura and Hanley (1975).

21. Some *miai* marriages do not involve the prior choice of a prospective bride or bridegroom by the parents, but *miai* is almost always used today when the parents are seriously involved in the arrangement of the match.

22. Shorter (1975:55) also argues that European peasant women subordinated their own needs to that of the male lineage.

23. Thomas (1941:41). Montgomery (1939:5–7) describes the system in similar terms. See Gaunt (1978) and Löfgren (1974) for discussions on the stem family system in Sweden.

24. Cited in Drake (1969:139). See Kälvemark (1977–1978) for a discussion of the Swedish marriage market in historical perspective.

PART III

The Evolution of Natality

CHAPTER 5

The Premodern Demographic Regime in Japan

5.1. Introduction

Part III of this book is devoted to examining the empirical basis for the theory using demographic data for Japan and Sweden. The main focus is on fertility, of course, because we have already discussed the evidence regarding household behavior. The data we shall consider in the next four chapters are areal data, that is, it represents averages for geographical entities, either for nations or for subunits of nations (e.g., prefectures, counties, cities, etc.). For this reason, the figures we shall consider are most appropriate to an examination of the model of aggregate population behavior developed in Sections 2.2, 2.5, and 2.6. In particular, Chapter 5 is devoted to examining the arguments of Section 2.5 for Japan, and Chapter 6 examines these same arguments for Sweden. Chapter 7 examines the arguments of Section 2.6 for Japan, and Chapter 8 looks at these points for Sweden. It should be emphasized here that the Swedish material has mainly been introduced for purposes of comparison; the primary focus is on Japan. The point of the comparison is to make appealing the argument that the framework for analyzing household behavior that we have developed can account for the evolution of natality wherever the assumptions of the model are met and that some of the diversity in fertility transitions are explicable in terms of this theoretical approach. It should also be kept in mind that because we are working with data for geographical units, the issue of "ecological fallacy" will always be a potential problem in the analysis undertaken in Part III.

The purpose in Chapter 5 is to present a variety of evidence that supports the interpretation given in Chapter 2 of Japan's premodern demographic regime, both its evolution over time and its characteristics as seen in a comparative prespective. The bulk of the statistical evidence offered is for the interwar period (mainly 1920–1930), a time when the fertility transition was commencing. However, we shall also extend the investigations back into the Tokugawa and Meiji periods, although, as we shall indicate, the relatively limited quality and quantity of the statistical materials for the period prior to 1920 precludes a detailed treatment of the pre-1920 situation.

The organization of this chapter is as follows. In the next section we discuss the nature of the functional forms that we utilize in statistical analysis. Then we review the major evidence that has emerged from studies of the Tokugawa period. This consists almost exclusively of findings for a small group of Tokugawa villages. Then we consider the Meiji period, and especially the estimates worked up from the scattered regional censuses of the Meiji period. Having established that the interpretation permits us to formulate a coherent and reasonable picture of the demographic situation in Japan before 1920, we consider an analysis of cross-sections and trends for the prefectures of Japan, 1920–1960. We devote a special section to the problem of dating the end of the premodern demographic regime in Japan with this data. Finally we discuss the results for the rural (*gun*) and urban (*shi*) sectors of the prefectures.

5.2. The Functional Forms

The basic relationships we are interested in examining in this chapter and the next chapter are similar to those given by Eq. (2.15) in Section 2.5. In particular, we shall explore these associations with several different functional forms with which we attempt to approximate the aggregate behavior described in Sections 2.2–2.5. The emphasis here is on the *structure* of the premodern demographic regime, i.e., on the association of nuptiality patterns with natural fertility and infant mortality. In Chapter 7 we shall consider some proxies for health conditions and relate these empirically to levels of natural fertility. We have adopted this strategy of presenting results because Chapter 7 is almost solely concerned with the determinants of marital fertility, and the level of natural fertility is a very important component of overall marital fertility before and during the early phases of the fertility transition.

To elaborate on this discussion, with an eye to presenting the empirical findings let us adopt a notation similar to that of Section 2.5, with A_f the average age at marriage for females; M the Coale–Trussell index of natural fertility; IMR the infant mortality rate; AD the adult death rate; and d the overall (crude) death rate. Then one elementary linear representation of Eq. (2.15) would be

$$A_f = a_0 + a_1 M + a_2 d + \epsilon \tag{5.1}$$

with the a priori expectation that $a_1 > 0$ and $a_2 < 0$. To bring the statistical model closer to the spirit of Eq. (2.3) of Section 2.3, we can decompose overall mortality into its components AD and IMR. That is, we can write

$$A_f = a_0 + a_1 M + a_2(IMR) + a_3(AD) + \epsilon \tag{5.2}$$

with the hypothesis that the signs of the coefficients are $a_1 > 0$, $a_2 < 0$, and $a_3 < 0$. This is the type of equation we shall work with in Chapters 5 and 6.

The reader may recall, from a perusal of Section 2.6, that we would expect a variety of influences other than those involving natural fertility and mortality to affect actual observed marriage patterns in a patriarchal stem family population. In particular, we would expect the sex ratio (a proxy for the number of marriageable males per marriageable female), proxies for the incidence of job opportunities for women outside of household labor, measures for the level of male wages, and the extent of male–female wage differentials to be significant in a statistical analysis of nuptiality in the populations under study here. Wherever possible in the empirical analysis of this chapter and the next, we attempt to introduce reasonable proxies for these influences.

Now let us consider a brief discussion of the Japanese evidence, proceeding chronologically (beginning with the Tokugawa period and working up to 1960).

5.3. The Tokugawa Period

Tokugawa government represented a compromise between centrist forces, which encouraged concentration of authority at the national level (the shogunate), and feudal tendencies, which demanded local autonomy for the *han* (the fiefdoms). As a result of the delicate political balance struck, the development of systematic population counts and the processing of vital statistics at the national level were hindered. Estimates of national population and population growth (and, consequently, given the virtually complete sealing off of the country to international migration, of the natural rate of population growth) have been worked up from a variety of sources,

TABLE 5.1

Measures of Fertility, Mortality, and Population Increase for Selected Premodern Japanese Villages[a]

Population and Date	Overall fertility	Nuptiality[b]		Marital fertility[c]							Mortality			Natural rate of population increase
							birth intervals (years)					$\mathring{e}_1$		
	CBR	*MAFMM*	*MAFMF*	*M*	*m*	*ALB*	average	0–1	1–2	2–3	*CDR*	Male	Female	*NRI*
Kandō-Shinden[d] (ca. 1800)	34.4	29.4	21.6	.95	.21	39.2	2.8	1.2	3.3	3.0	26.2	33.2	31.6	8.2
Yokouchi,[e] before 1700	35.3	26.0	18.8	.74	−.20	40.5	3.5	3.6	3.4	3.4	25.5	36.8	29.0	9.8
Yokouchi,[e] after 1800	22.2	28.0	21.7	.56	.34	33.6	3.3	2.0	4.5	3.8	18.9	n.a.	n.a.	3.3
Nakahara, 18th and 19th Centuries	36.3	27.1	19.6	.64	−.28	37.5	3.6	2.6	4.4	3.3	26.6	46.1	50.8	9.7
Fujito,[f] ca. 1800	15.4	n.a.	22.9	n.a.	n.a.	n.a.	3.6	n.a.	3.2	4.2	16.8	50.9	59.1	−1.4
Fukiage,[g] ca. 1683	31.0	n.a.	24.5	n.a.	n.a.	n.a.	4.2	n.a.	4.7	4.1	15.9	n.a.	n.a.	15.1
Fukiage,[g] ca. 1860	19.4	n.a.	24.6	n.a.	n.a.	n.a.	4.1	n.a.	4.2	4.1	22.2	n.a.	n.a.	−2.8

[a] From Smith (1977), Hanley and Yamamura (1977), and Hayami (1968, 1973). n.a. indicates that data were not available.

[b] *MAFMM* is the mean age at first marriage for marriage for males; *MAFMF* is the mean age at first marriage for females.

[c] *ALB* is the age of mother at last birth; 0–1 birth interval is from marriage to first birth. Birth intervals are in years and are all simple averages (means).

[d] *CBR, CDR,* and *NRI* are for 1838–1842, the earliest period for which Hayami gives *CDR*s. $\mathring{e}_1$ is for persons who died between 1838 and 1869.

[e] *CBR, CDR,* and *NRI* for "before 1700" are for period 1671–1700. For "after 1800" they are for 1776–1871. $\mathring{e}_1$ is for 1671–1725 period. The figure on age at last birth is based on a small sample of observations.

[f] *CBR, CDR,* and *NRI* for 1800–1804. $\mathring{e}_1$ is for 1800–1805. There are figures on age at last birth given for Fujito, but examination of the underlying methods of calculation suggests that the average figures may not be representative.

[g] *CBR, CDR,* and *NRI* for "ca. 1683" are for 1683–1700. For "ca. 1860" they are for 1854–1860. There are figures on age at last birth for Fukiage, but examination of the methods of calculation suggests that the average figures may not be representative.

however, and can be seen in the accompanying tabulation. Although totals for individual years may be somewhat inaccurate, the consistency of the figures from estimate to estimate suggests that the overall picture is probably a reasonable approximation. A few of the resulting figures clearly indicate the general pattern (the population figure is for the year given and the population growth figure is for the trend period).[1] What strikingly emerges from these figures is the picture of a population that expands considerably in numbers during the seventeenth century and then reaches a plateau, about which it fluctuates. Such a stationary population balance for the eighteenth and nineteenth centuries could be struck only if the crude birth and death rates were approximately equal (given the international isolation of Japan at the time). Thus the question that has tantalized historical demographers is as follows: at what levels of mortality and fertility was the balance struck, and why did the vital rates reach these levels during the eighteenth and nineteenth centuries?

Year	Estimated population (1000s)	Trend period	Rate of (natural) population growth (annual rate)
1660	18500	1600–1721	.28
1721	26064	1721–1750	−.02
1774	25991	1756–1786	−.13
1822	26602	1822–1828	.37
1852	27201	1834–1846	−.05

As already indicated, there are no reliable national figures on birth and death rates for the Tokugawa period. However, there are local village records, themselves a byproduct of the Tokugawa exclusionary policy. Concerned with Western meddling in the internal affairs of Japan and particularly with the subversion of loyalty to the shogunate that conversions to Christianity might encourage, the shogunate banned Christianity and required each household in the population to register all of its members at one of its local (village) Buddhist temples. The resulting religious records are called *shūmon-aratame-chō,* and these have been utilized by scholars trained in family reconstitution techniques to measure vital events in Tokugawa villages. There are problems with the *shūmon-aratame-chō,* however, that the reader should be aware of in evaluating their accuracy. First, in some villages, marriages were not formalized until a child had been born, or was about to be born. (This apparently was the case for Fujito and Fukiage, reported in Table 5.1). And, second, it was common to register newly-born infants at only one time of the year (the beginning of the Japanese new year). Thus it is probable that many infants perished prior to registration, either eliminated by natural causes or through deliberate infanticide.

In any event, the figures that have emerged through family reconstitution are of considerable interest. In Table 5.1 we present findings for a variety of these villages.[2] There is some variation, but the general picture that these data project is evident enough. First, levels of natural fertility tend to be low (compare the values of M and the protracted interbirth intervals).[3] Second, males appear to wed at relatively advanced ages, whereas females appear to wed at very youthful ages. These two observations suggest that the Japanese premodern demographic regime was characterized by poor health conditions and the attendant circumstances for nuptiality and natural fertility.[4]

There is one perplexing problem with these village data that concerns the question of parity-specific control. For none of the villages are there exceptionally large values for m, although the figure for Yokouchi after 1800 is above .3. Because the figures for Yokouchi after 1800 are based on a small sample of households, however, in this instance the reliability of the estimates for both M and m is open to question. More problematic are the figures on age at last birth (*ALB*) for mothers. Although the figures for Kandō-Shinden and Yokouchi are around 39–40 and, consequently, perfectly consistent with what we know for Western European populations prior to their fertility transitions, the figures for Nakahara and Yokouchi after 1800 are relatively low. We should not reject the idea that these villages were natural fertility populations on the basis of these data, however. First, the age gaps between the spouses in these villages are substantial, and the husband's infertility may account for the relatively early ages of terminal reproduction. Second, tuberculosis was very common in Japan before World War I, and some forms of this disease cause permanent sterility in women (the documented response of tuberculosis to improvements in living standards is one reason why we would expect natural fertility levels to improve as per capita income is enhanced in a population). Third, the early age of last birth may be partially attributed to unregistered infants dying after the final registered births. Fourth, Smith (1977:72) suggests that relatively early ages at marriage for women in Japan may have allowed subfecund couples, who in a late marriage setting such as eighteenth-century Western Europe might have no offspring at all, to have at least one birth. Fifth, there is the problem of small sample sizes that, at least in the case of Yokouchi after 1800, make it difficult to credit the precise numerical estimates presented. All in all, we need not reject the notion that the Tokugawa villages were natural fertility populations.

Special attention must be devoted to one issue regarding the interpretation of the Tokugawa data concerning mortality and marital fertility—infanticide. The historical literature on Tokugawa Japan refers to *mabiki,* or infanticide, in many places. Infanticide was undoubtedly a strategy resorted to by the Tokugawa peasant for at least two reasons: selection of sex of offspring and elimination of infants who appeared weak or deformed and whose survival chances appeared dim. Hanley and Yamamura (1977) suggest that infanticide in some of the villages they studied was especially directed against females, and this would fit in with the discussion on the relative value of children in an environment of low income when a patriarchal stem family system is adhered to. We have also shown (in Mosk, 1978a) how the alternating sex ratio of births T. C. Smith (1977) finds in his Nakahara data is consistent with the type of behavior we describe. An alternating strategy (whereby the couple attempts to have males follow females, so that as the children matured there were both males and females who could step in and take up the sex-differentiated tasks performed by the husband and by his wife) is consistent with the data that show infanticide having a slight bias against females (i.e., a tendency to prefer males and to accept males more readily, even if successive births are male). Indeed in the relatively small data sets generated by family reconstitution methods, it may be difficult to separate out the two effects or to clearly discern either because the number of observations are too slight. In sum, the evidence on infanticide, which often is cited in discussing Tokugawa demographic history, is consistent with the model we have elaborated, in which parents are concerned with the future labor services of their offspring and with the viability of infants and children.

A second issue, which is not central to our focus here but that must be touched on in passing, concerns the question of movements in the level of income per head during the Tokugawa period. We have nothing like the wealth of Meiji quantitative evidence (utilized in Chapter 3) for the Tokugawa period, so that most of the figures available have been derived from local sources, which are notoriously difficult to draw generalizations from (the qualitative evidence is mixed, at best, on the one hand there are reports of famines and peasant revolts, on the other hand there is evidence of conspicuous consumption of luxuries by some classes). Quantitative work for selected regions of Japan (e.g., Nishikawa, 1978; Akimoto, 1981) suggests that average per capita income improved gradually toward the end of the Tokugawa period and that this trend was mainly attributed to investment. Four points should be kept in mind regarding these findings. First, they show moderate growth at best. The rates calculated by scholars are far smaller than the rates documented for the Meiji economy. Second, positive growth rates that occurred in a few selected regions do not prove the case for the nation as a whole. The Hitotsubashi University national figures on income per head (i.e., the LTES data used in Chapter 3) are much more comprehensive than the scattered regional data available for late Tokugawa, and the Meiji data suggest that income per head was very low at the beginning of Meiji for the nation as a whole; of course, these figures may mask regional variations that probably obtained at that time. Third, income per head may have risen for some social groups and have remained stationary or even fallen for others during the Tokugawa period because of changes in income distribution (e.g., a greater concentration of assets and income in the hands of merchants and well-to-do peasant families). After the Meiji Restoration, growth rates in income per head were so high that any changes in income distribution that may have occurred almost certainly could not outweigh the benefits of growth for the bulk of the peasantry and workers. That is, it is highly unlikely that the mass of people lost ground or remained stable in terms of the standard of living during the period 1870–1940 (in any event, evidence on income distribution suggests that it was not greatly skewed during the interwar period). Finally, the fourth and last point to draw from this discussion is that even *if* we accept that income per head rose gradually for the bulk of the populace during the late Tokugawa period, this does not disprove the basic argument: relatively minor increases in the standard of living may not affect infant mortality and natural fertility at all. The much more momentous increases in the standard of living experienced by the Meiji population almost surely did, but that is a different story altogether.

Thus the demographic evidence for Tokugawa Japan, albeit scanty, tends to support the general interpretation we have given.[5] That my framework also accounts for the apparent rise in fertility during the Meiji period is documented in the next section.

5.4. The Meiji Period

In 1871 the new Meiji government introduced the *koseki* system as a means of consolidating control over the population and of keeping track of vital events and total human numbers.[6] A *koseki* is a family registration book, which is kept in the government office that has jurisdiction over the legal place of domicile of the family (the *honseki*). By law, one of the family members must report to the governmental office within a specified time any birth, death, marriage, or divorce that occurs. In theory, the *koseki* statistics should provide a complete count of the national population and the vital rates (regional statistics would not necessarily be accurate, even in theory, however, because it was common to migrate and not move one's *honseki* when one did). However, the government was aware of the possibility that families would fail to register, or delay the registration, of vital events (e.g., in the instance of marriage, where couples often delayed registering the union until a child was born, or in the case of births for which death occurred soon after delivery, so that neither birth nor death was recorded); and it sought to develop a census, a de facto count, of the population to secure a reliable record of age structure, marital status, labor force status, and the like. However, although the national government did commission a pilot census in 1879 (administered in Yamanashi prefecture), it did not conduct a nationwide census until 1920. Thus, in the first instance, we must turn to the figures generated from the *koseki* system because, on a national scale, there is no other set of figures for the period 1875–1920 that was systematically collected and published at regular intervals. After 1920 we are fortunate to have both the enumerative census and the statistics produced from the *koseki* system, so it is possible to adjust one with the other and secure very accurate measures.[7] This, however, does not help us with the national data for 1875–1919.

Out of the *koseki* data, the Japanese government published five "censuses" *Nihon teikoku jinkō seitai tōkei* (for 1898, 1903, 1908, 1913, and 1918) and vital statistics (*Jinkō dōtai tōkei*) on an annual basis from 1899 on (see Appendix 3 and the References). It also prepared a retrospective account of vital events for 1875–1899. Because the degree of underregistration of birth and infant death diminished over time (as people became more accustomed to the use of the *koseki* and more literate and the government more active in insuring that registration was attended to), we would expect some artificial increase in birth and death rates for this reason alone. However, as shown in Table 5.2, the official statistics show a dramatic rise in both rates, especially in the birth rate. It is difficult to credit problems of registration for all of this expansion in the crude rates. This is especially so in light of our previous discussion of the Tokugawa village figures, which show a relatively uniform low fertility. A complicating issue involving registration should also be noted here. Abandonment of deliberate infanticide, which presumably never involved registration, could explain some of this rise. The issue, then, is why families relinquished this practice. As a hypothesis consider the following: families abandon this practice as survival chances for infants and youths improve and as the relative economic value of males and females changes.

The suspicion that the official figures are seriously marred by a trend in the degree of underregistration has encouraged a number of Japanese demographers to offer alternative estimates, each alternative calculation involving slightly different working assumptions. These estimates are presented in Table 5.2. The estimates of Okazaki and Yasukawa-Hirooka both involve backward projection of the 1920 census figures on population grouped by age and sex, under assumptions about the trend in life expectancy of persons of the various cohorts.[8] Technically, the Yasukawa-Hir-

TABLE 5.2

Estimates of *CBR*s, *CDR*s and Life Expectancies ($\mathring{e}_0$), Japan, 1875–1920[a]

Authority, year (s)	*CBR*	*CDR*	$\mathring{e}_0$[b]	
			Males	Females
Official				
1875	25.4	18.5	—	—
1880	26.0	18.1	—	—
1890	30.4	20.9	42.80	44.30
1900	34.1	21.2	43.97	44.85
1910	36.2	21.5	44.25	44.73
1920	36.3	24.5	42.06	43.20
Morita				
1872–1876	31.1	23.6	—	—
1877–1881	32.1	23.7	—	—
1887–1891	29.2	22.8	—	—
1897–1901	32.6	23.1	—	—
1907–1911	32.2	23.1	—	—
1917–1921	34.6	22.6	—	—
Okazaki				
1875	36.3	31.3	—	—
1880	36.4	31.3	—	—
1890	33.7	28.3	—	—
1900	36.3	27.0	—	—
1910	37.0	25.3	—	—
1920	33.2	22.3	—	—
Mizushima				
1891–1898	—	—	35.29	36.86
1899–1903	—	—	37.80	38.20
1909–1913	—	—	40.22	40.82
1921–1922	—	—	41.48	42.49
Matsuura				
1891–1898	—	—	37.10	39.40
1899–1903	—	—	37.10	40.90
1911–1912	—	—	41.30	42.60
Yasukawa-Hirooka				
1875	34.37	26.11	35.76	37.89
1880	33.89	26.64	36.08	38.04
1890	32.16	25.26	36.89	38.50
1900	35.60	24.99	37.99	39.20
1910	36.81	24.17	39.51	40.46
1920	38.12	21.79	41.61	42.50

[a] Yasukawa and Hirooka (1974), Mizushima (1961), and Mosk (1977). The dash indicates that data were not available.

[b] For $\mathring{e}_0$ the figure for 1890 is for 1891–1898; for 1910 it is for 1899–1903; for 1910 it is for 1909–1913; and for 1920 it is for 1921–1925.

ooka estimates are the most convincing because they are based on an exceedingly detailed and thoroughly systematic method of backward projection. Their estimates suggest that fertility rose somewhat but mortality dropped. The decline in mortality is also part of the pattern revealed by the Okazaki backward projection, although it shows a slight fall in the birth rate as well. If we accept the Yasukawa-Hirooka figures, and we shall present additional evidence in support of them, they suggest that either natural fertility improved or else the age at marriage of females declined and the proportion married rose during the Meiji period, whereas the infant mortality rate probably declined somewhat (because illegitimacy was of relatively minor importance and there appears to have been almost no parity-specific control before World War I or so).

Because the question of whether natural fertility improved or the proportion married rose in the face of declining mortality is so crucial to the model, which predicts that the age of marriage for women and natural fertility would rise as infant mortality falls, it is imperative that we attempt to ascertain which trend did in fact occur. As we shall show, regional data that are of considerable reliability strongly supports the hypothesis that it was a rise in natural fertility that accounts for the trend in overall natality, but it is useful to explore this issue with the national figures as well. We have calculated, from the *koseki* figures on percentage women married by age group in 1918 and the de facto percentages in the 1920 census, adjustment ratios that capture the underregistration of marriage in 1918 for the *koseki* system and applied the same adjustment ratios to the early *koseki* data.[9] The results, as captured by percentages married and the Hutterite index I_m, are shown in the accompanying tabulation. They suggest that the age of mar-

Year	Hutterite index, I_m	Percentage married females 15–19	20–24	25–29
1886	.79	38	73	88
1898	.75	33	72	86
1908	.70	21	64	81
1913	.71	19	67	84

riage of women must have risen during the Meiji period, and, consequently, because illegitimacy was not of major importance at any time, that marital fertility (presumably natural fertility, given the absence of control in 1925 and the Tokugawa period) increased as well.[10]

Before closing out this discussion of the official vital statistics, however, it is useful to display graphically the general trends in a number of the crucial

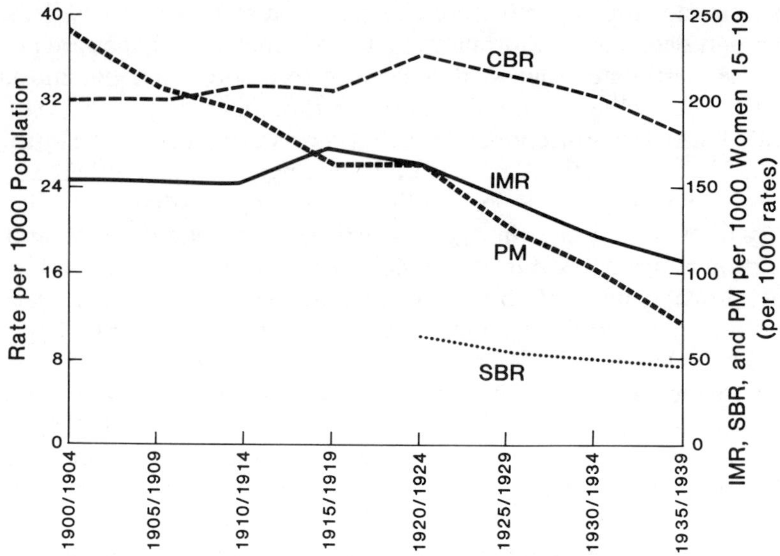

Fig. 5.1. Crude birth rate (*CBR*), infant mortality rate (*IMR*), stillbirth rate (*SBR*), and proportion women 15–19 married (*PM*): Japan, 1900–1939 (five-year averages for all variables except *PM*, which is for a selected date in each period).

demographic variables of the model. This is done in Figure 5.1. This diagram shows, for the first 4 decades of the twentieth century, the trends in nuptiality, infant mortality, the stillbirth rate (for 1920–1939), and the crude birth rate. The crude birth rate figures are adjusted for the period after 1920, but they are official figures for the period 1900–1919. The nuptiality estimates are based on the estimates discussed previously (see Mosk, 1980a). The still birth and infant mortality rates are taken from unadjusted data (so that the slight upward trend in the infant mortality rate prior to 1920 is probably an artifact of improvements in the completeness of registration of births that resulted in infant deaths). As a whole, these figures tend to support the view that fertility rose during the late Meiji period, and this rise is attributable to a pronounced increase in marital fertility accompanied by a simultaneous rise in the age at first marriage of females, both trends responding to improvements in the survivorship rate for infants.

Relying on the official *koseki* statistics to substantiate this argument, however, is clearly insufficient. Ideally, working from figures secured from a de facto census is preferable because the prewar census takers in Japan were careful to count every person (including newborn infants), actual unions whether registered in a *koseki* or not, and the like. Fortunately, as noted previously, the Meiji government did carry out one enumerative census,

TABLE 5.3

Measures of Fertility for Yamanashi Prefecture and its Subdistricts in 1879 and 1925[a]

Area	1879				1925				
	I_f	I_g	I_m	M[b]	I_f	I_g	I_m	M	MSE
Yamanashi *Ken* (Kai no Kuni)	.327	.467	.701	.548	.457	.674	.662	.890	.001
Kōfu *shi*	n.a.	n.a.	n.a.	n.a.	.299	.497	.587	n.a.	n.a.
Nishi Yamanashi (including Kōfu *shi* in 1879)	.322	.461	.699	.539	.475	.723	.641	n.a.	n.a.
Higashi Yamanashi	.366	.460	.795	.542	.431	.627	.670	n.a.	n.a.
Higashi Yatsushiro	.314	.450	.698	.529	.519	.779	.650	n.a.	n.a.
Nishi Yatsushiro	.397	.526	.755	.613	.523	.716	.712	n.a.	n.a.
Minami Koma	.318	.436	.731	.509	.482	.663	.709	n.a.	n.a.
Naka Koma	.328	.494	.664	.682	.459	.704	.636	n.a.	n.a.
Kata Koma	.367	.508	.723	.596	.500	.692	.705	n.a.	n.a.
Minami Tsuru	.320	.460	.695	.539	.481	.717	.654	n.a.	n.a.
Kita Tsuru	.353	.497	.710	.582	.475	.711	.651	n.a.	n.a.

[a] Mosk (1979b). n.a. indicates that data were not available.

[b] Calculated from data on total legitimate births and married women in the quinquennial age classes using the method described in Mosk (1981a).

TABLE 5.4

Aspects of Nuptiality, Marital Fertility, Mortality, and Population Increase for the Agricultural Prefectures of Japan, 1908 and 1925[a]

	Overall fertility		Marital fertility						Nuptiality	Mortality		Population increase
Prefecture	*CBR*	I_f	I_g	M^e	m^e	*MSE*	*SBR*	Percentage women born ca. year married at least 20 years who are childless (*CL*)[b]	I_m	*CDR*	*IMR*	*NRI*[d]
Circa 1908												
Aomori	36.7	.404	.504	.626	n.e.[c]	n.e.[c]	69	7.3	.798	21.9	197.1	14.8
Iwate	33.5	.369	.462	.545	n.e.	n.e.	114	5.5	.796	20.6	180.1	12.9
Akita	32.8	.364	.433	.495	n.e.	n.e.	123	5.9	.837	19.4	184.6	13.4
Yamagata	34.7	.376	.517	.672	n.e.	n.e.	86	6.0	.724	21.7	195.8	13.0
Ibaraki	30.8	.329	.440	.547	n.e.	n.e.	186	6.1	.743	22.0	201.8	8.8
Shimane	27.1	.297	.400	.551	n.e.	n.e.	113	11.3	.729	21.5	146.6	5.6
Oita	26.1	.277	.391	.458	n.e.	n.e.	55	10.5	.706	21.4	130.2	4.7
Miyazaki	24.1	.264	.370	.433	n.e.	n.e.	74	8.6	.708	19.1	118.8	5.0
Kagoshima	24.8	.256	.382	.451	n.e.	n.e.	21	8.3	.670	16.7	98.4	8.1

Circa 1925												
Aomori	43.0	.515	.633	.815	.274	.001	49	6.1	.790	22.2	180.8	20.8
Iwate	40.2	.455	.564	.721	.080	.002	73	5.2	.792	20.7	147.8	19.5
Akita	41.9	.472	.591	.694	−.059	.001	71	5.2	.784	20.4	149.9	21.5
Yamagata	38.8	.459	.630	.847	.246	.001	54	6.6	.706	20.2	141.9	18.6
Ibaraki	36.9	.461	.617	.781	.113	.000	76	5.2	.728	18.4	144.3	18.5
Shimane	30.9	.382	.483	.673	.336	.001	65	7.5	.745	23.2	143.4	7.7
Oita	33.8	.413	.553	.644	−.063	.000	45	7.7	.719	20.1	118.5	13.7
Miyazaki	36.1	.428	.553	.639	−.076	.000	51	7.6	.736	16.9	99.9	19.2
Kagoshima	35.4	.435	.641	.692	−.248	.001	37	7.8	.662	17.7	96.7	17.7

[a] Mosk (1979b); Taeuber (1958); Nihon Naikaku Tōkeikyoku (various years), *Jinkō dōtai tokei;* and Japan. Office of the Prime Minister. *Bureau of Statistics.* (various years), *1970. Population Census of Japan. Vol. 5. Part 2. Divisions 2–6.*

[b] For "circa 1908" refers to women aged 65–69 in 1970 who were married at least 20 years; for "circa 1925" refers to women ages 50–59 in 1970 who were married at least 20 years.

[c] n.e. = not estimated.

[d] *NRI* calculated by subtracting *CDR* in Table from *CBR.*

[e] Values for 1908 calculated as *M* values for Yamanashi prefecture in 1879 (see Table 5.3, note b) are computed.

directed by the well-known statistician Ryōji Sugi.[11] This was conducted in the prefecture known then as the province of Kai (*kai no kuni*) and currently by the name Yamanashi prefecture. Working with the figures on children aged 0, and adjusting them with various assumptions about the infant death rate to arrive at estimates of births, we secured the values reported in Table 5.3. As the reader can see from a comparison of the estimates for 1879 and 1925, the Hutterite index of marital fertility I_g (and the approximation to the Coale–Trussell index of natural fertility M) rose sharply both in the prefecture as a whole and in each of the counties (*gun*) that made up the prefecture. Also, the Hutterite index of nuptiality fell. In addition, the result of this rise in marital fertility and fall in proportions married was an *increase* in I_f, the index of overall fertility. This is consistent with what Yasukawa and Hirooka (1974) found on the national level and with the demography of the model used here. In short, Table 5.3 offers useful support for the framework of the model.

The findings presented in Table 5.3 can be bolstered with evidence for the prefectures that, although not as solid as the census data, is probably superior to the *koseki* figures. Beginning in early Meiji, the police were instructed to make annual enumerations of the households and individual members who resided in their jurisdiction. In 1908 and 1913 the government published tabulations of these data for each prefecture. Thus we were able to secure Hutterite indices and the Coale–Trussell parameters of natural fertility M from these data for 1908, which was at the close of the Meiji era (see Mosk, 1979b, 1980a). In Table 5.4 we present these estimates for 1908 and 1925 for the predominantly agricultural prefectures of Japan (classified as such on the basis of the 1930 census), so that we can compare the late Meiji situation with that obtaining in the early interwar period when the fertility transition was commencing. Only two of these measures require explanation here: the stillbirth rate (SBR) is defined as the stillbirths per 1000 live births and the percentage childless (CL) is defined as the percentage of women married 20 years or over who had no children as of 1970.[12]

The findings reported in Table 5.4 are useful. They indicate that a pronounced rise in natural fertility took place between 1908 and 1925, as well as a concomitant drop in infant mortality. With minor exceptions, the proportion married I_m drops in tandem with the observed trends in natural fertility and infant mortality. Moreover, the natural rate of increase of this population tends to be enhanced by this process of adjustment of nuptiality to the capacity of producing surviving offspring (although to the extent that concomitant improvements in income encourage farmers to reduce their reliance on a pure demographic strategy and substitute hired labor for family labor, permitting dowries and the age at which women marry to drift even further upward than the demographic strategy would suggest, the increase in population growth rates may be muted).

To summarize: The scanty evidence for Meiji that is sufficiently solid to merit serious discussion tends to support the theoretical perspective we have laid out. Although nothing conclusive can be said on the basis of this data, it (together with the figures presented previously for the Tokugawa era) does appear to support the argument we have laid out in Chapter 2 concerning the demographic adjustment mechanism—nuptiality responding to changes in infant mortality, natural fertility, and the level of per capita income. Now let us direct our attention to the data available after 1920, which is of sufficient quality to permit detailed statistical analysis.

5.5. The Structure of the Premodern Demographic Regime and Its Disappearance: The Prefectures of Japan, 1925–1960

In this section, data for the prefectures of Japan for the years 1925, 1930, 1950, and 1960 are used to test, using regression techniques, whether models of the sort described by eq. (5.2) are consistent with the data. To carry out these statistical explorations, an extensive data set for the Japanese prefectures has been assembled, which is briefly described in Appendix 3. Serious analysis is therefore confined to the cross-sections beginning with 1925 because this is the first year for which we have prefectural figures on age-specific births with which we can compute the Coale–Trussell parameters. This limitation on the data necessarily raises the question as to whether we are restricted to a period that is too late, in the sense that the fertility transition was already well underway by 1925. This certainly is an issue, but it is not nearly as serious as one might anticipate. Consider Table 5.5. This table gives us the principal measures of marital fertility that we have utilized in this study, for groups of the prefectures classified by the proportion of occupied males working in primary production in 1930.[13] The crucial points to be derived from these figures and the data for individual prefectures on which they are based are: (1) the index of parity-specific control m is not significantly greater than .2 (the cut-off value Coale and Trussell suggest that indicates the onset of parity-specific control) for more than a handful of prefectures in 1925; (2), the largest values of m do not appear in the figures for the industrial prefectures but rather in the data for the predominantly agricultural prefectures (in particular, for Tottori, Okayama, and Kōchi); the average for the group with *PPIM* falling between 55 and 60 percent being .26. We shall come back to this issue in Chapter 7 and suggest some

TABLE 5.5

Means and Standard Deviations for Measures of Marital Fertility for Groups of the Prefectures, 1920–1925, Defined in Terms of Percentage Occupied Male Labor Force in Primary Industry (*PPIM*) in 1930[a]

	Hutterite index I_g		Coale–Trussell indices	
Group	1920	1925	M	m
$PPIM \leq 29.9\%$	.53	.47	.66	.23
	(.04)	(.06)	(.03)	(.16)
$30\% \leq PPIM \leq 49.9\%$	.59	.54	.73	.25
	(.04)	(.04)	(.04)	(.08)
$50\% \leq PPIM \leq 54.9\%$	.62	.59	.78	.24
	(.03)	(.03)	(.05)	(.08)
$55\% \leq PPIM \leq 59.9\%$	.61	.59	.78	.26
	(.06)	(.06)	(.07)	(.13)
$60\% \leq PPIM$	.61	.59	.77	.23
	(.06)	(.05)	(.05)	(.08)

[a] Standard deviation is in parenthesis below the mean of the variable.

qualifications to this statement, but it is worth making note of here. Thus we are probably safe in assuming an analysis of the relationships that emerge in the 1925–1930 data captures relatively well the closing period of the pure premodern demographic regime in Japan (i.e., the period prior to the fertility transition), although, as we shall show, the basic structure of the Japanese premodern demographic regime persists down through the 1950s.

Before we begin to discuss the regressions that relate nuptiality to infant mortality, natural fertility, and other variables, it is useful to consider the variability in nuptiality patterns across the prefectures in 1925. This is done in Table 5.6, again using 1930 census figures to classify the prefectures by type. Two points deserve mention regarding this table and the raw data on which this table is based. First, although the proportions married (I_m) are relatively low in the five most industrial prefectures (Tokyo, Kanagawa, Kyōto, Ōsaka, and Fukuoka) and the singulate mean ages at marriage of females (*SMAMF*) comparatively old, the industrial districts are not alone in having these characteristics. Consider Kagoshima, one of the most agricultural prefectures in Japan in 1930, it has one of the lowest values of I_m and one of the highest values for the singulate mean age at marriage of females. Also Shiga, Gumma, Saitama, Yamanashi, and Nagano prefectures, all relatively agricultural, have comparatively low values of I_m and high values of *SMAMF*. Indeed, what is striking about the data reported in Table 5.6 is, first, the great diversity of nuptiality patterns *within* each of the

TABLE 5.6

Means and Standard Deviations for Measures of Nuptiality for Groups of the Prefectures, 1920–1925, Defined in Terms of Percentage Occupied Male Labor Force in Primary Industry (*PPIM*) in 1930[a]

	Hutterite index, I_m		Singulate mean age at marriage			Age gap at marriage at exact age of wife, 1920	
			SMAMF		*SMAMM*		
Group	1920	1925	1920	1925	1925	Age 20	Age 25
PPIM ≤ 2.9.%	.66	.68	21.8	21.7	26.1	3.1	4.4
	(.02)	(.03)	(.5)	(.4)	(.6)	(.3)	(.4)
30% ≤ *PPIM* ≤ 49.9%	.72	.72	20.7	20.7	25.0	3.5	4.9
	(.03)	(.03)	(.6)	(.6)	(.4)	(.8)	(.6)
50% ≤ *PPIM* ≤ 54.9%	.70	.71	21.0	21.0	24.8	3.2	4.7
	(.05)	(.04)	(1.1)	(1.0)	(.8)	(1.2)	(1.1)
55% ≤ *PPIM* ≤ 59.9%	.70	.70	21.3	21.3	24.4	2.3	3.8
	(.04)	(.04)	(1.1)	(1.1)	(.8)	(.6)	(.7)
60% ≤ *PPIM*	.74	.74	20.0	20.2	23.7	2.9	4.2
	(.04)	(.04)	(1.1)	(1.0)	(.6)	(.8)	(.6)

[a] Standard deviation is in parenthesis below the mean of the variable.

classification groups as opposed to variation between the groups; for example, the singulate mean age at marriage of females in the most agricultural group of prefectures ranges between 18.6 and 21.7 in 1920 (see the standard deviations). In short, a model that attempts to account for the rise in the mean age of marriage in terms of industrialization or urbanization will not be of help here. Second, the ages at which males wed are associated—but apparently not in a tight fashion—with the ages at which females wed. This point, which can be seen from a perusal of the figures on the singulate mean age at marriage of males and females in 1925, or more strikingly perhaps in the estimates of the age gap at marriage, is worth emphasizing because it bears on the contention that the factors determining male nuptiality are to some extent different from those shaping marriage patterns for women.

One last preliminary observation concerning the areal variations in nuptiality and marital fertility is useful to make before plunging into the analytical discussion. That concerns the regional clustering of nuptiality customs and levels of (natural) marital fertility (and infant mortality), due largely to the regionality of environmental conditions that surrounded the development of agriculture. (See Appendix 1 for a discussion of the regions). The diffusion of high productivity techniques in Meiji agriculture was not uniform across regions, partly because differences in soil, the length of the

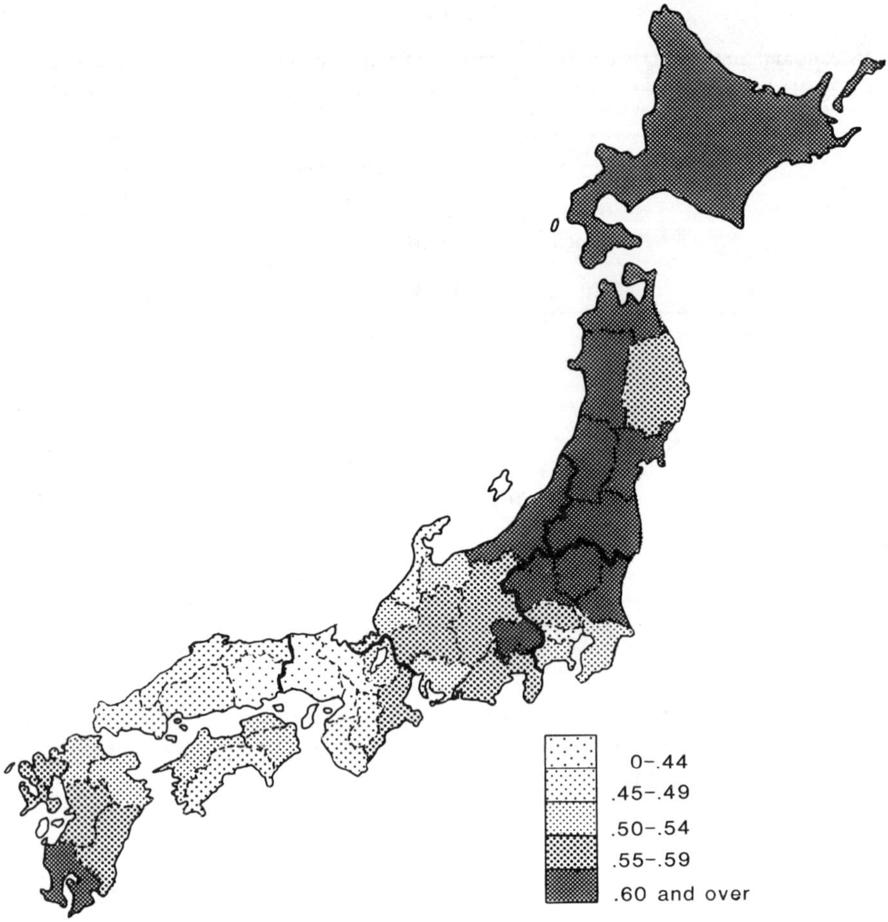

Fig. 5.2. I_g, 1930 Japan.

growing season, the harshness of the winter, and propinquity to industrial zones was not uniform. Seed varieties conducive to enhancements of production in Kinki were not necessarily useful in Tōhoku and Kyūshū. Thus improvements in the standard of living, as well as levels of infant mortality and natural fertility, tended to be regionally concentrated. This is reflected in the farm family household statistics displayed in Table 4.8. It is also reflected in the regionality of the demographic patterns just stated, a point that is documented statistically in Mosk (1978b) and visually in Fig. 5.2 and 5.3. The point is, however, that the regional concentration is explicable in terms of considerations the model takes into account, and we need not fall

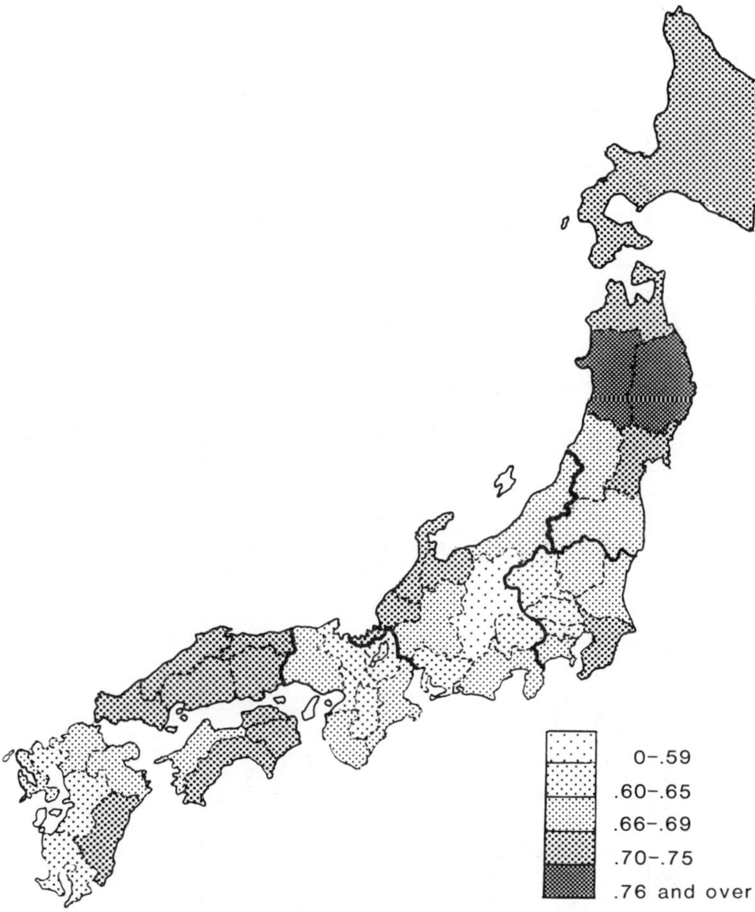

Fig. 5.3. I_m, 1930 Japan.

back onto a vague notion of unspecified "cultural" factors to make them comprehensible.

With this preliminary discussion completed, we can turn to the analytical discussion of the hypothesis, commencing our endeavors with Table 5.7. This table provides us with means and standard deviations for the principal variables utilized in the regressions for 1925, 1930, 1950, and 1960. These figures should be of use to the reader in evaluating questions of the magnitude of the impact of given variables and the like. We shall use some of them in the discussion that follows.

Our analytical work focuses around Table 5.8, with which we attempt to capture the structure of the premodern demographic regime in Japan.[14] We

TABLE 5.7

Means and Standard Deviations for Variables on the Prefectures of Japan, 1925–1960

Variable	1925 Mean	1925 Standard deviation	1930 Mean	1930 Standard deviation	1950 Mean	1950 Standard deviation	1960 Mean	1960 Standard deviation
Singulate mean age at marriage: females (*SMAMF*)	20.93	.97	21.57	.94	23.37	.78	24.67	.76
Coale–Trussell M	.75	.07	.73	.07	.88	.04	.91	.04
Coale–Trussell m	.25	.10	.27	.10	.82	.19	2.27	.33
Hutterite index I_g	.56	.06	.55	.07	.50	.06	.29	.03
Life expectancy of males aged 42 (*ALEM*)	23.79	1.09	24.37	1.07	28.99	.84	30.70	.89
Infant mortality rate (*IMR*)	143.1	23.8	127.3	20.2	62.8	11.3	33.3	5.8
Proportion males in primary industry (*PPIM*)	n.e.[a]	n.e.	.51	.14	.46	.14	.33	.12
Female employment ratio (E_f)	.36	.10	.38	.08	.34	.07	.51	.10
Female–Male wage differential (*FMWD*)	n.e.	n.e.	.49	.09	.61	.08	.61	.09
Real male wages (*RWM*)	n.e.	n.e.	2.20	.55	2.90	.62	3.38	.85
Real female wages (*RWF*)	n.e.	n.e.	1.04	.16	1.74	.21	2.00	.26

[a] n.e. = not estimated.

TABLE 5.8

The Structure and Disappearance of the Premodern Demographic Regime in Japan: The Prefectures of Japan

Year	Dependent variable	Constant	Independent variables: Demographic variables: Coale–Trussell parameters M	m	Hutterite index I_g	Infant mortality rate *IMR*	Life expectancy for males, aged 42 *ALEM*	Structural variables: Proportion males in primary industry[a] *PPIM*	Density D	Sex ratio *SR*	Labor force variables: Female employment ratio E_f[b]	Female–Male wage differential *FMWD*	Real male wages *RWM*[c]	R^2	Adjusted R^2
[1] 1925	*SMAMF*	16.3[e]	10.4[d]	1.1	n.e.	−.02[d]	−.01	−3.3	.3	−5.6[d]	1.4	3.9[e]	1.4[e]	.68	.59
[2] 1925	*SMAMF*	19.9[d]	n.e.[g]	n.e.	3.4	−.02[e]	.04	−4.7	−.02	−5.7[d]	3.3[e]	4.4[e]	1.4[f]	.55	.44
[3] 1930	*SMAMF*	23.7[d]	6.6[d]	.7	n.e.	−.02[d]	−.08	−3.8[e]	.01	−2.1	3.4[e]	1.2	1.1	.75	.68
[4] 1930	*SMAMF*	27.6[d]	n.e.	n.e.	3.3[f]	−.03[d]	−.12	−2.8[f]	−.2	−2.1	4.7[e]	1.5	1.2	.71	.64
[5] 1950	*SMAMF*	24.5[d]	7.8[d]	−.06	n.e.	−.04[d]	−.04	−2.7	n.e.	−4.5[f]	−1.0	2.2	.9	.68	.60
[6] 1950	*SMAMF*	33.8[d]	n.e.	n.e.	1.5	−.06[d]	−.11	−2.8	n.e.	−5.8[f]	−1.8	4.2[e]	1.1	.57	.47
[7] 1960	*SMAMF*	17.1[d]	3.9[d]	−.8[e]	n.e.	−.03	.18	−2.4	n.e.	−.3	−1.8	2.5[f]	1.2	.52	.40
[8] 1960	*SMAMF*	19.4[d]	n.e.	n.e.	6.7[f]	−.06[e]	.13	−1.1	n.e.	−.4	−1.2	2.4	2.1	.42	.30

[a] In the case of 1925 this refers to the proportion of occupied males engaged in agriculture (in 1920). Possible problems involving effects due to multicollinearity can be seen from the following correlations of variables with *PPIM* in 1930: *PPIM* and M: +.62; *PPIM* and I_g: +.59; *PPIM* and E_f: −.47. The correlation between *IMR* and *ALEM* in 1930 is −.32.

[b] The values in the 1925 regression are for 1930.

[c] Estimated nominal daily wages for males in 1930 deflated by a price index with all urban prices in Japan in 1950–1951 = 100. See Appendix 3.

[d] Significant at the 1 percent level. (All are one-tailed tests except for the test on *PPIM* and *RWM*, which are two-tailed tests.)

[e] Significant at the 5 percent level.

[f] Significant at the 10 percent level.

[g] n.e.: Not entered as an independent variable in the regression.

TABLE 5.9

Variables Utilized in the Quantitative Analysis of the Premodern Demographic Regime in Japan and Their Interpretation

Variable	Expected sign	Rationale for expectation about sign
M (Coale–Trussell index of natural fertility	Positive	Model of premodern demographic regime (see Section 5.2)
m (Coale–Trussell index of parity-specific control)	Negative	Efficiency of control over reproduction (see Section 2.6)
I_g (Hutterite Index of Marital Fertility)	Positive	See previous discussion of *M* and *m*.
IMR (Infant Mortality Rate)	Negative	Model of premodern demographic regime (see Section 5.2)
ALEM (Life Expectancy Rate for Males Aged 42)	Positive	The higher *ALEM* is the patriarchs will die (or retire) later. The theory in Section 2.3 suggests that *ALEM* should be positively associated with the *SMAMF*.
PPIM (Proportion Males in Primary Industry)	No a priori expectation	Proxy for degree of patriarchal control. Pure effect is unclear.
D (Density)	Positive	The higher *D* is the harder it is for noninheriting males to find positions in peasant farming. If there is some direct relationship between male and female ages at marriage (not specified in the simple version of the model given in Chapter 2) it may appear here.
SR (Sex ratio: males 15–29 divided by females 15–29)	Negative	Relative availability of potential spouse in marriage market
E_f (Female Employment Ratio)	Positive	Relative availability of jobs outside of primary production
FMWD (Female–Male Wage Differential: Female Wages Divided by Male Wages)	Positive	Relative value of female labor as compared with male labor. The greater the *FMWD* is the more valuable an unmarried daughter is to the patriarch.
RWM (Real Male Wages)	No a priori expectation	Proxy for income per capita (a factor expected to undermine the premodern demographic regime).

shall also use these results to say something about structural breaks, that is, about the timing of the disappearance of the premodern demographic regime in Japan, although we shall go into this issue concerning timing in greater detail in the next section. Before we review the empirical results, something must be said about the precise functional forms examined here. In Table 5.8 we present two variants of the regression for each year: one utilizes I_g as a measure of marital fertility and—for 1925 and 1930 at any rate—also as a proxy for natural fertility; the other variant utilizes the direct estimate of natural fertility, the Coale–Trussell index M, and also includes the index m. As noted in Appendix 7, there are a number of special problems in measuring m and M, and so the use of I_g may seem preferable. However, for Japan the fits of the Coale–Trussell model are sufficiently good that M and m are measured very well. Moreover, I_g is not a good measure of natural fertility once parity-specific control becomes significantly diffused throughout a population. So for these reasons we wish to direct the reader's attention particularly to the regressions having M and m in them. The specifications employed are simple linear expressions with the singulate mean age of marriage for females *SMAMF* as the principal dependent variable and a group of independent variables whose expected coefficients are given in Table 5.9. With this preliminary discussion completed, let us turn to the results revealed in the Table 5.8.

First, let us consider the major life-cycle variables and their interrelationship: *SMAMF* (nuptiality), M (natural fertility), and *IMR* (infant mortality). Table 5.8 suggests that up through 1950 there was a structural relationship that accords with the a priori hypotheses laid out previously, and that this appears to have weakened considerably between 1950 and 1960 (the coefficient on M for 1960 is considerably smaller than it is for 1925–1950, and the coefficient on the *IMR* is not significant in 1960). Life expectancy for adult males is not significant in the regression (nor is density). The labor force variables (female employment ratio, male–female wage differentials) have the expected signs when they are significant, suggesting perhaps that market forces were cutting into the operation of the demographic adjustment mechanism. Finally, the measures of labor force structure (*PPIM*) and standard of living (*RWM*) appear to be significant in only a few cases.[15] The implication of the combined force of these two variables is as follows: as economic development takes place in Japan, in the twin senses of industrialization and a rise in per capita income, the age at marriage for females is enhanced; that is, this tendency reinforces the mechanism associated with the demographic adjustment mechanism (M rising and *IMR* falling) and, consequently, the *SMAMF* increases as development occurs. In interpreting these results, however, we must keep in mind that interprefectural migration (whose impact is not directly estimated in the equations because of data

TABLE 5.10

β Coefficients and Elasticities for Selected Variables from Regressions for 1925, 1930, and 1950 in Table 5.8

Year and equation number	Variables					
	Coale–Trussell M		Infant mortality rate, IMR		Female employment ratio, E_f	
	β	Elasticity	β	Elasticity	β	Elasticity
[1] 1925	.70	.38	−.39	−.11	.16	.03
[3] 1930	.48	.22	−.50	−.14	.29	.06
[5] 1950	.44	.29	−.58	−.11	−.09	−.01

limitations) may be a factor in producing the particular results we have secured from Table 5.8, although, presumably, the variables representing the female employment ratio and the sex ratio capture most of its impact.

It is useful to extend our discussion of Table 5.8 by assessing the magnitude—the social importance—of the major effects pinpointed by Table 5.8. Table 5.10 helps us to do this for the three most prominent variables in the regression M, IMR, and E_f using β coefficients and elasticities. First, note that the elasticity on M is quite substantial in absolute value. Second, note that the elasticity on the IMR is not particularly great in absolute value but that, because the infant mortality rate fell dramatically in percentage terms from 1920 to 1960, the implied impact of the decline of infant mortality in raising the mean age at first marriage for females over the period 1920–1960 is considerable. The β coefficients also suggest that M and IMR are of considerable import in terms of the magnitude of their effects. For example, the standard deviations of the infant mortality rate are relatively large in these samples compared with the means of this variable. This, combined with the β coefficients, suggests that infant mortality is a major shaper of nuptiality patterns in the samples for 1925, 1930, and 1950.

This completes our initial examination of the basic structural equation for the premodern demographic regime in Japan. Now we wish to turn to a more systematic study of the structural break, i.e., to the question of when the ending of the premodern demographic regime occurred.

5.6. The Timing of the Structural Break in Japan

In this section we utilize some standard methods of econometrics to statistically examine the question of when the premodern demographic regime ended. Elsewhere in this book we have argued that we can date this break to the period of the 1950s. Some simple statistical tests discussed here suggest that this is indeed a reasonable interpretation.

The method we utilize involves pooling the four cross sections examined in Table 5.8. Step one, on the pooled data set (consisting of 184 observations) we estimate the structural equation of Table 5.8. Step two, then we reestimate the structural equation on the pooled data set with the addition of three dummy variables representing the years other than 1925—one for 1930, one for 1950, and one for 1960. With this second regression, in effect we let each year have its own intercept term but imposed no further restrictions. Step three, we carry out a third estimation of the structural equation with the addition of the three dummy variables marking the years and an extra twelve variables—three for the interaction of M (natural fertility) with the three dummy time variables; three for the interaction of IMR (infant mortality) with the three dummy time variables; three for the interaction of E_f (female employment ratio) with the three dummy time variables; and three for the interaction of RWM (real male wages) with the three dummy time variables. In this third specification we allow each of the four variables M, IMR, E_f, and RWM to take on different coefficient values for the four different years.

We report the results for the third specification in Table 5.11. In comparing Table 5.11 with Table 5.8, it should be noted that all variables were excluded that lacked data for all four years. The coefficients for 1930, 1950, and 1960 represent the *differences* between the estimated parameter values for 1925 (the base year) and 1930, 1950, and 1960, respectively. Standard significance coefficients are attached to these parameter estimates.

Standard F statistics were calculated to see whether there was a significant difference in the results as one moved from a totally unrestricted pooled regression (Step 1) to a regression with time dummies (Step 2) and finally to a regression with time dummies and interaction terms (Step 3). An F test that tested for the joint significance of the introduction of the three time dummies yielded $F^{3}_{171} = 5.4$, significant at the 1 percent level; an F test that tested for the joint significance of the introduction of the twelve interaction variables yielded $F^{12}_{159} = 2.7$, significant at the 1 percent level. Finally, an F test that tested for the simultaneous introduction of the three time dummies and the twelve interaction variables yielded $F^{15}_{159} = 3.5$, significant at the 1 percent level. So the F tests do suggest that there was some structural break between 1925 and 1960, with reference in particular to the two life-cycle variables M and IMR and the two labor variables E_f and RWM.

Examination of the results for individual coefficients in Table 5.11 bears out this contention. The findings suggest two breaks: a partial break between 1930 and 1950 and a more sweeping break between 1950 and 1960. Because

TABLE 5.11

Results for Pooled Time-Series–Cross section Regressions of the Form Used in Table 5.8, in Which There Is an Intercept for Each Year and *M*, *IMR*, E_f and *RWM* Are Allowed to Interact with the Dummy Variable for Each Year

			Independent variables[a]								
			Demographic variables				Structural variables			Labor force variables	
Year	Dependent variable	Constant for 1925; difference between 1925 value and value for other years for 1930, 1950 and 1960	Coale–Trussell parameters *M*	Coale–Trussell parameters *m*	Infant mortality rate *IMR*	Life expectancy for males, aged 42 *ALEM*	Proportion males in primary industry *PPIM*	Sex ratio *SR*	Female employment ratio E_f	Female–Male wage differential *FMWD*	Real male wages *RWM*
1925	*SMAMF*	17.3[c]	7.8[c]	−.4[c]	−.02[c]	.01	−2.9[c]	−2.4[d]	3.1[c]	2.3[c]	.6[d]
1930	*SMAMF*	2.8	−2.1	0[b]	−.004	0[b]	0[b]	0[b]	.5	0[b]	−.2
1950	*SMAMF*	3.5	.1	0[b]	−.02[d]	0[b]	0[b]	0[b]	−3.3[e]	0[b]	−.6[e]
1960	*SMAMF*	9.9[c]	−5.6[d]	0[b]	−.05[d]	0[b]	0[b]	0[b]	−4.2[c]	0[b]	−.5[e]

[a] Coefficients for variables for 1925; differences between coefficient for 1925 and given year for other years. All tests are two-tailed. $R^2 = .91$ and adjusted $R^2 = .89$.

[b] Identically equal to 0 (not estimated).

[c] Significant at the 1% level.

[d] Significant at the 5% level.

[e] Significant at the 10% level.

the four variables M, IMR, E_f and, RWM represent the influences that we have highlighted in the qualitative discussion of a structural break (i.e., of the collapse of the premodern demographic regime in Japan), this evidence does appear to support the general position. The only really anomalous result to emerge here concerns the change in the coefficient on the infant mortality, which *increases* in value between the interwar period and 1960. For this finding we have no satisfactory explanation. It should be emphasized, moreover, that the tests conducted here do reflect the particular specifications chosen for the analysis.

Now we would like to turn to a discussion of the empirical impact of certain variables indicative of social structure on the structure of the premodern demographic regime in Japan.

5.7. Social Status and the Premodern Demographic Regime: The Rural and Urban Districts of Japan, 1925

In this section we attempt to deal empirically with the question as to whether or not the distribution of assets and income (i.e., social structure) affected the operation of the premodern demographic regime in Japan. The foray into these issues is exploratory only, both in the sense of the theoretical model (which does not really incorporate these considerations directly into it) and in terms of the empirical analysis we are able to conduct. Although the treatment is necessarily constrained by the limited amount of relevant data available, some progress can be made in addressing these issues. As it turns out, the most fruitful approach discovered involves separate treatment of the rural and urban sectors of the Japanese prefectures and, in particular, analysis of figures for individual counties (*gun*) and cities (*shi*) that make up the rural and urban sectors, respectively, of the prefectures.[16] In addition, these data help us to explore further the question of how much impact modernization was having on the operation of the patriarchal stem family system. Let us commence our discussion with some comparative results for the rural areas, which will put the subsequent analysis into perspective.

To begin, let us consider the nuptiality and marital fertility of the rural sectors of the prefectures relative to that obtaining in the urban sectors of the prefectures. This is done in Table 5.12, which provides us with averages for groups of the prefectures defined in terms of the structure of their labor force. These data, and the raw figures on which they are based, clearly show that (1) average marital fertility for the rural districts of Japan was greater than that for the urban districts and (2) both males and females tended to marry at slightly higher ages in the rural districts than in the urban areas. But

TABLE 5.12

Means and Standard Deviations for Measures of Marital Fertility and Nuptiality for the Rural and Urban Sectors of the Prefectures and the Urban to Rural Relatives, 1925, for Groups of the Prefectures Defined in Terms of Percentage Occupied Male Labor Force in Primary Industry (*PPIM*) in 1930[a]

	Marital fertility			Nuptiality				
	Hutterite index I_g		Urban I_g divided by rural I_g	Hutterite index I_m		Urban I_m divided by rural I_m	Difference between singulate mean age at marriage in urban and rural areas	
Group	Rural	Urban		Rural	Urban		Males	Females
PPIM ≤ 29.9%	.52	.41	.80	.70	.66	.94	.97	.43
	(.06)	(.04)	(.10)	(.02)	(.05)	(.09)	(.30)	(.78)
30% ≤ *PPIM* ≤ 49.9%	.57	.43	.75	.73	.66	.90	.97	1.02
	(.04)	(.05)	(.04)	(.03)	(.03)	(.03)	(.47)	(.35)
50% ≤ *PPIM* ≤ 54.9%	.60	.47	.78	.72	.61	.85	.84	1.28
	(.03)	(.02)	(.04)	(.04)	(.05)	(.06)	(.54)	(.38)
55% ≤ *PPIM* ≤ 59.9%	.60	.48	.80	.71	.60	.85	1.24	1.26
	(.07)	(.07)	(.08)	(.05)	(.02)	(.05)	(.63)	(.58)
60% ≤ *PPIM*	.60	.49	.82	.76	.61	.80	1.96	2.09
	(.05)	(.07)	(.08)	(.04)	(.04)	(.02)	(.56)	(.36)

[a] The standard deviation is in parenthesis below the mean of the variable.

having recognized this point—and we shall come back to this again in discussing the relatives for urban areas—and although these conclusions do follow, the most impressive fact to emerge from a perusal of Table 5.12 is the closeness of the averages for the rural and urban sectors of the same prefecture. That is, the impression given by Table 5.12 is of a high correlation between the rural and urban averages for these demographic variables.[17] Given the marked variability of nuptiality and marital fertility between the prefectures as noted in Table 5.12 and Tables 5.5 and 5.6, this suggests that the marriage markets in rural and urban sectors of each prefecture were closely linked. For instance, one such linkage would develop if male migrants from rural areas moved to cities close by in search of employment, worked a while to build a secure economic foundation for marriage, and then married a woman hailing from the region from which he had moved. Given the patriarch's role in the arrangement of marriages, that is, the importance of family connections, this would stand to reason. Although this does not bear very heavily on the analysis of the premodern demographic regime in rural districts, it is important in explaining the urban patterns (their connection with the rural patterns), and so it is useful to make note of these points here.

The core of the discussion of rural and urban districts is contained in Table 5.13. The table provides various separate estimates (specifications) of the structure of the premodern demographic regime for various subgroups of the approximately 500 *gun* (counties) of interwar Japan and for the cities (*shi*).[18] The reader should not, referring to Appendix 4, that m is estimated for individual *gun* and *shi* under assumptions about M in these areal units and is, perhaps, not a very accurate estimation. Thus the equations involving the Hutterite index I_g are preferable for drawing inferences. The following two variables, the proportion of arable land owned (*PCHO*) and the proportion of occupied women in domestic service (*PDSFO*), are the variables we wish to put special attention on in assessing the importance of social structure. It is reasonable to infer that the degree of land ownership measures the prevalence of socially subordinate tenants (who are relatively lacking in capital assets), and the proportion of occupied women in domestic service (crudely) measures both the extent to which income and wealth are skewed and the average level of income per head, poorer families giving over their daughters into service for wealthier families. It is these proxy variables, albeit flawed, that aid us in evaluating the role of social structure.

As the reader can gather from Table 5.13, the demographic life-cycle mechanism (involving nuptiality, natural fertility, and infant mortality) is clearly revealed in the data for those rural areas in which agriculture is the main source of livelihood and/or tenancy is relatively uncommon. Where tenancy is prevalent, the life-cycle mechanism seems to be of less impor-

TABLE 5.13

Social and Economic Structure and the Premodern Demographic Regime: Regressions of Measures of Female Nuptiality on a Number of Variables for Groupings of *Gun* (Counties) and *Shi* (Cities) in Japan, 1925[a]

				Independent variables									
Data set	Number of observations	Dependent variables	Constant	Coale–Trussell index of parity-specific control m	Hutterite index of marital fertility I_g	Percent occupied women in domestic service *PDSFO*	Sex ratio *SR*	Infant mortality rate *IMR*	Density *D*	Female employment index E_f	Percent male labor force in primary industry *PPMI*	Percent cultivated land owned *PCHO*	R^2
All *gun*	546	I_m	.655[c]	Ex.[b]	−.176[c]	−.140[d]	.134[c]	.0006[c]	−.0005	−.249[c]	.048[d]	−.007	.510
			(337.591)		(42.616)	(4.063)	(74.986)	(75.315)	(.184)	(105.674)	(3.745)	(.178)	
Agricultural *gun*	122	I_m	.595[c]	Ex.	−.139[c]	.446	.178[c]	.0008[c]	−.004	−.313[c]	.009	.001	.439
			(23.856)		(6.006)	(2.572)	(12.728)	(31.575)	(.926)	(12.954)	(.005)	(.001)	
gun with $m \leq .4$	475	I_m	.678[c]	Ex.	−.199[c]	−.165[d]	.132[c]	.0007[c]	−.002	−.265[c]	.030	.004	.532
			(301.745)		(42.292)	(3.895)	(62.114)	(86.614)	(1.775)	(101.918)	(1.131)	(.049)	
Agricultural *gun*	122	I_m	.528[c]	.032[d]	Ex.	.376	.187[c]	.0009[c]	−.002	−.367[c]	−.038	.016	.427
			(19.157)	(3.332)		(1.821)	(13.861)	(31.557)	(.138)	(17.135)	(.087)	(.239)	
Agricultural *gun* with $PCHO \geq .54$	72	I_m	.357[d]	.023	Ex.	.201	.222[c]	.001[c]	.0000	−.266[d]	.107	Ex.	.476
			(5.593)	(1.081)		(.265)	(11.238)	(29.708)	(.0000)	(5.445)	(.419)		

Agricultural *gun* with $PCHO < .54$	50	I_m	.992[c]	.064[d]	Ex.	.451	.071	.0003	.002	−.618[c]	−.363	Ex.	.427
			(23.815)	(5.355)		(.690)	(.690)	(1.174)	(.405)	(17.632)	(2.905)		
Cities (*shi*)	98	I_m	.620[c]	.029[d]	Ex.	−.217[d]	.117[c]	.00001	.0000	−.218[c]	.173	−.049	.498
			(97.519)	(3.332)		(4.257)	(32.525)	(.003)	(.188)	(16.828)	(2.433)	(1.185)	
All *gun*	546	*SMAMF*	20.104[c]	Ex.	4.726[c]	2.251	−1.327[c]	−.016[c]	.012	5.000[c]	−.768	.443	.418
			(567.193)		(55.024)	(1.885)	(13.069)	(88.619)	(.185)	(75.807)	(1.683)	(1.325)	
gun with $m \leq .4$	475	*SMAMF*	19.346[c]	Ex.	5.010[c]	3.149	−1.258[c]	−.018[c]	.051	5.860[c]	−.045	.209	.458
			(419.917)		(46.240)	(2.434)	(9.712)	(94.928)	(2.469)	(85.117)	(.004)	(.257)	
Agricultural *gun*	122	*SMAMF*	20.819[c]	Ex.	3.297[d]	−17.833[c]	−1.125	−.020[c]	.057	10.073[c]	−.472	.027	.428
			(43.092)		(5.014)	(6.062)	(.747)	(26.636)	(.251)	(19.788)	(.020)	(.0009)	
Agricultural *gun*	122	*SMAMF*	22.403[c]	−.647	Ex.	−15.663[d]	−1.373	−.020[c]	.702	11.261[c]	.718	−.342	.413
			(50.810)	(2.041)		(4.651)	(1.098)	(26.883)	(.331)	(23.738)	(.046)	(.156)	
Agricultural *gun* with $PCHO \geq .54$	72	*SMAMF*	28.171[c]	−.291	Ex.	11.435	−1.586	−.025[c]	−.785	7.526[c]	−5.359	Ex.	.466
			(58.376)	(.260)		(1.437)	(.968)	(28.486)	(.315)	(7.313)	(1.781)		
Agricultural *gun* with $PCHO < .54$	50	*SMAMF*	8.243	−1.731[d]	Ex.	−18.051	.281	−.008	−.014	19.287[c]	13.652[d]	Ex.	.473
			(2.148)	(5.103)		(2.273)	(.014)	(1.022)	(.004)	(22.441)	(5.374)		
Cities (*shi*)	98	*SMAMF*	22.573[c]	−.529[d]	Ex.	3.218[d]	−1.416[c]	−.005	−.0000	2.619[c]	−2.373	Ex.	.372
			(491.745)	(4.153)		(3.556)	(18.140)	(2.230)	(.168)	(9.203)	(1.742)		

[a] F statistics given in parenthesis below coefficient estimate.
[b] Ex.: excluded from regression.
[c] Significant at the 1% level (two-tailed test).
[d] Significant at the 5% level (two-tailed test).

tance, although this inference is admittedly based on a very tight, and perhaps somewhat exaggerated, interpretation of the relatively small differences between the equations. However, the statistical significance of the variable involving female domestic servants suggests somewhat more forcefully that social structure makes a difference. In the equations involving I_m as a dependent variable, the coefficient on the domestic servant variable is negative—when it is significant—implying that a high standard of living and/or a relatively skewed distribution of assets and income encourages later marriage. The results involving the singulate mean age at marriage tend to run against this interpretation, however; only in the instance of the *shi* (city) data are the two coefficients (in the equations involving I_m and *SMAMF*) both consistent in sign and significant. But in the urban districts it is plausible to assume that the domestic service variable is a proxy for the standard of living because many of the domestic servants migrated into the cities from the countryside to work in the homes of the wealthy.[19] In any event, the thrust of the tentative findings, on the one hand, is that social structure per se does not appear to have played a *major* role in modifying the dependence of populations on the life-cycle strategy. On the other hand, the results also suggest that in cities the life-cycle strategy was of little importance; income, female job opportunities, and the associated sex ratio dominated the picture. This suggests dowry (and perhaps, in some districts, education as well) was assuming paramount importance in the arrangement of marriages.

Now let us return to Table 5.12 and examine the extent of the rural–urban differentials in marital fertility, comparing them with differentials in nuptiality. As can be gleaned from the table, the differentials in marital fertility are far greater than differentials in nuptiality customs. This confirms the previous deductions we have made concerning the marriage market, namely, arrangements tended to be forged by patriarchs on the basis of family connections, and because a substantial proportion of the male urban dwellers hewed from the rural districts, so did their brides. Given the relevant life-cycle considerations of the rural farming family, we would expect patriarchs to actively engage in the arranging of marriages for their daughters when they were approximately the same age, regardless of whether the daughter was to go into a rural household or an urban household. Presumably the patriarch would tend to arrange the matches of his younger daughters to farming families, who favored the bride's youth over dowry, and of older daughters to men who lived in the cities and were principally concerned (along with their fathers) with dowry.[20] The relatively small differential in nuptiality customs between rural and urban districts of the same prefecture testifies to the influence of the rhythm of the agricultural village's life cycle on nearby city populations. However, as we have already argued, the life-cycle strategy was of little consequence to most urban families — particularly to houses headed by wage earners — so we would not expect *their* levels of marital fertility and infant mortality (the latter probably a function of the density, water, sewage, and public health conditions peculiar to the city and largely independent of the conditions obtaining in the villages from which brides migrated) to correspond to the nuptiality patterns prevailing among them. This argument will take on added force after we have shown, in Chapter 7, that populations abandoning the life-cycle strategy altogether attempted to reduce overall marital fertility by suppressing natural fertility (M) as well as by engaging in parity-specific control. But the details of this argument should properly be postponed until Chapter 7, which deals with the Japanese fertility transition.

To summarize: In this section we have attempted to explore statistically the role of social structure and to probe further the impact of modernization of labor markets on the premodern demographic regime. The findings are tentative, but they point to a relatively narrow influence of social structure, as contrasted with a more marked impact of labor markets, the structure of employment, and the standard of living.

5.8. Conclusion

In this chapter we have presented a variety of statistical evidence for the Tokugawa, Meiji, Taishō, and Shōwa periods with which we have attempted to document the model of the premodern demographic regime that we have developed. We now wish to consider the Swedish premodern demographic regime to demonstrate that similar forces appear to be operating there.

Notes to Chapter 5

1. From Mosk (1979c:Table 2, p. 47). For an extensive discussion of the estimates of national population statistics for Tokugawa Japan, see Hanley and Yamamura (1977) and Smith (1977). Professor Akira Hayami has pointed out in conversation that the estimates given here exclude the *samurai* class and, in the case of some *han,* children as well. He estimated the total Tokugawa population in 1600 as about 12 million (plus or minus 2 million) and the population around 1770 as 30–32 million.

2. See Smith (1977), Hanley and Yamamura (1977), and Hayami (1968, 1973) for figures concerning other villages.

3. There appears to be one exception to these generalizations about natural fertility: Minami Ōji, an outcaste (*eta*) village studied by Morris and Smith (1979). Unlike Kandō-Shinden, which had a fluctuating value of M (Table 6.1 gives a relatively high value of M for Kandō-Shinden), Minami-Ōji apparently remained relatively high over the period 1758–1869, the time interval Morris and Smith concentrated their analysis on. However, the social and

economic conditions (and perhaps the standard of living and diet) that obtained in Minami Ōji, where farming was not of great importance, were very different from those characterizing the predominantly agrarian villages that are captured in Table 6.1, so the inferences we draw are not contradicted by the Minami Ōji findings. This would be particularly true if the standard of living, and especially the consumption of animal protein, was more substantial in Minami Ōji than in the other villages heretofore analyzed, a possibility that the Morris–Smith discussion does not rule out.

4. Smith (1977), and Hanley and Yamamura (1977) offer different explanations of the patterns pointed to in Table 6.1. Smith argues that the desire to keep the property intact was paramount, so that families employed infanticide as a means of holding down completed household size. Hanley and Yamamura (1977) argue that families attempted to maximize their income and bolster their standard of living by eliminating children through infanticide. For a detailed critique of Smith's interpretation see Mosk (1978a), and for a critique of the Hanley and Yamamura view see Mosk (1979a). In addition to the specific problems raised regarding these authors' interpretations of the Tokugawa data, there is the additional issue of explaining how and why the Meiji population grew as it did. Neither Smith's nor Hanley and Yamamura's interpretation lends itself to an explanation of why this occurred. Inheritance customs did not change; nor, presumably, was there a diminution in the household's desire to "maximize" the household's standard of living. In their theory, Hanley and Yamamura rule out the possibility that a positive income elasticity of demand for children could account for this trend because they argue households *increased* their incomes per head during the later Tokugawa period and simultaneously decreased their fertility. They also appear to accept the official Meiji figures at face value.

5. An interesting question raised by the Tokugawa population figures is why population grew during the seventeenth century before it reached the plateau of the eighteenth and nineteenth centuries. Part of the explanation lies in the age of marriage of men and women; under the joint family system characteristic of early Tokugawa, presumably, men were not constrained by the need to secure an inheritance, as they were in the stem family system that gradually evolved out of the joint system. As the joint family strategy gave way to the stem family pattern, ages at nuptiality (for both sexes) rose, and this reduced fertility somewhat. It is also possible that the standard of living fell during the seventeenth century, bringing natural fertility down and increasing the risks of infant death.

Something should be said at this juncture about another possible interpretation of the relationship between nuptiality, natural fertility, and infant mortality. It is theoretically possible that marital fertility and/or infant mortality adjust to the age at marriage, rather than the reverse. It is impossible to rule out this theory on statistical grounds because statistical tests cannot establish causation. But there are some a priori grounds for suspecting this interpretation. An argument of the sort that explains behavior about birth spacing and infant mortality in terms of the age at marriage would constitute some sort of "target fertility" thesis: the notion is that couples develop a target desired surviving family size once their union is established, and they adjust birth intervals and/or let infant mortality affect survivorship rates to secure (but not substantially exceed) this target. The argument against this view is that this is an unlikely strategy, parity-specific control being a far more efficient means of obtaining a target. Because parity-specific control is eventually adopted in these populations (historically for Europe and Japan in the absence of modern contraceptive devices), it is a fair implication that these populations would have developed a parity-specific control strategy over the centuries prior to the fertility decline if it had been an attractive alternative to the natural fertility strategy.

But why does a parity-specific control strategy make more sense than one based on controlling fertility through choice of marriage age if we suppose that the couple is aiming at a target? First, the older the women are at marriage, the greater is the variance in their completed surviving family sizes. There is probably also a greater risk of temporary or permanent sterility that would lead to a failure in meeting fertility targets. It would certainly make more sense to marry a young woman, discover her capacity for reproduction, and if she is fecund and capable of raising healthy offspring, reach one's desired target relatively early on and then cease bearing children. This is a far less risky strategy. Second, there is the question of what the target is. It is likely that in many cases the target is thought of in terms of a specific sex—say, so many males. Given the demand for males as heirs and potential sources of labor this is surely a reasonable inference. However, a strategy of marrying an older female would make such targets very hard to realize in practice because in a significant number of cases only females would be born at the first several parities. For this reason a strategy of marrying a young woman and stopping after the male target is achieved makes far greater sense.

The second major type of reason for doubting the target fertility hypothesis is that there is little evidence for replacement of deceased infants in observed populations, either historical populaces or ones in the present day. The failure of the replacement hypothesis suggests that either targets are vague or ill-defined and poorly conceived or that most households typically fail to achieve their targets. In short the target fertility view of nuptiality has logical and empirical weaknesses.

6. For a discussion of the *koseki* system and the delays in conducting a national census, see Taeuber (1958).

7. We adjusted all of the data on births for the period 1920–1955 utilizing the census data on infants aged 0 and the *koseki* data on infant deaths. We compared these estimates with the official figures on births to estimate the degree of underregistration of births. From these tabulations it appears that the degree of underregistration of births (and presumably of infant deaths) declined sharply over time, and that by the 1950s there was very little underregistration. We followed Taeuber (1958) in making these adjustments and in some cases actually took these figures from the original worksheets prepared by Taeuber and her colleagues.

8. For a useful discussion of these various estimates, see Ohbuchi (1976).

9. See Mosk (1980a, 1980b). If underregistration and late registration of nuptiality declined over time, as seems likely and is documented by the figures for the period after 1899 concerning delayed registration of marriage, then this method would tend to underestimate the rise in the age at marriage. It should be noted that the Meiji data do not give figures on women who are single, as does the census, for the vital statistics pick up women when they entered the married state as far as nuptiality status is concerned.

10. On illegitimacy during the Meiji period see Hayami (1980) and Mosk (1978c).

11. Nihon Tōkeiin (1882: reprinted 1968). During late Meiji (1908–1910) certain regional and local governments commissioned enumerative censuses. These were the cities of Tokyo, Sapporo, Kobe, and Sado county (*gun*) in Niigata prefecture. In addition there are police count figures for Meiji, which are discussed subsequently. The staff of the documentation section of the Institute of Economic Research at Hitotsubashi University is currently engaged in assembling all of the police count figures for Meiji. Official national publication of tabulations for the prefectures and major cities only occurred in 1908 and 1913. For a discussion of these data see Mosk (1980a).

12. See Mosk (1981a) and Appendix 3. It should be noted that we use the same variable *CL* in the regressions reported in Table 8.4 but there use a different acronym to describe it [i.e., *STER*—the index of permanent sterility].

13. The 1930 census is used throughout this book for the classifications of the prefectures by type in Chapters 5 and 7. The 1920 census data on industrial classification are difficult to use because they fail to distinguish between "occupation" and "industry," and industrial developments during the 1950s tended to reduce only slowly the relative proportions of occupied persons engaged in primary production (i.e., in agriculture, fishing, and forestry) for the

prefectures. That is, as industrialization occurred throughout the period 1920–1960, the tendency was for the population leaving the agricultural districts to work in industry to migrate to the industrial prefectures, so that the declines in proportions dependent on primary industry for the prefectures change gradually over the interwar period and the 1950s. The groups are as follows: (a) *PPIM ≤ 29.9%:* Tokyo, Kanagawa, Kyōto, Ōsaka, and Fukuoka; (b) *30% ≤ PPIM ≤ 49.9%:* Hokkaidō, Ishikawa, Fukui, Shizuoka, Aichi, Hyōgo, Nara, Wakayama, Hiroshima, Yamaguchi, and Nagasaki; (c) *50% ≤ PPIM ≤ 54.9%:* Tochigi, Toyama, Gifu, Mie, Shiga, Kagawa, and Saga; (d) *55 ≤ PPIM ≤ 59.9%:* Miyagi, Fukushima, Gumma, Saitama, Chiba, Niigata, Yamanashi, Nagano, Tottori, Okayama, Tokushima, Ehime, Kōchi, and Kumamoto; (e) *60% ≤ PPIM ≤ 100%:* Aomori, Iwate, Akita, Yamagata, Ibaraki, Shimane, Oita, Miyazaki, and Kagoshima.

14. See Chapter 7 for a discussion concerning the problems of multicollinearity encountered in working with these data.

15. The coefficient on real male wages, the proxy for earning potential of household heads, is always positive but insignificant except for 1925.

16. See Appendix 4 for a discussion of the data concerning the *shi* and *gun.* The data used in the regressions reported in Table 5.13 are primarily for 1925, although some of the figures are for 1929 and 1930 (labor force structure, density, and type of land farmed) and, in the case of the infant mortality rate, for 1938.

17. In this regard see Mosk (1977, 1979a, 1980b) where this is shown. This issue will be picked up again in Chapter 7 in considerable detail.

18. An "agricultural" *gun* is one in which at least 70% of *both* the male and the female occupied labor forces are engaged in primary industry (which was primarily agriculture).

19. It should be noted, however, that the category "domestic servants" in the 1930 Japanese census includes employees in inns and hotels.

20. For males the father's chief effort was devoted to the arrangement of permanent positions as in-adopted sons or employees at the time of the transmission of the headship. He had a secondary commitment of arranging the marriage of each son, but because the primary commitment of the patriarch was job placement, he tended to postpone this until the son had acquired sufficient skill and security at work to warrant the patriarch's active participation in his marriage arrangement. Because the inheriting son usually married soon after he acquired the headship, about the time the other sons were entering jobs, and because urban mean ages exceeded those in rural areas, the cross-prefectural correlation between rural and urban singulate mean ages at marriage is explicable in terms of these considerations. And of course, as noted previously, the relative wages of males and females in the labor market, distortions in the sex ratio, etc., would also affect the equilibrium ages of marriage somewhat.

CHAPTER 6

Comparison with the Premodern Demographic Regime in Sweden

6.1. Introduction

In the previous Chapter we set out a broad range of evidence for Japan that is consistent with the model of the premodern demographic regime in patriarchal stem family peasant societies. However, it is certainly true that the empirical evidence adduced may be consistent with any one of a variety of alternative hypotheses. Although it is never possible definitely to counter this objection, it is possible to provide a useful and stringent check on the interpretation. As we have seen in Chapter 4, the basic assumptions of the model hold for both Japan and Sweden. Thus if Swedish data are also consistent with the model, they will provide strong support for the approach. Although one or several alternative hypotheses might explain both cases (this possibility cannot be ruled out on logical grounds), the procedure we follow considerably reduces the likelihood of this being the case. Moreover, it permits us to explore more deeply the questions raised in Chapter 5 concerning social structure, the standard of living, and the premodern demographic regime. And, finally, it helps us address the question of why there is diversity in fertility transitions, that is, it helps us address the problem raised in the introduction to this book.

The organization of this chapter is as follows: In the next section we briefly explore some evidence for the period 1700–1800. Then we consider a cross-sectional analysis of statistics for the 24 countries of Sweden (excluding Stockholm City), devoting a special section to the question of the dating of the structural break in Sweden. And, finally, we turn to a discussion of social structure. As the reader will see, the figures lend credence to the hypothesis that a demographic life-cycle strategy was operating in preindustrial Sweden and that it disappeared rapidly as modern economic growth commenced. The contrast of this rapid decay in the Swedish premodern demographic regime with the Japanese case will serve to tell us much about the nature of the patriarchal stem family system and its demographic implications.

6.2. The Period 1700–1800

Sweden has one of the oldest systems of population registrars, systematically collecting figures on births, marriages, and deaths from about the middle of the eighteenth century.[1] Originally a responsibility of the clergy, the collection and tabulation of population figures were gradually taken over by professionals in the central statistical offices that were created in the government (the clergy still are responsible for registration of the population, although they no longer tabulate the figures), and by the mid-nineteenth century the Swedish demographic figures are generally considered to be of exceptionally fine quality. Unfortunately, the government did not publish figures on population classified by quinquennial age class and sex until 1870, and thus our statistical knowledge of the details of Swedish nuptiality and marital fertility prior to 1870 is seriously hampered. The prominent statistician Gustav Sundbärg undertook to estimate the composition of the entire Swedish population by marital status, age, and sex, and these approximations, although based sometimes on arbitrary and perhaps indefensible assumptions, have been widely utilized by scholars. However, we need not rely exclusively on these data in forming a picture of the Swedish premodern demographic regime before 1880. For there are now in print the findings of a number of family reconstitution studies for Swedish parishes, and these permit us to gather substantial, detailed information about the demographic history of Sweden in the preindustrial era.[2] To simplify the presentation of this material, it is useful to review the evidence from national estimates first, and then turn to the parish findings. Having done this, we can outline some tentative generalizations and suggest an interpretation that fits the evidence reviewed here.

The national estimates of birth and death rates, population increase, and

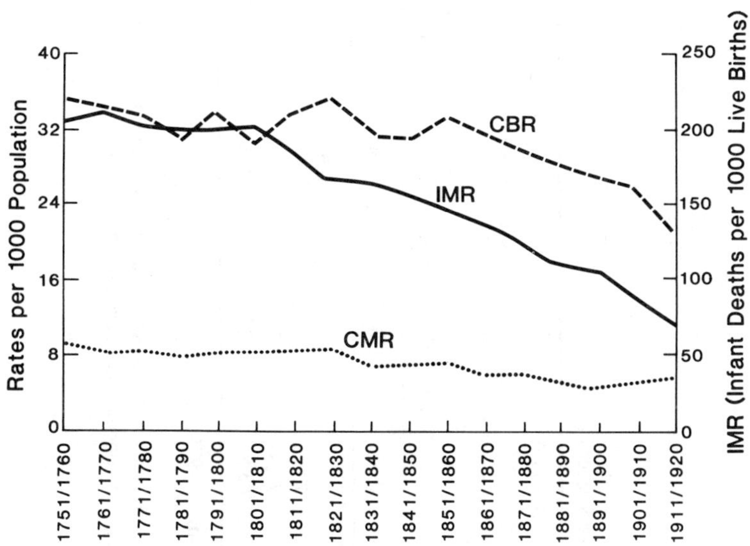

Fig. 6.1. Crude birth rate (*CBR*), crude marriage rate (*CMR*), and infant mortality rate (*IMR*) for Sweden, 1750–1920 (decade averages).

nuptiality reported in Table 6.1 and Fig. 6.1 suggest that a number of trends characterized the Swedish premodern demographic regime during the eighteenth and nineteenth centuries. First, the birth rate appears to have risen somewhat between 1736 and 1850, although the rate for 1850 is lower than that for 1750. Second, the death rate shows a sustained decline after 1750; all authorities attribute this to a rather sharp reduction in the infant mortality rate.[3] Third, the age at marriage of women seems to have risen over the century 1750–1850. [Figure 6.1 gives figures on the marriage rate (marriages per 1000 population), admittedly a poor indicator of the age at marriage. Unfortunately, series of more appropriate vital rates representing nuptiality, such as the mean age at first marriage for females, do not extend back into the eighteenth century, and the census figures on proportion married are only available for a few benchmark years.]

Evidence that further supports the preceding claims can be culled from the Swedish parish family reconstitution studies. In Table 6.2 we present a sample of the results this literature has produced.[4] It should be emphasized that the small size of the parish populations and the relatively small number of parishes sampled make definite conclusions extremely difficult to make and comparison with other figures (e.g., national averages) problematic. The first point that is of interest concerns nuptiality. The table suggests that in the earlier period (16th and 17th centuries), females married at earlier ages

TABLE 6.1

Various Demographic Figures and Rates for Sweden, 1736–1850[a]

		Crude rates			Nuptiality, females			
					Percentage women single			Singulate mean age at marriage
Year	Population	Crude birth rate *CBR*	Crude death rate *CDR*	Natural rate of population increase *NRI*	20–24	30–34	45–49	*SMAMF*
1736	1708	29.8	27.0	2.8	n.a.[b]	n.a	n.a.	n.a.
1750[c]	1781	33.6	27.4	6.2	72.7	25.9	10.4	26.4
1800[c]	2347	32.2	23.9	8.3	77.6	29.7	11.7	27.3
1850[c]	3483	30.0	19.0	11.0	83.5	28.9	12.3	27.7

[a] Sweden Statistiska Centralbyrån (1969: Tables 2, 27, 28); and Hofsten and Lundström (1976: Table 2.7).

[b] n.a. = not available.

[c] Crude vital rates and natural rates of increase are for fifty-year periods. 1750 figure is for period 1751 to 1800; figure for 1800 is for 1801 to 1850; figure for 1850 is for 1851 to 1900. Percentages women single, singulate mean age at marriage, and population figures are for exact year.

TABLE 6.2

Characteristics of Fertility and Mortality for Selected Premodern Swedish Parishes[a]

Population and Date	Nupiality				Marital fertility						Mortality
			Celibacy[d] (%)				Birth intervals				
	MAFMM[b]	*MAFMF*[c]	Males	Females	*M*	*m*	Average	0–1	1–2	2–3	*IMR*[e]
Alskog,[f] (1745–1820)	n.a.	24.5	n.a.	n.a.	.79	.15	2.0	1.1	n.a.	n.a.	n.a.
Möklinta,[g] (1650–1680)	29.1	25.4	n.a.	n.a.	.83	−.04	2.5	1.6	2.2	2.3	n.a.
Dala,[h] (1776–1830)	28.7	25.9	n.a.	n.a.	.90	.10	n.a.	n.a.	n.a.	2.2	212
Kolbäck, (1581–1610)	36.6	20.0	0	12	n.a.	n.a.	n.a.	n.a.	n.a.	n.a.	n.a.
Kolbäck, (1671–1700)	30.1	28.7	3	9	n.a.	n.a.	n.a.	n.a.	n.a.	n.a.	n.a.

[a] Alskog figures from Gaunt (1973: 41–57). Möklinta figures from Åkerman (1978: 40–43). Dala figures from Winberg (1978: 177, 179–181). Kolbäck figures from Gaunt (1978: 80).

[b] *MAFMM* is the mean age at first marriage for males. n.a. means that data were not available.

[c] *MAFMF* is the mean age at first marriage for females.

[d] Percentage unmarried after age 50. Precise method of calculation varies from study to study.

[e] *IMR* is the infant mortality rate.

[f] Figures for the *MAFMF* and 0–1 birth interval are for averages of subperiods. The 0–1 birth interval is for women married between 20 and 25. The average birth interval figure is for 1745–1769.

[g] Average birth interval is average for birth intervals 0–1 to 6–7. *MAFMM* and *MAFMF* are median values, not means.

[h] *MAFMM* and *MAFMF* are for peasants only. Birth interval for 2–3 interval average of several groups defined according to mortality experience of 1st and 2nd born. *IMR* for free holders only.

than they did in the eighteenth and nineteenth centuries. This means the trend in Swedish nuptiality stretches back into the 17th century. Second, the estimates of natural fertility (birth intervals and the Coale–Trussell parameter *M*) point to somewhat lower levels than those calculated for Sweden in the 1870s (see Table 2.9). By way of contrast with the Japanese village reconstitution findings, however, it should be noted that females marry at relatively late ages and the interbirth intervals are comparatively short, even in the seventeenth century. That is, if the Swedish premodern demographic regime was characterized by trends in marital fertility, nuptiality, and mortality in the 17th–19th centuries similar to those for Meiji Japan, the initial level when we pick up the trends was different from that characterizing Tokugawa Japan. Whether the Swedish patterns looked similar to those of premodern Japan further back in time or in certain regions is a tantalizing question that the discussion and the data assembled here cannot attend to. In any event, we wish to concentrate on interpreting the findings we can actually document.

At the outset it should be noted that the trends in nuptiality, natural fertility, and infant mortality fit the model and are roughly consistent with what we found for Meiji Japan. However, it should also be recalled that (1) Swedish income per head in the 17th and 18th century probably exceeded that of late Tokugawa Japan and (2) that the century of population growth between 1750 and 1850 took place in an environment in which there was little industrialization to speak of. Thus as demonstrated in Chapters 3 and 4, prepetuation of the stem family system stimulated downward social mobility during this period, and many sons of peasants and crofters moved into landless classes with only the most tenuous claim to the land. Kälvemark (1977–1978) argued that this "proletarianization" of the Swedish countryside had a far greater impact on the nuptiality of landless groups than on farming households, encouraging later marriage and permanent celibacy, especially among the daughters of the lower strata. For these women would secure long-term employment as domestic workers on the farms of peasants who were relatively well-to-do, and they would attempt to save and build a dowry, postponing marriage until their own financial prospects were sufficiently (if ever) attractive to justify a match to a male that had access to land and economic security. It should be noted that this argument hinges on the standard of living of a broad range of the rural peasantry that was sufficiently affluent so as to allow them to hire servants. However, the continued population pressure on land worked against the consumation of many of these marriages because increasing numbers of men found it impossible to secure a land holding. Although the creation of the *statare* system did encourage some members of this class both to wed earlier than they might otherwise and to avoid permanent celibacy, the increase in numbers did tend to generate substantial numbers of permanent celibates, primarily among the landless. [It should be noted that the extent of population pressure during this period on the land and its purported impact on economic and social conditions is a matter of some debate. See Winberg (1975) for the thesis that population pressure was not exceptionally great.] Moreover, with the reduction in transit costs of international migration after the 1850s, owing in part to the introduction of the steamship driven by the screw propellor, many landless rural Swedish laborers (especially males) emigrated to the United States and Canada, skewing the sex ratios against women and further intensifying the difficulties women faced in locating spouses. In short, the stem family system remained intact, and population growth, because of dropping infant mortality and perhaps increasing marital fertility, tended to drive up the number of spinsters and the mean age at marriage for women beyond the ages that the pure demographic life-cycle mechanism model would predict. Kälvemark (1977–1978) and others emphasize that nuptiality patterns were considerably different in the 17th century, the incidence of celibates being considerably lower and marriage ages earlier, and this fits this interpretation. What she observes about peasants also fits well into the interpretation we use, for she notes their marriage ages also increased (though celibacy did not), and this is what we expect on the basis of the life-cycle adjustment mechanism, given declining infant mortality rates and enhanced natural fertility.[5]

But why did infant mortality rates decline and natural fertility improve? Smallpox vaccination, made compulsory in 1815, may account for these trends to a degree, but Fridlizius (1975) argued that the introduction and wide spread use of the potato was a major factor. He points out that the wide spread use of the potato had two effects on production and consumption of agrarian households. First, it reduced the chance of complete crop failure (in contrast to rye, barley, and wheat), and, consequently, it helped ward off the chance of malnutrition. Second, it provided a more balanced diet and a better range of nutrients than hitherto characterized standard Swedish diet, and in particular added vitamin C to the nutritional intake. Moreover, Fridlizius points to institutional changes, specifically to the enclosures that we discussed in Chapter 3, as encouraging some productivity gain. In short, this view would support the following tentative generalization: food intake began to improve in the eighteenth century, encouraging reductions in infant mortality (and hence shortening of interbirth intervals and enhancing natural fertility). In turn this generated population growth that, under a stem family system, tended to eventually increase the number of permanently landless and celibate men and women. Slow institutional changes and the wide spread use of new crops, themselves partially a response to population increase, as we saw in Chapter 3, kept the standard of living from falling in a secular sense (short-term fluctuations certainly occurred) as population grew throughout the century before modern economic growth commenced. Nuptiality patterns responded to these evolving environmental conditions: the relatively late marriage and substantial celibacy of Sweden in the 1870s were reflected in the low infant mortality, high natural fertility, moderate standard of living, and substantial proportion landless that characterized it during the period just preceding industrialization and modern economic growth.

Before we proceed to a discussion of the cross-sectional evidence for Sweden, 1880–1900, it is important to emphasize that although the patriarchal stem family system survived into the early period of modern economic growth in Sweden, the developments that took place during the eighteenth and nineteenth centuries undoubtedly weakened it. Patriarchs among the lower classes of rural society undoubtedly experienced a loss in leverage over their sons and daughters as population growth reduced the number of local opportunities and cottages available and made marriages to persons who had access to land increasingly difficult to arrange. And the swelling of labor markets by unmarried single women probably encouraged the development of ideologies and viewpoints hostile to the woman's role in the patriarchal stem family system. In addition, the opening up of reasonably cheap transportation to the Americas after the 1850s further weakened the patriarchs' positions, for a son or daughter seeking employment in the United States would not necessarily be able to rely on his or her parents for contacts in arranging jobs. These points should be kept in mind throughout the discussion of the statistical evidence for 1880 and after, for the early disappearance of the Swedish premodern demographic regime is most readily understood in terms of the points just noted.

6.3. The Premodern Demographic Regime and Its Disappearance: The Counties of Sweden, 1880–1960

As noted in the previous discussion of the availability of Swedish demographic data, reliable figures on nuptiality status cannot be secured for the period prior to 1870. And age-specific marital fertility rates for the counties are not available until 1880 (1881 to be precise), see Appendix 6 for details. Thus we restrict the discussion in this chapter and Chapter 8 to the period 1880–1960, for which the list of demographic data available for the counties is complete, in the sense that we can measure the Hutterite indices, the Coale–Trussell parameters M and m, and the singulate mean age at marriage. That this choice of dates does not prevent us from analyzing the Swedish situation cross sectionally before the fertility transition com-

TABLE 6.3

Means and Standard Deviations for Measures of Marital Fertility for Groups of the Counties of Sweden Defined in Terms of Percentage Male Labor Force in Primary Industry (*PPIM*) for 1900

	Hutterite index[a] I_g		Coale–Trussell indices, 1880	
Group	1880	1900	*M*	*m*
PPIM ≤ 39.9%	.69	.62	.93	.20
	(.06)	(.07)	(.06)	(.18)
40% ≤ *PPIM* ≤ 59.9%	.70	.65	.90	.11
	(.08)	(.09)	(.06)	(.08)
60% ≤ *PPIM*	.72	.69	.90	.09
	(.10)	(.10)	(.09)	(.10)

[a] Hutterite indices calculated with averages of the births for five years centered around the census date. The standard deviation is in parenthesis beneath the mean for the variable.

menced is shown by Table 6.3, which presents figures for groups of the counties defined in terms of percentage male labor force in primary industry in 1900.[6] The raw figures on which the averages displayed in Table 6.3 are based reveal that the index of parity-specific control is substantially different from 0 (i.e., significantly above .2, the Coale–Trussel "cut-off" level) in only one of the counties in 1880: Stockholm City. In two other counties (Uppsala and Gotland) it is slightly above .2, but basically the description of Sweden outside Stockholm City as a natural fertility population in 1880 is valid. It should be emphasized that we exclude observations for Stockholm City in the county level regression results reported on subsequently. Table 6.3 also documents the slowness of the fertility decline before 1900. In most of the counties I_g is approximately the same in 1900 as it is in 1880, the declines being gradual during the last quarter of the nineteenth century. An interesting aspect of the state of marital fertility in Sweden before 1900 concerns areal variations in natural fertility. This was wide-ranging, as a perusal of the standard deviations on the indices I_g and *m* for the three groups in Table 6.3 suggests. For example, the Stockholm value of *M* in 1880 is 1.01 but that for Gotland is .70, and there is a distinct clustering of values in the middle .90s.

The impression conveyed by Table 6.3 and the surrounding discussion that there was little systematic variation of natural fertility with respect to labor force structure (the variations being principally *within* these groups) is reflected in figures on nuptiality given in Table 6.4. This table presents figures on singulate mean ages at marriage, the Hutterite index of nuptiality for 1880 and 1900, and age gaps at marriage for 1900 for the groups of the

TABLE 6.4

Means and Standard Deviations for Measures of Nuptiality for Groups of the Counties of Sweden, 1880–1900, Defined in Terms of Percentage Adult Male Labor Force in Primary Industry (*PPIM*) for 1900

	Hutterite index, I_m		Singulate mean age at marriage			Age gap at marriage at exact age of wife, 1900	
			SMAMF		*SMAMM*		
Group	1880	1900	1880	1900	1900	Age 20	Age 25
PPIM ≤ 39.9%	.39	.40	27.7	27.4	29.0	.70	1.72
	(.08)	(.08)	(1.2)	(1.3)	(1.1)	(.16)	(.13)
40% ≤ *PPIM* ≤ 59.9%	.45	.45	26.8	26.7	28.8	.83	2.06
	(.03)	(.03)	(.7)	(.7)	(.6)	(.13)	(.24)
60% ≤ *PPIM*	.40	.40	27.8	27.7	29.8	.81	1.91
	(.04)	(.03)	(.9)	(.7)	(.5)	(.41)	(.56)

[a] The standard deviation is in parenthesis under the mean for the variable.

Swedish counties used in Table 6.3. As with the Japanese data in the interwar period, nuptiality patterns show considerable variation even *within* each of the three groups of counties, suggesting that shifts in the structure of the labor force do not alone account for the variations we see. For example, in the first group the lowest value of the *SMAMF* in 1880 is 26.1 and the highest is 28.8; in the second group this variable ranges between 25.7 and 27.7; and in the third group it ranges between 26.4 and 28.7. Moreover, age gaps at marriage, although considerably smaller than those characterizing interwar Japan, show considerable variability as well, pointing to differential determinants in the decision to marry of males and females; this casts doubt on the view that there is an ideal age gap at marriage that couples aim for, with economic and demographic constraints operating only on men, and female ages at marriage emerging as a resultant.

Moreover, as with the Japanese premodern demographic regime, there is significant regionality displayed by the Swedish patterns. This can be seen clearly in Figure 6.2, which displays the Hutterite indices I_g and I_m for 1900, see Appendix 2 for the Swedish regions. Statistical tests also support the thesis that there is a geographical clustering of patterns in nuptiality and marital fertility for the Swedish premodern demographic regime. However, as will be shown in this chapter, the areal concentration is explicable in terms of environmental conditions, and we need not fall back on the vague notion of "culture" to account for this phenomenon.

Now let us turn to the analytical findings. In setting up the Swedish data for statistical testing, we attempted to replicate as nearly as possible (for the Swedish county figures) the equations utilized for the Japanese prefectures. The definitions of the variables are the same as those reported in Table 5.8, the two exceptions being the density variable (*D*), here it is persons per square kilometer, and the measure of infant mortality employed to probe the Swedish data. Because illegitimate fertility is relatively pronounced in the Swedish case (see Table 3.8) and the infant mortality rate of illegitimate offspring is substantially greater than for legitimate infants, we deemed it useful to restrict the proxy for infant mortality risks to those characteristic of married couples, under the presumption that nuptiality decisions would most likely revolve around the expectations about events within marriage that prospective brides, bridegrooms, and their families hold.

As in the previous analysis of the Japanese regression results concerning the premodern demographic regime, we shall commence the discussion with a presentation of the means and standard deviations for the relevant variables (for convenience we also give values for a variable concerning schooling that will play a role in the analysis of marital fertility in Chapter 8). The figures appear in Table 6.5. As with the comparable figures given in Chapter 5, the reader should find these data useful in exploring the magni-

TABLE 6.5

Means and Standard Deviations for Variables on the Counties of Sweden, 1890–1960

Variable	1890		1910		1920		1930		1960	
	Mean	Standard deviation	Mean	Standard deviation	Mean	Standard deviation	Mean	Standard deviation	Mean	Standard deviation
Singulate mean age at marriage: females (*SMAMF*)	25.70	1.06	25.53	.78	25.33	.70	26.57	.46	22.91	.45
Coale–Trussell *M*	.90	.05	.87	.07	.78	.09	.58	.08	.61	.03
Coale–Trussell *m*	.11	.11	.29	.14	.41	.13	.91	.11	1.40	.14
Legitimate infant mortality rate (*IMRL*)[a]	98.22	17.52	66.17	9.44	51.84	9.68	51.20	9.25	15.37	2.98
Adult mortality rate for males (*ADMR*)[b]	10.04	1.28	8.55	1.18	7.01	.86	6.13	.70	2.68	.22
Hutterite index (I_g)	.68	.08	.59	.08	.40	.08	.33	.07	.25	.02
Proportion males in primary industry (*PPIM*)	.58	.09	.51	.11	.46	.10	.43	.10	.22	.09
Sex ratio (*SR*)	1.02	.04	1.02	.04	1.04	.04	1.06	.05	1.05	.05
Female employment ratio (E_f)	.38	.07	.44	.09	.60	.11	.63	.13	.67	.08
Female–male wage differential	.51	.04	.54	.03	.68	.06	.68	.04	n.e.[c]	n.e.
Real male wage	3.31	.34	4.99	.35	3.88	.53	5.92	.52	n.e.	n.e.
Real female wage	1.66	.41	2.69	.22	2.63	.41	4.03	.38	n.e.	n.e.
Proportion of pupils in primary school who are full-time, 1920 (*PFTES*)	n.e.	n.e.	n.e.	n.e.	.75	.19	n.e.	n.e.	n.e.	n.e.

[a] Infant mortality rate in 1890.

[b] Death rate for men aged 40–49. Generally rate given for date refers to death rate about a decade earlier.

[c] n.e. means not estimated.

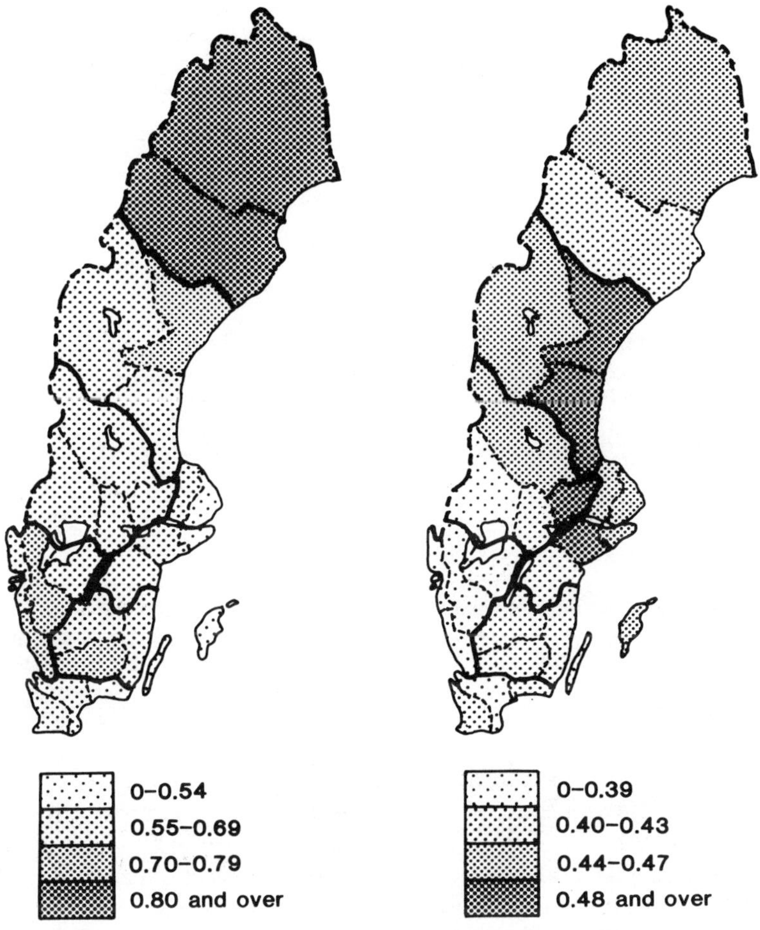

Fig. 6.2. I_m and I_g for counties of Sweden, 1900.

tudes of various effects that are estimated in the regressions concerning the structure of the premodern demographic regime in Sweden.

Before we examine the regression results, something should be said regarding our a priori expectations about the signs on the coefficients. Our expectations are identical to those we had with reference to Table 5.8 in Section 5.5 for Japan. The reader is asked to consult that section for the relevant discussion. The findings appear in Table 6.6. As with Table 5.8, the regressions come in pairs, those with M and m preceding those with I_g for each year, as with the Japanese results. For technical reasons discussed in Appendix 7, the fits for the Coale–Trussell parameters appear to be far

TABLE 6.6

Year	Dependent variable	Constant	Independent variables[a] — Demographic variables — Coale–Trussell, parameters *M*	*m*	Hutterite index I_g	Legitimate infant mortality rate *MRL*	Adult male mortality rate *ADMR*
[1] 1890	*SMAMF*	28.9[b]	7.6[d]	−2.8[d]	n.e.	−.04[b]	−.05
[2] 1890	*SMAMF*	29.3[b]	n.e.	n.e.	8.2[b]	−.04[b]	−.07
[3] 1910	*SMAMF*	35.5[b]	5.0	−2.3[d]	n.e.	.02	−.5[b]
[4] 1910	*SMAMF*	35.9[b]	n.e.	n.e.	7.1[b]	.02	−.5[b]
[5] 1930	*SMAMF*	24.3[c]	2.4	− .0001	n.e.	−.02	−.2
[6] 1930	*SMAMF*	23.7[c]	n.e.	n.e.	1.9	−.02	−.1
[7] 1950	*SMAMF*	32.0[b]	.3	− .4	n.e.	−.02	.3
[8] 1950	*SMAMF*	31.1[b]	n.e.	n.e.	−1.3	−.01	.3
[9] 1960	*SMAMF*	26.7[b]	−5.3	−1.8[c]	n.e.	−.02	.6[d]
[10] 1960	*SMAMF*	24.2[b]	n.e.	n.e.	−4.1	−.003	.9[c]

[a] There are significant intercorrelations of some of the independent variables in 1890 and 1910. For instance, for 1890, the correlation between *ADMR* and *IMRL* is .51, between *M* and *SR* is .46. For 1910 the correlation between *M* and *FMWD* is .57, and between *ADMR* and *IMRL* it is .69. All are one tailed tests except those for *PPIM* and *RWM*, which are two-tailed tests. n.e. means not estimated.

poorer for the Swedish counties, particularly for the years after 1890, than for the Japanese prefectures. Thus I_g is probably preferable to *M* as a measure of natural fertility in the period, say up to 1900, when there was relatively little parity-specific control in Sweden. As can readily be gleaned from the table, the Hutterite index of marital fertility and the legitimate infant mortality rate in the earliest year (1890) have the expected signs (as does the Coale–Trussell parameter *M*) and are statistically significant (*M* is not nearly as significant as I_g but, as noted, I_g is probably a better measure of natural fertility for the Swedish counties in 1890 than is *M*). The sign on the coefficient for the adult male mortality rate also has the expected sign, although the coefficient is not significant for 1890 (it is in 1910). This supports the thesis that life-cycle factors were operating in the Swedish premodern demographic regime as they were in the Japanese case. Other regressions, not reported here, show similar results for the counties in 1880 and 1900. The second point that strikes us in perusing the findings for the demographic component of the model is the early disappearance of the life-cycle relationships: it would appear that beginning with 1910 the infant mortality rate ceases to be significant and the results for 1930, 1950, and

The Structure and Disappearance of the Premodern Demographic Regime in Sweden

Independent variables[a]							
Structural variables			Labor force variables				
Proportion males in primary industry *PPIM*	Density *D*	Sex ratio *SR*	Female employment ratio E_f	Real male wage *RWM*	Female–male wage differential *FMWD*	R^2	Adjusted R^2
3.5[d]	.02[c]	−7.5[c]	2.1	.2	−4.5	.92	.86
3.4[c]	.03[b]	−7.0[c]	2.2	.2	−3.7[d]	.91	.84
−.7	.001	−5.2	.04	−.6	−4.5	.77	.59
.8	.0001	−5.5[d]	.4	−.6	−4.7	.75	.59
6.7	−.01	−6.2[c]	1.7	1.2	−2.2	.45	.02
7.2[d]	−.01	−5.8[d]	1.5	1.2	−1.4	.40	.01
2.5	.001	−9.7[c]	−1.7	n.e.	n.e.	.59	.38
3.1[c]	.001	−9.3[c]	−1.5	n.e.	n.e.	.59	.41
1.1	−.005	−1.6	3.3	n.e.	n.e.	.58	.36
.7	−.002	−1.6	−1.6	n.e.	n.e.	.42	.18

[b] Significant at the 1 percent level.
[c] Significant at the 5 percent level.
[d] Significant at the 10 percent level.

1960 suggest that the life-cycle relationships had completely ceased to be important by the interwar period and after. This implies that the basic structural mechanism of the premodern demographic regime ceased to operate with great force in Sweden around the turn of the century, a full fifty years prior to its erosion in most of Japan. In Chapter 2 we sketched out theoretical grounds for why we would expect this result; to pursue the question more thoroughly, however, we must turn to the economic and social factors included in the regressions, and also, in the next section, to a more systematic examination using pooled time-series cross-sectional methods.

Recall that the argument is that the patriarchal stem family system gives way early on in Swedish modern economic growth, patriarchs finding their leverage in the job and marriage markets seriously weakened as industrialization commences. Carlsson (1978:226) refers to this process in describing circumstances toward the close of the nineteenth century: "The agrarian distribution of sex roles became more and more foreign to growing parts of the population, and the family increasingly lost its importance as a productive, working unit. Girls coming from the peasantry and proletarian groups began to voice their demands for additional education and more remunerative employment." By the close of the century women were entering the labor market largely on their own initiative and contracting marriages by personal contacts rather than by relying on their parents. In interpreting the empirical results involving the economic and social factors, we wish to avoid the "ecological fallacy" (we have already attempted to avoid those pitfalls in reading the Japanese results) and so considerable care must be exercised in the analysis. The findings, however, appear to point in the following direction: population pressure in the agricultural zones (note the density variable *D*) and the requirement of inheriting sons to wait for the patriarch to reach old age before acquiring the land, kept marriage ages in the rural areas high. Those sons and daughters who did not expect to stay in agriculture, however, entered labor markets at comparatively early ages and increasingly on their own terms because education was becoming an effective screening device for job placement and income per head was high to begin with, having already encouraged robust labor markets to develop in the rural areas during the eighteenth and nineteenth centuries. Thus a man would commonly work and save over a number of years, beginning from his graduation from school, until his resources appeared adequate to enter the marriage market and attract a woman with a dowry: his notion of a desirable dowry being formed on the basis of what girls in the locale he grew up in typically raised and what he could expect from the experience of his peers. These arguments may account for why the variables representing the sex ratio and structure of the labor force (*PPIM*) take on the signs they do in the equations. In an environment in which the number of marriageable women is small relative to the men looking for brides, there is a "squeeze" in the marriage market faced by the men, and they settle for more youthful brides who bring dowries less substantial than those in markets with a sex ratio more favorable to men (see Norman, 1974). It should be emphasized that this argument concerning the importance of dowry and the savings a woman accumulates *prior* to marriage hinges on the notion that people perceive it is difficult for a married woman to work outside the home and generate income flow during married life once she begins bearing children because parity-specific control is hard to achieve during the early stages of the fertility transition (without an international market for effective contraceptives, see Chapter 8). In short, the results are consistent with the thesis that the Swedish premodern demographic regime was rapidly giving way to market forces with modernization.[7]

Before leaving this discussion of the structure of the Swedish premodern demographic regime as captured in regressions concerning female nuptiality, it is useful to examine β coefficients and elasticities for some of the crucial variables in Table 6.6. The relevant figures appear in Table 6.7. For

TABLE 6.7

β Coefficients and Elasticities for Selected Variables from Regressions for 1890 and 1910 in Table 6.6

Year and equation number	Hutterite index I_g β	Hutterite index I_g Elasticity	Legitimate infant mortality rate *IMRL* β	Legitimate infant mortality rate *IMRL* Elasticity	Adult male mortality rate *ADMR* β	Adult male mortality rate *ADMR* Elasticity
[2] 1890	.61	.21	−.61	−.14	−.09	−.03
[4] 1910	.75	.17	.25	.06	−.78	−.17

1890 the β coefficients and elasticities are roughly the same in value as those that we secured for Japan 1925–1950 (see Table 5.9). Because they take on values of this magnitude it implies—when taken together with the means and standard deviations in Table 6.5—both that natural fertility and infant mortality seem to have had major impacts on the age of female first marriage, as estimated in the structural equations presented in Table 6.6 and that these findings parallel closely our findings for Japan.

Now let us take up in slightly more detail the question of the timing of the structural break (i.e., the ending of the premodern demographic regime) in Sweden.

6.4. The Timing of the Structural Break in Sweden

In the discussion of the ending of the premodern demographic regime in Japan, we utilized pooled time-series cross-sectional methods in attempting to date the structural break for Japan. In this section we employ the same methods for Sweden. Table 6.8 gives Swedish results paralleling those for Japan as presented in Table 5.10. In comparing Table 6.8 with Table 6.6, the reader should note that, because we lack data on real wages for the counties of postwar Sweden, we did not enter real male wages (*RWM*) or female–male wage differentials (*FMWD*) into the regression as independent variables.

As with the Japanese pooled regressions, F tests were carried out to see whether the introduction of the time dummies (cf. the differences for the constant term) and/or introduction of interaction variables between M, *IMRL*, and E_f and the time dummies were statistically significant (see Steps 1–3 of the analysis in Section 5.6). The F statistics for introducing the

TABLE 6.8

Results for Pooled Time-Series–Cross Section Regressions of the Form Used in Table 6.6, in Which There Is an Intercept for Each Year and M, IMR, and E_f Are Allowed to Interact with the Dummy Variable for Each Year[a]

			Independent variables[b]							
			Demographic variables				Structural variables			Labor force variable
Year	Dependent variable	Constant for 1890; difference between 1890 value and value for other years for 1910, 1930, 1950, and 1960	Coale–Trussell parameters M	Coale–Trussell parameters m	Legitimate infant mortality rate $IMRL$	Adult male mortality rate $ADMR$	Proportion males in primary industry $PPIM$	Density D	Sex ratio SR	Female employment ratio E_f
1890	*SMAMF*	20.6[d]	12.4[d]	.0001	−.04[d]	−.2[e]	1.9[e]	.002	−4.01[d]	6.5[d]
1910	*SMAMF*	4.0	− 5.8[e]	0[c]	.03[d]	0[c]	0[c]	0[c]	0[c]	−5.9[d]
1930	*SMAMF*	9.9[d]	−11.4[d]	0[c]	.05[d]	0[c]	0[c]	0[c]	0[c]	−7.1[d]
1950	*SMAMF*	6.0[f]	−11.3[d]	0[c]	.04	0[c]	0[c]	0[c]	0[c]	−8.2[d]
1960	*SMAMF*	13.3[d]	−21.2[d]	0[c]	.01	0[c]	0[c]	0[c]	0[c]	−8.0[d]

[a] R^2 = .95; Adjusted R^2 = .94.

[b] Coefficients for variables for 1890; differences between coefficient for 1890 and for given years for other years. All tests are two-tailed tests.

[c] Identically equal to 0 (not estimated).

[d] Significant at the 1% level.

[e] Significant at the 5% level.

[f] Significant at the 10% level.

dummy variables representing 1910, 1930, 1950, and 1960 is $F^{4}_{107} = 45.2$, significant at the 1 percent level; for introduction of the twelve interaction variables corresponding to *M, IMR,* and E_f, the *F* statistic is $F^{12}_{95} = 5.3$, significant at the 1 percent level; and for introduction of the four time dummies and the twelve interaction variables, the F statistic is $F^{16}_{95} = 20.7$, significant at the 1 percent level. All of these results testify to the existence of at least one structural break between 1890 and 1960 in Sweden.

Perusal of the coefficients in Table 6.8 suggests that the break took place between 1890 and 1910 (at least as far as *M, IMRL,* and E_f are concerned). It would not be wise to place great weight on this interpretation, however, because the test for structural break used here undoubtedly reflects the specification utilized in the analysis. The finding, however, is consistent with the arguments advanced as to why the premodern demographic regime gave way at an earlier date in Sweden than in Japan.

Now let us briefly consider some findings for the rural and urban sectors of the Swedish counties to delve into the possible impact of variables representing differentials in social status on the Swedish premodern demographic regime.

6.5. Social Structure and the Premodern Demographic Regime in Sweden: The Rural and Urban Sectors of the Counties, 1880–1900

Following the approach taken in studying the impact of social structures on the premodern demographic regime for Japan, we shall address this issue by studying the rural and urban sectors of the Swedish counties separately (Stockholm City has only an urban sector). Table 6.9 provides a useful place to commence the discussion. The table provides an illuminating contrast to Table 5.11 for Japan, for the uniform tendency of Japanese urban marriage ages to exceed those in the correspondingly rural sectors is not at all evident in Swedish data. The proportions married are always higher in the rural sectors because many women who stay permanently single are attracted to cities where relatively remunerative jobs are available, but the ages at marriage do not correspond to the Hutterite indices here. The closeness of the rural I_g values to those for the county as a whole are also noteworthy. The implication of Table 6.9 is that rural and urban populations in Sweden just prior to the fertility transition enjoyed similar levels of natural fertility. It should be emphasized, however, that we cannot measure the equivalent variables for the Japanese prefectures for a date at the inception of the Japanese transition, as we can for Sweden in 1880. Another interesting facet of Table 6.9 is that the excesses or decrements in marriage ages between the

TABLE 6.9

Means and Standard Deviations for Measures of Marital Fertility and Nuptiality for the Rural and Urban Sectors of the Counties and the Urban to Rural Relatives, 1925, for Groups of the Counties Defined in Terms of the Percentage Occupied Male Labor Force in Primary Industry (*PPIM*) in 1880[a]

	Marital fertility			Nuptiality				
	Hutterite index I_g		Urban I_g divided by rural I_g	Hutterite index I_m		Urban I_m divided by rural I_m	Difference between singulate mean age at marriage in urban and rural areas	
Group	Rural	Urban		Rural	Urban		Males	Females
$PPIM \leq 39.9\%$	.68	.67	1.02	.43	.35	.88	.53	−.14
	(.06)	(.05)	(.06)	(.06)	(.04)	(.11)	(.22)	(.64)
$40\% \leq PPIM \leq 59.9\%$	.70	.68	.97	.46	.36	.78	.33	1.04
	(.04)	(.07)	(.07)	(.03)	(.04)	(.06)	(.61)	(.73)
$60\% \leq PPIM$	.72	.68	.96	.41	.32	.78	−.43	.75
	(.10)	(.06)	(.15)	(.04)	(.04)	(.13)	(1.22)	(1.43)

[a] Based on averages of births for five years about census date. Calculated by subtracting the rural values from the urban value. Male figure is for 1900. The standard deviation is in parenthesis under the mean for the variable.

rural and urban zones are not the same for males as for females. All of this underscores the argument advanced in the previous section that the patriarchal influence over nuptiality had diminished considerably in Sweden by 1880, so that the regular type of pattern observed for Japanese rural and urban sectors did not emerge with industrialization and urbanization in Sweden.

Now let us delve into the question of social status with analytical results for the rural sectors. These appear in Table 6.10. The results support the view that the distribution of income and assets and the associated differentials in social status do make a difference. The coefficient for proportion of rural dwellers dependent on agriculture who are *statare* is significant in this regression and negative in sign (the proportion who are farm and estate owners also has a negative coefficient), suggesting that where estates are relatively large and the lower social strata numerous, early nuptiality is encouraged because state owners preferred the married *statare* to the unmarried hired hand: for the owner could secure some of the benefits accruing to the patriarch from the family labor of the *statare*'s wife and

TABLE 6.10

Social Structure and the Premodern Demographic Regime for the Rural Sectors of the Counties of Sweden, 1880 and 1900

			Independent variables										
			Demographic variables		Structural variables					Labor force variables			
								Percentage in agriculture in 1910					
Variable	Year	Constant	Hutterite index I_g	Infant mortality rate[a] *IMRL*	Sex ratio *SR*	Density *D*	Percentage of population dependent on primary industry *PPI*	*Statare* *PSI*	Farm and estate owners *FEO*	Real male agricultural wage *RAWM*	Female–Male differential in agricultural wages *FMAWDS*	R^2	Adjusted R^2
Singulate mean age at marriage, females													
SMAMF	1880	29.2[c]	6.1[c]	−.04[c]	−3.1	.0003[c]	n.e.[b]	n.e.	n.e.	− .02	− .4	.74	.64
SMAMF	1900	36.4[c]	− .06	−.02[d]	−5.0	−.02	3.3	−.2[c]	−.03	− .9[d]	3.1[e]	.86	.78
Singulate mean age at marriage, males													
SMAMM	1900	39.4[c]	n.e.	n.e.	−5.5	−.02	−1.1	−.2[c]	−.04	−1.1[c]	1.6	.69	.55

[a] Infant mortality rate (*IMR*) in 1880 (i.e., not restricted to legitimate births).

[b] n.e. = not entered into regression as an independent variable.

[c] Significant at the 1% level (two-tailed test).

[d] Significant at the 5% level.

[e] Significant at the 10% level.

children by taking on the *statare.* The other results worthy of note in this table concern male wages and female – male wage differentials.[7] By 1900 the patriarchal system had decayed to a considerable degree, and we should not interpret male real wages as representing the per capita living standards of patriarchs and their ability to hire workers because the patriarchal system was already weakened. Thus the level of male real wages may perhaps best be understood as an (inverse) indicator for the length of time a man would need to work to acquire financial resources sufficient to enter the marriage market and attract a woman with a dowry, and, consequently, the negative coefficient implies that rapid accumulation of resources did encourage men to wed relatively youthfully (see Martinius, 1977). The capacity of women to accumulate resources and a dowry (the wage differential) also fits into this general argument, which emphasizes the ability of prospective partners to save and build a capital stock prior to matrimony. That life-cycle forces were also important among some sectors of the rural populace—especially in 1880—is confirmed by the coefficients on I_g and the infant mortality rate (the 1880 data do not classify infant deaths by legitimacy status, so we cannot use the legitimate infant mortality rate for that year). We would expect that the demographic life-cycle adjustment mechanism would persist longer in the predominantly agricultural rural areas, especially among the peasantry; these results suggest that this was the case, although it appears that market forces (and of course emigration and the development of rural industry) were playing a major role in shaping the nuptiality patterns of the rural districts by the turn of the century.

6.6. Conclusions

In this Chapter, we provided evidence that suggests that the empirical structure of the premodern demographic regime that we discovered for Japan also characterized Sweden at the onset of modernization. We also attempted to demonstrate that the hallmarks of premodern demographic regime, those involving the demographic life-cycle adjustment mechanism, ceased to be of consequence in shaping Swedish nuptiality patterns by the early twentieth century. These results all fit in well with the model of the evolution of fertility in societies that, prior to modernization, maintain a patriarchal stem family system. The empirical contrast between the early decline of the premodern demographic regime in Sweden and its persistence in Japan is, indeed, one of the strongest results that we adduced in favor of the general approach.

Notes to Chapter 6

1. For a detailed discussion of the Swedish population statistics, see Hofsten and Lundström (1976:150–168; Appendix 1).

2. See Mosk (1979e) for a discussion of family reconstitution studies in Denmark, Sweden, Norway, and Finland.

3. See, for example, Öhngren (1979:2). Other studies of the decline of infant mortality in Sweden include Lithell (1981b) and Norman (1977).

4. See Mosk (1979e) for a discussion of results from other Swedish family reconstitution studies.

5. On this point also see Carlsson (1978). Carlsson writes (1978:224),

> "This investigation has shown that the 'European marriage pattern' was already quite apparent in Sweden in the eighteenth century as far as the upper and middle classes were concerned. However among the broader social strata, especially the peasantry, there was another pattern, characterized by a very high nuptiality. Eventually, however, these groups were also influenced by the 'European' pattern. . . ."

6. In this table and elsewhere in the volume we rely on the 1900 census figures in classifying the Swedish counties by industrial type. This is because the primary concern is with that period of the Swedish fertility transition that occurred between 1880 and 1930, and 1900 represents an approximate midpoint. Moreover, the 1900 census figures on labor force appear to be very accurate. See Chapter 5 for the choice of the 1930 census in classifying the Japanese prefectures.

The counties in these groups are as follows: (a) $PPIM \leq 39.9\%$: Sodermandland, Malmöhus, Gothenburg and Bohus, and Stockholm Stad (City); (b) $40\% \leq PPIM \leq 59.9\%$: Stockholm Län, Uppsala Län; Ostergötland, Jönkoping, Kalmar, Blekinge, Örebro, Vastmandland, Kopparberg, Gälveborg, Vasternorrland, and Norbotten; (c) $PPIM \geq 60\%$: Kronoberg, Gotland, Kristianstad, Hallands, Älvsborg, Skaraborg, Värmland, Jämtland, and Vasterbotten.

7. The sign on the female–male wage differential is negative, a result that is surprising. It may reflect the composition of industrial employment in the counties, however, because the county level composite wages for males and females that I constructed rely heavily on the relative distribution of employment for each sex in each county. Low wages were associated with domestic oriented industries (like textiles) in which females predominated and high wages with export oriented industries (like machine making, iron and steel, and production of wood products) in which males dominated employment. That this argument is reasonable is suggested by the findings in Table 6.10 for the rural sectors of the counties, in which the wage differential used is only for agriculture and the sign on the coefficient—when significant—is positive.

CHAPTER 7

Fertility Transition in Japan

7.1. Introduction

The purpose in this chapter is to demonstrate that the model of the patriarchal stem family system developed here accounts empirically for the Japanese fertility transition. To accomplish this task we shall focus attention on statistical analyses of data for the Japanese prefectures and their rural and urban sectors, over the period 1925–1960. The findings yield considerable support for the approach used here because they demonstrate the importance of education for both males and females in explaining Japan's fertility transition, and they show that the relationship of transformations in the labor market to changes in natality follows along the theoretical lines laid out in Chapter 2. In addition, we shall offer some evidence in this chapter concerning the relationship of health conditions to levels of natural fertility.

The reader should note that the findings occasionally contradict assertions advanced by other scholars.[1] For instance, we show that wages play a complicated role in explaining the reduction of marital fertility. The discrepancies between these results and those of others generally stem from two circumstances. First, we assembled a data set for both prewar and postwar Japan and, in consequence, were able to carry out a statistical analysis for both periods. Previous analytical studies have concentrated almost exclusively on postwar trends and cross-sections. Second, the specifications for the behavioral relationships tested were often considerably different from those utilized by previous scholars because the theoretical position does not coincide with theirs. However, the reader should note that we include in the analysis almost every variable that other researchers incorporated into theirs, and a considerable number of other variables as well. Thus we attempted to include proxies for all of the factors other studies have pointed to but gave them an interpretation that, occasionally, they do not receive in these other analyses. Because the model is general in terms of the variety of factors it pinpoints as playing a role in the fertility transition, it is natural that the list of variables incorporates those used by others.

The organization of this chapter is as follows. In the next section we provide an overview of Japan's fertility transition and point to a number of features of that historical evolution that we wish to concentrate on. Then we briefly discuss the functional forms used in testing the theories statistically. In the two sections following that we draw on cross-sectional evidence, as well as material concerning trends, in substantiating the theories for Japan. Finally, we drew all of the findings together and make note of the most important results in the conclusion to the chapter.

7.2. The Japanese Fertility Transition: An Overview

In Chapter 3 we briefly outlined the main characteristics of Japan's fertility transition: a gradual decline in marital fertility during the interwar period and a dramatic drop in the decade of the 1950s. As we shall argue, the speed and duration of the Japanese transition must be understood in terms of a number of factors. One of these should properly be discussed at the outset because it provides a background necessary to the comprehension of all the other results. The factor referred to is governmental policy toward, and legislation concerning, the use of contraceptives and the practice of birth control. During the interwar years the Naimushō (Ministry of Home Affairs) outlawed the discussion of birth control methods in books, magazines, and public gatherings. In general, the government was pursuing a pronatalist policy at the time, and the ban on the public airing of issues concerning contraception fit well into that policy.[2] After the ending of the Second World War, however, defeat and occupation at the hands of an enemy, the drop in the standard of living compared with the 1930s, and the prodding of the occupation authorities all combined to encourage a wholesale reversal in the government's birth control policy. The Diet passed the National Eugenics Law of 1948 rendering abortion legal "if the health of the mother is endangered by the continuation of pregnancy or the delivery due to physical or economic reasons." Abortion, a certain, albeit somewhat dangerous, means of regulating reproduction, now became available to the entire population virtually without restriction. In addition to legalizing abortions, legislation was also passed that established governmental birth control clinics designed to provide the population with abortions performed under supervised conditions at a low fee and to disseminate contraceptive devices. Within half a dozen years knowledge about the law and clinics to assist persons in securing abortions and contraceptives spread throughout Japan. Although the rapidity of the postwar fertility decline as contrasted with the slowness of the prewar trend cannot be completely explained by this change in governmental position, an issue we shall take up at a later point in this chapter, there is little doubt that it reduced the costs of fertility regulation and, consequently, sped up the decline that was already well underway.

We are now set to explore the dynamics of the transition itself. Table 7.1 provides us with an initial point of reference. It offers us figures on the Coale–Trussell parameters M and m for the prefectures of Japan, as classified by composition of labor force, at three dates during the fertility transition (1960 represents the conclusion of the fertility decline).[3] From this table we can draw three observations that will be invaluable to us in focusing our subsequent statistical analysis. First, in the prefectures that were relatively industrial in 1930 ($PPIM \leq 29.9\%$), M appears to be low in 1930. This suggests that populations in *some* of the prefectures, namely, the nonagricultural districts, were consciously reducing marital fertility (i.e., regulating reproduction with the purpose of limiting surviving family size) by purposively lengthening birth intervals beyond what considerations of health and the guaranteeing of survivorship for offspring would dictate.[4] Second, in 1930 the age-specific values of m show a pattern that differs rather markedly from that displayed by the figures for 1950 and 1960. Specifically the values for 1930 tend to decline (or do not demonstrably increase) with the age of mother; whereas in 1950 and 1960, the values of m increase with age. From these findings we can infer that the availability of relatively cheap and efficient methods of regulating reproduction in the 1950s encouraged those couples who wished to regulate fertility to concentrate their reproduction in a few years right after marriage and then to cease having children altogether afterwards. Because regulating couples were sure they could control their fertility, they were willing to opt for such a strategy. This stands in contrast to the prewar situation, where the costs of controlling reproduction were high and the efficacy of existing methods (permanent abstinence, which involves tremendous psychological costs, excepted) highly uncertain, so such a strategy would tend to be perceived as too risky. Third, m reaches substantial levels in a number of prefectures by 1930 (the particular prefectures are Kyōto, Ōsaka, Fukui, Tottori, Okayama, Kōchi, and Shimane; but see the averages for the more industrial prefectures). It is interesting that only two of these prefectures are largely industrial in composition in 1930; or to state the same matter in a slightly different manner, in

TABLE 7.1

Means and Standard Deviations[a] for the Coale–Trussell Parameters of Natural Fertility and Parity-Specific Control (Average and for Individual Age Groups) for Groups of the Prefectures of Japan [Groups Defined in Terms of Percentage Occupied Male Labor Force in Primary Industry (*PPIM*) in 1930]: 1930, 1950, and 1960

	1930						1950						1960					
			m						*m*						*m*			
Group	*M*	*m*	25–29	30–34	35–39	40–44	*M*	*m*	25–29	30–34	35–39	40–44	*M*	*m*	25–29	30–34	35–39	40–44
$PPIM \leq 29.9\%$	.65	.32	.33	.30	.30	.34	.85	.93	.89	.79	.85	1.01	.89	2.33	1.74	1.95	2.36	2.43
	(.03)	(.12)	(.10)	(.11)	(.10)	(.13)	(.02)	(.15)	(.13)	(.13)	(.15)	(.17)	(.05)	(.14)	(.15)	(.19)	(.15)	(.15)
$30\% \leq PPIM \leq 49.9\%$	.70	.30	.39	.29	.27	.31	.86	.88	.83	.78	.82	.94	.89	2.35	1.85	2.15	2.42	2.37
	(.05)	(.09)	(.10)	(.06)	(.08)	(.10)	(.04)	(.21)	(.18)	(.16)	(.19)	(.23)	(.05)	(.35)	(.30)	(.28)	(.35)	(.38)
$50\% \leq PPIM \leq 54.9\%$	.75	.27	.34	.26	.23	.28	.88	.88	.88	.76	.83	.94	.93	2.48	1.98	2.24	2.51	2.54
	(.06)	(.07)	(.08)	(.06)	(.06)	(.09)	(.06)	(.13)	(.11)	(.11)	(.13)	(.14)	(.09)	(.31)	(.27)	(.33)	(.33)	(.31)
$55\% \leq PPIM \leq 59.9\%$	.76	.26	.31	.26	.24	.27	.89	.80	.76	.72	.77	.84	.91	2.22	1.79	2.05	2.22	2.26
	(.07)	(.12)	(.14)	(.10)	(.11)	(.13)	(.05)	(.19)	(.16)	(.16)	(.19)	(.21)	(.09)	(.24)	(.29)	(.32)	(.25)	(.26)
$60\% \leq PPIM$	.77	.23	.29	.22	.22	.25	.89	.66	.69	.57	.64	.70	.90	2.07	1.67	1.99	2.11	2.07
	(.06)	(.08)	(.10)	(.07)	(.08)	(.09)	(.02)	(.16)	(.11)	(.21)	(.15)	(.17)	(.08)	(.41)	(.25)	(.36)	(.41)	(.44)

[a] The standard deviations are in parenthesis under the means for the variables.

four of these low fertility prefectures, at least half of their male labor force is engaged in primary industry in 1930. This suggests that the prewar reduction of fertility and the diffusion of parity-specific control were not because of the introduction of new methods and technology emanating from industrial and urban districts but were occurring with traditional methods like *coitus interruptus* and abstinence in the isolated agricultural districts where desired fertility was falling considerably below natural fertility. To summarize the points concerning Table 7.1, we must look to desired fertility in explaining how and why the Japanese transition got underway. However, the availability of means of controlling fertility *did* condition to an extent the dynamics of the fertility transition.

Now let us turn to the evolution of nuptiality that took place during the Japanese fertility transition. This is captured in Table 7.2. The striking feature of these data can be grasped quickly. Without serious exception, the trends in female nuptiality that accompanied the fertility decline involved a rising age at marriage and a corresponding decline in proportions married. It is remarkable that this occurred everywhere in Japan, regardless of the occupational structure of individual prefectures. The importance of these trends will become more evident in the analysis carried out in the following two sections as well as in the discussion of the Swedish patterns that are demonstrably different.

TABLE 7.2

Means and Standard Deviations[a] for Measures of Nuptiality, 1930–1960, for Groups of Prefectures Defined in Terms of Percentage Occupied Male Labor Force in Primary Industry (*PPIM*) in 1930

	Hutterite index I_m			Singulate mean age at marriage, females *SMAMF*		
Group	1930	1950	1960	1930	1950	1960
PPIM ≤ 29.9%	.65	.58	.54	22.3	24.1	25.5
	(.03)	(.02)	(.03)	(.3)	(.6)	(.5)
30% ≤ *PPIM* ≤ 49.9%	.69	.60	.60	21.4	23.2	24.4
	(.02)	(.03)	(.03)	(.6)	(.6)	(.5)
50% ≤ *PPIM* ≤ 54.9%	.69	.60	.60	21.6	23.2	24.8
	(.04)	(.04)	(.03)	(.9)	(.8)	(1.0)
55% ≤ *PPIM* ≤ 59.9%	.68	.58	.60	21.9	23.6	24.8
	(.04)	(.03)	(.03)	(1.0)	(.9)	(.8)
60% ≤ *PPIM*	.72	.61	.63	20.9	23.0	24.3
	(.04)	(.03)	(.02)	(1.0)	(.6)	(.5)

[a] The standard deviations are in parenthesis under the means for the variables.

In short, the evidence assembled in this section points toward the following tentative generalizations, which we will pursue further in the subsequent analysis: the impetus for the Japanese fertility decline is social and economic change that affects desired fertility; but the timing, duration, and speed of the transition were probably partly shaped by the legal and political circumstances of the period. In particular, passage of the National Eugenics Law and the subsequent establishment of birth control clinics undoubtedly contributed to the speed of the precipitous postwar drop in marital fertility by reducing the costs of controlling reproduction.

7.3. Functional Forms Utilized in the Analysis of Marital Fertility

The discussion in Section 2.6, and in particular, Table 2.1, is designed to provide a framework for our empirical analysis of the determinants of marital fertility in this chapter and the next. Let X be the ith variable ($i = 1, \ldots, N$) that represents one, or a component of one, of the influences delineated in Table 2.1. Now consider the Hutterite index I_g as one major proxy for marital fertility. We can represent the relationships described in Table 2.1 in a linear fashion with the following specification:

$$I_g = a_0 + \sum_{i=1}^{N} a_i X_i + \epsilon \tag{7.1}$$

A second approach is to use a (logarithmic) proportional specification. When one suspects nonlinearities (e.g., threshold effects, etc.) are present, this is a useful alternative procedure for setting up regressions. in this context we can write

$$I_g = a_0 \prod_{i=1}^{N} X_i^{a_i} e^{\epsilon} \tag{7.2}$$

where e^x is the exponential function. Taking logarithms of both sides of (7.2) we have

$$\begin{aligned} \ln(I_g) &= \ln(a_0) + \sum_{i=1}^{N} a_i \ln(X_i) + \epsilon \\ &= \overline{a}_0 + \sum_{i=1}^{N} a_i \ln(X_i) + \epsilon \end{aligned} \tag{7.3}$$

where $\overline{a}_0$ is the natural logarithm of a_0. This latter specification is of a log–linear type and we shall refer to it below as the "logarithmic" specification.

In the analysis in Chapters 7 and 8, we shall utilize equations of the form of (7.1) and (7.3) in a number of places. It is desirable, however, that we attempt to also estimate equations with the Coale–Trussell parameters m and M as dependent variables. In doing so, however, we enter into a host of problems that we touched on previously (and that Appendix 7 considers in detail). The approach taken here is a simple one, and we should note that in earlier versions of this work we did try other more complicated methods (e.g., simultaneous equation estimation techniques such as two- and three-stage least squares and a graphical methodology based on analysis of residuals).

We work with the following specifications. Let $Y, i = 1, \ldots, N,$ be the variables that we suppose influence m and $Z_i, i = 1, \ldots, N_2$, the variables we suppose influence M. Then we write

$$m = b_0 + \sum_{i=1}^{N_1} b_i Y_i + \epsilon \tag{7.4}$$

and

$$M = c_0 + \sum_{i=1}^{N_2} c_i Z_i + \epsilon \tag{7.5}$$

The operating assumption is that the household (the patriarch through a bargaining process with other household members) arrives at a joint decision about m and M (i.e., there is a single decision of which m and M are outcomes), and averages of these decisions produce the figures on m and M for areal units that we work with in the analysis of prefectural and county data. It should be noted that this approach differs from an approach that assumes levels of m and M determine each other (in conjunction with the influence of other independent variables), the latter approach leading logically to simultaneous estimation methods (e.g., two- and three-stage least squares). The method utilized here permits us to restrict our attention to simple ordinary least squares regressions. In point of fact, the work done using the simultaneous equation approach and a graphical methodology (too complicated to explain here) is demonstrative that one can find similar results using a variety of methodologies. In any event the assumptions about joint determination of m and M seem to be the most reasonable on the basis of theoretical grounds, so we shall utilize specifications of the form of (7.4) and (7.5) in the analysis of m and M [we shall also use logarithmic specifications similar to Eq. (7.3) in places, replacing Eqs. (7.4) and (7.5) with variants in which the logarithms of all the variables are entered into the regressions].

It should also be noted in reference to the regressions on M that in analyzing the influence of health conditions on the capacity to produce

TABLE 7.3

Various Aspects of Economic and Social Development for the Prefectures of Japan, for Groups Defined in Terms of Percentage Male Labor Force in Primary Industry (*PPIM*) in 1930: For 1920–1960 (Means and Standard Deviations[a])

	Demographic			Labor force characteristics													Education	
	Infant mortality rate *IMR*			Real male wages[b]			Real female wages[b]			Female–male wage differential		Female employment ratio E_f			Percentage of persons aged 55–64 in 1970 who completed some advanced education[c]	
Group	1920	1950	1960	1930	1950	1960	1930	1950	1960	1930	1960	1930	1950	1960	Males	Females
PPIM ≤ 29.9%	184.4	48.2	24.0	3.44	4.03	5.12	1.35	1.85	2.33	.39	.46	.45	.42	.61	.40	.30
	(24.8)	(6.0)	(2.6)	(.38)	(.67)	(.52)	(.19)	(.21)	(.15)	(.03)	(.04)	(.06)	(.04)	(.08)	(.06)	(.04)
30% ≤ *PPIM* ≤ 49.9%	161.2	61.7	32.0	2.42	3.28	3.83	1.04	1.86	2.07	.44	.54	.39	.39	.57	.28	.21
	(25.5)	(10.3)	(4.1)	(.43)	(.34)	(.48)	(.13)	(.19)	(.31)	(.09)	(.07)	(.09)	(.08)	(.11)	(.05)	(.06)
50% ≤ *PPIM* ≤ 54.9%	168.6	67.3	35.2	2.02	2.87	3.32	1.05	1.85	2.09	.52	.64	.39	.37	.55	.25	.18
	(15.1)	(8.2)	(3.3)	(.15)	(.28)	(.43)	(.07)	(.16)	(.15)	(.04)	(.05)	(.03)	(.03)	(.05)	(.03)	(.03)
55% ≤ *PPIM* ≤ 55.9%	158.3	60.4	33.6	1.90	2.56	2.95	.98	1.65	1.95	.52	.67	.40	.31	.49	.27	.19
	(20.8)	(6.9)	(4.5)	(.14)	(.29)	(.36)	(.08)	(.18)	(.14)	(.08)	(.06)	(.08)	(.04)	(.05)	(.05)	(.05)
60% ≤ *PPIM*	162.7	72.8	37.9	1.85	2.39	2.59	.97	1.61	1.75	.53	.68	.30	.26	.40	.24	.16
	(38.4)	(12.7)	(6.2)	(.14)	(.31)	(.34)	(.14)	(.22)	(.18)	(.06)	(.06)	(.07)	(.03)	(.05)	(.05)	(.04)

[a] The standard deviations are in parenthesis under the means for the variables.

[b] Estimated nominal wages for each prefecture deflated by a price index for the prefecture (based on three-year averages of prices and wages centered about census dates). The price index sets = 100 the average price level of the urban areas of Japan in 1950–1951. Thus figures are for real wages in 1950–1951. See Appendix A.3 for further details.

[c] Education beyond elementary school. See Appendix 3.

surviving children an alternative approach to the one adopted here would be to treat $s = (1000 - IMR)/1000$ as a survivorship function capturing survival probabilities from birth to age 1 (the *IMR* is expressed as infant deaths per 1000 live births). Then one could analyze *sM* rather than simply *M*. Although this might bring the analysis concerning health constraints closer to that implicit in the model of household behavior it complicates the discussion of the determinants of overall marital fertility, so we have eschewed it here. What we did instead was to treat the infant mortality rate as one proxy for the risks of death to infants, and to enter it into regressions on *M* as a determinant of *M*. This is certainly not an ideal solution to the problem of empirically relating *M* to the risks of infant demise (in light of the formulation of the model of household behavior), but it does help us capture some important aspects concerning the determination of *M*.

This completes the general discussion of the functional forms with which we carried out the analysis in this chapter and Chapter 8. Now let us turn to the results.

7.4. Education, Wages, and the Fertility Transition: Cross Classifications and Regressions for the Prefectures, 1925–1960

The thesis of this book is that evolution of conditions in the labor market, and especially the relationship of education to job placement, is crucial to the demise of the patriarchal stem family system, the diminution of desired fertility, and the diffusion of parity-specific control. In this section we attempt to verify the propositions concerning fertility, working with data for the Japanese prefectures over the period 1925–1960. In the next section we shall extend and enrich the findings with results for the rural and urban sectors of the prefectures considered separately.

Between the early interwar period and 1960, Japan experienced a remarkable transformation in infant mortality, the structure of the labor market, and education. Some traces of this can be captured in the vital statistics, industrial figures, and censuses that cover the period 1920–1960. Table 7.3 is designed to capture a few of the most salient aspects of this process for the prefectures of Japan classified by composition of the labor force. It is useful to read the table both cross-sectionally (i.e., along the columns) as well as in a trend sense (along the rows) because both approaches tell us much about the character of Japanese modernization. Let us commence our investigations with infant mortality, which serves as a useful indicator of education, public health, and the standard of living. Two points are demonstrated in the table. First, infant mortality rates were still relatively pronounced around 1920 but they dropped quickly to very low levels by 1960.[5] This was not an isolated phenomenon for it seems to have taken place in every prefecture regardless of its industrial composition. Second, examination of the successive cross-sections indicates that the risks of infant death were not simply related to the standard of living, education, and public health alone (climate, for example, probably played a role). For instance, consider the variation within each of the groups of prefectures: in the group of the most highly industrial prefectures the rates vary from 160.5 (Kanagawa) to 223.8 (Ōsaka). In most agricultural prefectures the rates vary from 102.5 (Kagoshima) to 211.1 (Aomori). Examination of data for each prefecture suggests that these real variations are not explicable in terms of real wages or education alone. In light of the rather extreme climatic differences between Hokkaidō and Aomori in the Northeast and Kagoshima in the Southeast (the former districts experiencing long and harsh winters and the latter a relatively warm, more benign climate), it is undoubtedly true that wide differentials in infant mortality characterized Japan before modernization and the introduction of conditions that reduced it so effectively. (The relatively high infant mortality rates of prewar Northeastern Japan may also stem in part from problems of transportation. This was definitely the case in Northern Sweden, which prior to the development of railroads occasionally suffered from food shortages, even when the Southern districts were enjoying surpluses.) It is noteworthy that the general national decline in infant mortality tends to narrow, reverse, or eliminate these premodern differentials so that although real variation still exists in 1960, it is hardly a mirror image of the situation existing just after World War I.

Now let us explore the labor market over this period as revealed by the table. First, consider wages. The table shows several facets of the improvement in real wages germane to our inquiry. First, over the period 1930–1960 real daily wages for both male and female workers increased significantly. This trend was nationwide though most pronounced, perhaps, in the more industrial districts. Second, there was a tendency for female–male wage differentials to contract. It is interesting and noteworthy that this contraction is least in the most industrial prefectures, where manufacturing wages are far more significant in determining the overall level of daily remuneration, and appears most salient in the agricultural prefectures, where the wage for farming work dominates the average wage for the district as a whole. The structure of employment opportunities is certainly a factor here because men and women both compete for relatively similar jobs in the villages (especially after men began leaving the villages for industrial employment in the late 1900s) whereas jobs in the large firms of cities during this period tended to be wholly stratified by sex, women entering short-term employment that they would hold until marriage and men securing permanent positions.[6] Moreover, the rural labor market during this period probably permitted more flexible reentry of women who had finished childbearing because jobs were near the home and skills less likely lost during the period of greatest attention to children. Third, the figures on the female employment ratio (E_f), which is defined as the ratio of women employed outside of primary industry to women age 20–44, indicate that the incidence of female employment was increasing in all prefectures between 1930 and 1960, although the E_f ratio is obviously considerably higher in the more industrial districts at each date. It is interesting to note regarding this last point, however, that by 1960 the E_f ratios in many of the more agricultural prefectures exceed those for the most industrial prefectures in 1930. In short, the figures on the labor market indicate a general upward trend in real wages over the period 1930–1960, an increase in the labor force participation of women in jobs that are outside the home (i.e., outside agriculture), and a contraction in the female–male wage differential.

Finally, Table 7.3 speaks to the question of education. Figures for other cohorts (see Chapters 3 and 4 on this), which are not shown here, taken in conjunction with these data, reveal a cohort by cohort successive increase in the proportions securing advanced education. That is, the proportions for persons aged 35–44 are uniformly greater than those for persons aged 45–54. The figures reported in Table 7.3 also tell us a good deal about the relative levels of higher education obtained by persons in the industrial districts as opposed to the agricultural areas: in general more advanced schooling characterizes the areas that are urban and do not depend on primary production.[7] They also suggest that the sex differential in education is in absolute terms relatively uniform across the country (around 10 percent in absolute magnitude) although *relative* to the proportion of males receiving a higher education, the female proportions are larger in the districts where the proportion of males obtaining advanced education is higher.

In short, the figures in Table 7.3 offer support for the assertion made previously that between 1930 and 1960 Japan experienced substantial social and economic transformations—in labor markets, education, the standard of living, and public health. According to the logic of the model these are the most critical factors for the fertility transition. With this in mind let us systematically explore data for 1925 and 1960 to determine whether it supports the interpretation.

Before we commence our analysis of the regression results, however, we should present the means and standard deviations of those variables that prove to be crucial for our subsequent analysis and for which we have not yet presented for figures in Chapter 5 (see Table 5.7). This we do in Table 7.4. We shall define and discuss the new variables in the text accompanying the

TABLE 7.4

Means and Standard Deviations for Additional Variables on the Prefectures of Japan

Variable	Mean	Standard deviation
Stillbirth rate *SBR*, 1925[a]	.06	.01
Stillbirth rate *SBR*, 1930[a]	.05	.01
Index of permanent sterility *STER*[b]	9.95	2.33
Sex ratio at birth *SRB*, 1925[c]	1.03	.02
Sex ratio at birth *SRB*, 1930[c]	1.05	.01
Proportion of women 65 in 1970 who had not completed any school *PNEF*	.08	.03
Proportion of males in age group 55–64 in 1970 completing some schooling, who completed higher education *PEDHMA*	.28	.07
Proportion of females in age group 55–64 in 1970 completing some schooling, who completed higher education *PEDHFA*	.20	.06
Proportion of males in age group 45–54 in 1970 completing some schooling, who completed higher education *PEDHMB*	.41	.08
Proportion of females in age group 45–54 in 1970 completing some schooling, who completed higher education *PEDHFB*	.31	.09
Proportion of males in age group 30–34 in 1970 completing some schooling, who completed higher education *PEDHMC*	.52	.07
Proportion of females in age group 30–34 in 1970 completing some schooling, who completed higher education *PEDHFC*	.45	.09

[a] Stillbirths/(stillbirths and live births).

[b] Percentage of women aged 75–79 in 1970 and married at least 20 years who had no live births. Based on 1970 census data.

[c] Male live births/female live births (recorded births).

relevant tables; and we shall use these figures in interpreting the magnitudes of the effects of certain variables on marital fertility.

The focus is on explaining cross sections and trends in marital fertility and its components, using the Hutterite index I_g and the Coale–Trussell parameters as the dependent variables. We concentrate on cross sections for 1925, 1930, 1950, and 1960 and trends for the periods 1925–1950 and 1930–1950. In evaluating the results it is useful to keep in mind the problem of multicollinearity that definitely crops up with respect to these regressions. Some of the independent variables in the regressions we report are significantly correlated with each other. Methods like principal components analysis or factor analysis would certainly help in dealing with this problem in a purely formal statistical sense, but would not render much assistance to the job of interpreting the results because the composite variables one typically secures with such a procedure are notoriously difficult to define. To see what is involved we report the correlations between the independent

TABLE 7.5

Variables Utilized in the Quantitative Analysis of the Fertility Transition (in Marital Fertility) in Japan and Their Interpretation

Variable	Sign	Rationale
(a) Expectations on Coefficients for *M*		
IMR (infant mortality rate)	Negative	Proxy for risks of death to infants. Behavioral relationships specified in Section 2.3.
SBR (stillbirth rate)	Negative	Proxy for health of female population.
SRB (sex ratio at birth): $\frac{\text{male live births}}{\text{female live births}}$	Negative	Measure of degree to which parents resort to infanticide to select children (see Section 5.3).
STER (index of permanent sterility)	Negative	Measure of health conditions and perhaps especially the incidence of tuberculosis, which produces subfecundity.
ALEF (life expectancy of females aged 42)	Positive	Measure of health conditions for female population.
PPIM (proportion male labor dependent on primary industry)	Positive	Measure of demand for child labor services and represents degree of adherence to life-cycle strategy.
RWM (real wage for males)	Positive	Proxy for household income per capita (income constraint).
RWF (real wage for females)	No expectation until I_g is low; then negative.	This variable is expected to influence *M* when the patriarchal system has given way and women space births to stay in or leave the labor force at optimal times.
PNEF (proportion women 65+ in 1970 who have not completed any school)	Negative	Proxy for lack of knowledge (or ability to acquire knowledge) about public health techniques reducing infant mortality.
PEDHM (proportion of males in a certain age group in 1970 who completed higher education)[9]	Positive	Proxy for educational attainment of male children when the partriarchal system is still strong. As male children demand and receive more education they work less on the household enterprise, raising the value of female children, and discouraging infanticide against girls (infanticided births not being registered).
PEDHF (proportion of females in a certain age group in 1970 who completed higher education)	Negative	When the patriarchal system is still strong, a woman's education becomes crucial for arranging her marriage; the parents' leverage over her vis-a-vis the securing of her labor services is substantially diminished.

Table 7.5 continues

TABLE 7.5 (Cont.)

Variable	Sign	Rationale
(b) Expectations on coefficients for m		
IMR (infant mortality rate)	No expectation	See discussion in Chapter 2 and the rejection of the target fertility hypothesis.
PPIM (proportion male labor force dependent on primary industry	Negative	Proxy for demand for child labor services.
RWM (real wage for males)	Negative	Proxy for household per capita income (income constraint).
RWF (real wage for females)	No expectation until m is large	Proxy for opportunity cost of a woman's time only becomes significant when patriarchal system has collapsed.
PEDHM (proportion of males in certain age groups in 1970 who completed higher education)	Negative	Proxy for household per capita income (income constraint). Also as with discussion of this variable's influence on M previously, a proxy for factors increasing demand for daughters when patriarchal system is strong.
PEDHF (proportion of females in certain age groups in 1970 who completed higher education)	Positive	See discussion of influence of this variable on M.

(c) Expectations on coefficients on I_g

(i) *SBR, SRB, STER, PNEF,* and the *IMR* are all expected to be negatively associated with M, and they are not expected to influence m at all. Thus they should be negatively associated with I_g.

(ii) *ALEF* is expected to be positively associated with M and it has no expected influence on m, so it should be positively associated with I_g.

(iii) *PPIM, RWM,* and *PEDHM* are expected to raise M and lower m, so they should have a positive impact on I_g.

(iv) *PEDHF* and *RWF* are expected to lower M and raise m, so they should have a negative impact on I_g. (The latter variable should only have an impact when the transition in fertility is over or in a late phase.)

variables used in the regressions for 1925 at the foot of Table 7.6. This gives an example of the problems involved with multicollinearity.

Before we proceed to a discussion of the results let us briefly state in Table 7.5 the expectations about the coefficients estimated in the regressions and the rationale for these expectations in terms of the theory. First we state the expectations for the equations with M as the dependent variable, then for that with m as the dependent variable, and finally for that with I_g as the dependent variable.[8] Variables not utilized in the earlier analysis are defined in the footnotes to the accompanying tables. With this preliminary discussion of our expectations completed, let us turn to an analysis of the results, concentrating first on the prewar (interwar) period (i.e., 1925 and 1930) cross-sections when the patriarchal stem family system was still functioning strongly, especially in the rural districts.

The results are reported in Tables 7.6–7.9. The reader should check the results against the a priori hypotheses about the coefficients that were laid out in Table 7.5. The findings generally speak for themselves, and so we shall simply summarize them briefly. It should be noted, by the way, that we choose different cohorts for each date in measuring the proxies for the educational attainment of children because we wish to match as closely as possible the educational performance of people who were children at a certain date with the date for which other variables in the regression are measured (i.e., the regressions for 1930 use a different cohort's completed educational experience). Necessarily the match is crude, but it is a fair approximation.

On the one hand the results are largely consistent with the hypotheses concerning the coefficients. In particular the proxies for educational attainment (or lack of it for mothers) and labor force structure proved to be fully consistent with the hypotheses for both 1925 and 1930 and for the two different specifications. In general, with the major exception of the proxy for adult female life expectancy, results for the variables representing health conditions are also consistent with the hypothesized signs. On the other hand, the sign of the proxy for household income (real wages for males) was not consistent with the expected sign. However, the real male wage variable is undoubtedly a poor proxy for household income so it is difficult to place great weight on the results for this particular variable.

Before turning to a discussion of the postwar results (i.e., the cross-sections for 1950 and 1960) let us briefly examine β coefficients and elasticities for the most important variables in Tables 7.5 and 7.7 to evaluate the social significance of the results. We do this in Tables 7.10 and 7.11. What is particularly striking about the values presented here are the elasticities and β coefficients for the proxy for the daughter's education. The elasticity estimated for m is very large; and the β coefficients for this variable in all three regressions are also substantial.

In Tables 7.12 and 7.13 we present similar cross-sectional results for 1950 and 1960. The original aim in exploring the postwar data was to concentrate on the determinants of m because we felt the constraints on natural fertility had largely vanished by 1950. For this reason we did not collect data on stillbirth rates, indices of sterility, etc., for the postwar period, as a consequence nor do we present regressions on M. Our focus is on explaining variations in I_g and m. The basic findings that emerge from these tables can

TABLE 7.6

Marital Fertility, the Diffusion of Parity-Specific Control, and the Spacing of Births in the Prefectures of Japan: Cross Sections, 1925[a]

Constant and independent variables	Dependent variables		
	m	M	I_g
Constant	.6[j]	2.1[i]	2.0[i]
Independent variables			
Demographic variables			
Infant mortality rate *IMR*	1.3[j]	−.5	−.6[j]
Stillbirth rate[b] *SBR*	n.e.[h]	−.2	−1.1[j]
Sex ratio at birth[c]	n.e.	−1.0[j]	−.7[j]
Index of permanent sterility[d] *STER*	n.e.	−.01[i]	−.01[i]
Life expectancy of females aged 42 *ALEF*	n.e.	−.002	−.01
Labor force variables			
Proportion male labor force dependent on primary industry[e]	−.4	−.1	.1
Real wage for males[f]	−.1[j]	−.02	−.004
Real wage for females[f]	−.2	−.001	−.04
Education[g]			
Proxy for education of mothers			
Proportion women 65+ in 1970 who have not completed any school *PNEF*	n.e.	−.4[k]	−.1
Proxy for education of children			
Proportion of males in age group 55–64 in 1970 completing some schooling, who completed higher education *PEDHMA*	−1.0[j]	.5[j]	.4[j]
Proportion of females in age group 55–64 in 1970 completing some schooling, who completed higher education *PEDHFA*	1.9[i]	−1.0[i]	−.8[i]
R^2	.38	.77	.81
Adjusted R^2	.28	.69	.75

[a] All tests are one-tailed tests except for *IMR* in regression on m and for *RWF* in regressions on M and m. The significant correlations between the independent variables used in the preceding regression are as follows (the correlation is in the parenthesis following the pair of variables): *PNEF* and *PEDHFA* (−.63); *RWF* and *PEDHFA* (.60); *PEDHFA* and *PEDMA* (.94); *PNEF* and *PEDHMA* (−.58); *IMR* and *PPIM* (−.69); *RWF* and *PPIM* (−.93); *RWM* and *PPIM* (−.62); *RWM* and *PEDHMA* (.63).

[b] Stillbirths/(stillbirths + live births).

[c] Male live births/female live births (recorded births).

[d] Proportion of women aged 75–79 in 1970 and married at least 20 years who have had no live births. Based on 1970 census data.

[e] This based on the proportion of occupied persons in agricultural production.

[f] Estimated nominal daily wages deflated by a price index which sets the price index for "all urban Japan" in 1950–1951 equal to 100.

[g] These are based on 1970 census data. "Higher education" refers to graduation from any school above a prewar primary (elementary) school.

[h] n.e. = not entered into regression as independent variable.

[i] Significant at the 1 percent level.

[j] Significant at the 5 percent level.

[k] Significant at the 10 percent level.

TABLE 7.7

Marital Fertility, the Diffusion of Parity-Specific Control, and the Spacing of Births in the Prefectures of Japan, 1925: Logarithmic Specification[a]

Constant and independent variables	Dependent variables[b]		
	m	M	I_g
Constant	.9	−.4	.6
Independent variables			
Demographic variables			
Infant mortality rate *IMR*	.5[d]	−.7	−.1[e]
Stillbirth rate *SBR*	n.e.[f]	−.02	−.1[e]
Sex ratio at birth *SRB*	n.e.	−1.4[d]	−1.4[d]
Index of permanent sterility *STER*	n.e.	−.2[c]	−.25[c]
Life expectancy of females aged 42 *ALEF*	n.e.	.06	−.4
Labor force variables			
Proportion male labor force dependent on primary industry *PPIM*	−.4[e]	.06	.1[d]
Real wage for males *RWM*	−.9[c]	−.07	.01
Real wage for females *RWF*	−.6[e]	.03	.01
Education			
Proxy for education of mothers			
Proportion women 65+ in 1970 who have not completed any school *PNEF*	n.e.	−.05[d]	−.03
Proxy for education of children			
Proportion of males in age group 55–64 in 1970 completing some schooling, who completed higher education *PEDHMA*	−1.2[d]	.2[d]	.2[e]
Proportion of females in age group 55–64 in 1970 completing some schooling, who completed higher education *PEDHFA*	1.3[c]	−.3[c]	−.28[c]
R^2	.37	.77	.81
Adjusted R^2	.28	.70	.75

[a] The logarithms of every variable (dependent and independent) are entered rather than the variables themselves. When a variable takes on values close to 0, 1 was added to the variable (i.e., $1 + x$ where x is the variable) and then the logarithm was taken. See Table 7.6 for a discussion of the definitions of certain of the variables.

[b] All are one-tailed tests except for *IMR* in regression on m and for *RWF* in regressions on M and m.

[c] Significant at the 1 percent level.

[d] Significant at the 5 percent level.

[e] Significant at the 10 percent level.

[f] n.e. = not entered into the regression as an independent variable.

be stated briefly. First, the proxy for female education continues to play a relatively significant role in determining m and I_g, in line with our results for the prewar cross-sections. Second, by 1960, we secure findings for the labor market variables that are relatively consistent with the neoclassical "cost of

TABLE 7.8

Marital Fertility, the Diffusion of Parity-Specific Control, and the Spacing of Births in the Prefectures of Japan: Cross Sections, 1930

Constant and independent variables	Dependent variables[a]		
	m	*M*	I_g
Constant	.5[i]	.8[j]	1.03[h]
Independent variables			
Infant mortality rate *IMR*	2.2[h]	−.9[h]	−1.1[h]
Stillbirth rate[b] *SBR*	n.e.[g]	−1.6[i]	−2.0[h]
Sex ratio at birth[c] *SRB*	n.e.	.6	−.9
Index of permanent sterility[d] *STER*	n.e.	−.1[h]	−.01[h]
Life expectancy of females at age 42 *ALEF*	n.e.	−.01	−.01
Labor force variables			
Proportion male labor force dependent on primary industry *PPIM*	−.5[h]	.1	.2[i]
Real wage for males[e] *RWM*	−.1[h]	−.04	.07
Real wage for females[e] *RWF*	−.2[j]	−.01	.03
Education[f]			
Proxy for education of mothers			
Proportion women 65+ in 1970 who have not completed any school *PNEF*	n.e.	.07	.1
Proxy for education of children			
Proportion of males in age group 45–54 in 1970 completing some schooling, who have completed higher education *PEDHMB*	−.3	1.0[h]	.5[i]
Proportion of females in age group 45–54 in 1970 completing some schooling, who completed higher education *PEDHFB*	.9[i]	−1.2[h]	−.6[h]
R^2	.53	.82	.83
Adjusted R^2	.46	.76	.78

[a] All are one-tailed tests except for *IMR* in regression on *m* and for *RWF* in regressions on *M* and *m*.

[b] Stillbirths/(stillbirths + live births)

[c] Male live births/female live births (recorded births)

[d] Proportion of women aged 75–79 in 1970 and married at least 20 years who have had no live births. Based on 1970 census data.

[e] Estimated nominal daily wages deflated by a price index which sets the price index for "all urban" Japan in 1950–1951 equal to 100.

[f] These are based on 1970 census data.

[g] n.e. = not entered into regression as independent variable.

[h] Significant at the 1 percent level.

[i] Significant at the 5 percent level.

[j] Significant at the 10 percent level.

TABLE 7.9

Marital Fertility, the Diffusion of Parity-Specific Control, and the Spacing of Births in the Prefectures of Japan, 1930: Logarithmic Specification[a]

Constant and independent variables	Dependent variables[b] m	M	I_g
Constant	2.1[d]	.5	.4
Independent variables			
Infant mortality rate *IMR*	1.3[d]	−.2[d]	−.3[d]
Stillbirth rate *SBR*	n.e.[c]	−.1[e]	−.2[d]
Sex ratio at birth *SRB*	n.e.	1.0	−1.2
Index of permanent sterility *STER*	n.e.	−.2[d]	−.3[d]
Life expectancy of females at age 42 *ALEF*	n.e.	−.3	−.5
Labor force variables			
Proportion male labor force dependent on primary industry *PPIM*	−.6[d]	.06[e]	.1[d]
Real wage for males *RWM*	−.6[e]	−.1	−.3
Real wage for females *RWF*	−.8[e]	.03	.1
Education			
Proxy for education of mothers			
Proportion women 65+ in 1970 who have not completed any school *PNEF*	n.e.	−.002	.02
Proxy for education of children			
Proportion of males in age group 45–54 in 1970 completing some schooling, who have completed higher education *PEDHMB*	−1.2[e]	.4[d]	.4[d]
Proportion of females in age group 45–54 in 1970 completing some schooling, who completed higher education *PEDHFB*	1.5[d]	−.3[d]	−.4[d]
R^2	.58	.83	.84
Adjusted R^2	.51	.77	.80

[a] The logarithms of every variable (dependent and independent) are entered rather than the variables themselves. When a variable takes on values close to 0, 1 was added to the variable, and then the logarithm was taken. See Table 7.8 for a discussion of the definitions of certain of the variables.

[b] All are one-tailed tests except for *IMR* in regression on m and for *RWF* in regressions on M and m.

[c] n.e. = not entered into the regression as an independent variable.

[d] Significant at the 1 percent level.

[e] Significant at the 5 percent level.

time" interpretation of fertility determinants: the coefficients on female wages is significant and positive in the regression on m and significant and negative in the regression of M. The variable representing the product of male and female wages (introduced to look for nonlinearities in the relationship between income and fertility owing to complicating effects of male

TABLE 7.10

β Coefficients and Elasticities for Selected Variables from Regressions for 1925 in Table 7.6

	Variables									
	Infant mortality rate *IMR*		Index of permanent sterility *STER*		Proxy for mother's education *PNEF*		Proxy for son's education *PEDHMA*		Proxy for daughter's education *PEDHFA*	
Dependent variable	β	Elas-ticity	β	Elas-ticity	β	Elas-ticity	β	Elas-ticity	β	Elas-ticity
m	.29	.72	n.e.[a]	n.e.	n.e.	n.e.	−.66	−1.16	1.11	1.54
M	−.17	−.09	−.45	−.17	−.20	−.04	.54	.20	−.87	−.25
I_g	−.21	−.14	−.51	−.24	−.07	−.02	.44	.21	−.79	−.29

[a] n.e. = Variable not entered into the regression in Table 7.6.

and female wages in determining household income) has a negative sign in the regression on m and a positive sign in the regression on I_g (we experimented with this variable in the prewar regressions and never found it to be significant there). Only the sign on male wages is inconsistent with the standard neoclassical hypothesis. Our view—hinted at previously in the discussion of the results for 1925 and 1930—is that once the patriarchal system gives way and leverage over children ceases to yield net economic return, natural fertility gives way to parity-specific control and the degree of

TABLE 7.11

β Coefficients and Elasticities for Selected Variables from Regressions for 1930 in Table 7.8

	Variables									
	Infant mortality rate *IMR*		Index of permanent sterility *STER*		Proxy for mother's education *PNEF*		Proxy for son's education *PEDHMB*		Proxy for daughter's education *PEDHEB*	
Dependent variable	β	Elas-ticity	β	Elas-ticity	β	Elas-ticity	β	Elas-ticity	β	Elas-ticity
m	.46	1.0	n.e.[a]	n.e.	n.e.	n.e.	−.26	−.46	.78	.97
M	−.27	−.16	−.46	−.18	.03	.01	.94	.38	−1.06	−.34
I_g	−.35	−.26	−.48	−.24	.06	.02	.58	.35	−.84	−.36

[a] n.e. = Variable not entered into the regression in Table 7.8.

TABLE 7.12

Marital Fertility, the Diffusion of Parity-Specific Control, and the Spacing of Births in the Prefectures of Japan: Cross Sections, 1950 and 1960

Constant and independent variables	Dependent variable[a] and year			
	m (1950)	I_g (1950)	m (1960)	I_g (1960)
Constant	−.2	.9[e]	−1.6	.8[e]
Independent variables				
Demographic variables				
Infant mortality rate *IMR*	1.5	−1.4[f]	−3.6	−1.3[g]
Labor force variables				
Proportion male labor force dependent on primary industry *PPIM*	−1.2[f]	.2[f]	−.2	−.1
Real wage for males[b] *RWM*	.2	−.09	.7	−.1
Real wage for females[b] *RWF*	1.2[e]	−.3[f]	2.1[e]	−.2[e]
Product of male and female wages[c] *RWP*	−.2[g]	.6[g]	−.4[f]	.04[e]
Education[d]				
Proxy for education of children				
Proportion of males in age group 30–34 in 1970 completing some schooling, who completed higher education *PEDHMC*	−1.6[g]	.3	−.5	.4
Proportion of females in age group 30–34 in 1970 completing some schooling, who completed higher education *PEDHFC*	2.1[e]	−.5[f]	.7	−.2[g]
R^2	.44	.49	.45	.53
Adjusted R^2	.34	.39	.35	.44

[a] All are one-tailed tests except for *IMR* in regression on m.
[b] Estimated nominal daily wages deflated by a price index that sets the price index for "all urban Japan" in 1950–1951 equal to 100.
[c] $RWP = RWM \cdot RWF$.
[d] These are based on 1970 census data.
[e] Significant at the 1 percent level.
[f] Significant at the 5 percent level.
[g] Significant at the 10 percent level.

control is largely determined by the variables pinpointed by the neoclassical school.

We have now completed our discussion of the cross sections, and we can turn to an analysis of trends. We concentrate on trends in m and I_g because, as previously noted, we did not set up these data so that M could be properly analyzed (but, see Chapter 5 for evidence concerning trends in natural fertility). We felt more comfortable about using the educational proxies for 1950 than for 1960 (because many children born around 1960 had not yet

TABLE 7.13

Marital Fertility, the Diffusion of Parity-Specific Control, and the Spacing of Births in the Prefectures of Japan: Cross Sections, 1950 and 1960: Logarithmic Specification[a]

Constant and independent variables	Dependent variables[b] and year			
	m (1950)	I_g (1950)	*m* (1960)	I_g (1960)
Constant	.4	−1.3[c]	.4	−1.9[c]
Independent variables				
Infant mortality rate *IMR*	.2	−.2[c]	−.03	−.3[d]
Labor force variables				
Proportion male labor force dependent on primary industry *PPIM*	−.09	.05	.08	−.03
Real wage for males *RWM*	−.2	−.1	.01	−.07
Real wage for females *RWF*	.8	−.2	.9[c]	−.4[c]
Education				
Proxy for education of children				
Proportion of males in age group 30–34 in 1970 completing some schooling, who completed higher education *PEDHMC*	−.4	.1	−.02	.09
Proportion of females in age group 30–34 in 1970 completing some schooling, who completed higher education *PEDHFC*	.9[d]	−.4[d]	.2	−.3[d]
R^2	.34	.46	.47	.46
Adjusted R^2	.24	.38	.39	.38

[a] The logarithms of every variable (dependent and independent) are entered rather than the variables themselves. When a variable takes on values close to 0, 1 was added to the variable, and then the logarithm was taken. See Table 7.12 for a discussion of the definitions of certain of the variables.

[b] All are one-tailed tests except for *IMR* in regression on *m*.

[c] Significant at the 1 percent level.

[d] Significant at the 5 percent level.

completed their education by 1970 when the information was secured by the census takers) and so attention was restricted to trends between 1925 and 1950 (Table 7.14) and trends between 1930 and 1950 (Table 7.15). The results must be treated with caution because it was difficult to match trends in all the variables satisfactorily (e.g., the proxies for education), but it is worth briefly going through the findings. The results for female education are consistent with the thesis—trends in the proportion of females securing advanced education tend to be positively associated with trends in *m* and negatively associated with trends in I_g (when the coefficients are significant). The results involving dependence on primary industry are also consistent with the thesis (note that trends in *PPIM* tend to be negative). The results

TABLE 7.14

Trends[a] in Marital Fertility and the Diffusion of Parity-Specific Control: Prefectures of Japan, 1925–1950

			Demographic variable	Labor force variables			Education			
							Proportion of children receiving higher education[d]			
Trend period	Dependent variable	Constant	Infant mortality rate *IMR*	Proportion of male labor force in primary industry *PPIM*[b]	Real male wage *RWM*[c]	Real female wage *RWF*[c]	Males	Females	R^2	Adjusted R^2
Linear specification										
1925–1950	m	.09	−3.2[e]	−.72[f]	.11	−.09	−.63	1.28[e]	.48	.40
1925–1950	I_g	−.01	−.58	−.02	−.02	.03	−.49	.12	.18	.06
Logarithmic specification										
1925–1950	m	.81[f]	−.04	−.86[e]	.36	−.76	−.47	.95[e]	.38	.28
1925–1950	I_g	.14	.06	.05	−.17	.15	−.43	−.21[f]	.24	.12

[a] Trends in each variable are computed as $(X_{t_2} - X_{t_1})$, where X_{t_1} and X_{t_2} are the values of the variable X_t in year $t = t_1$ and t_2, $t_2 > t_1$. All variables have been entered as trends in the regressions in linear specification; their logarithms are entered in logarithmic specification. All tests are one tailed.

[b] The figure for 1925 is actually for 1920 and was taken from the 1920 census, when this trend was calculated.

[c] Trends in nominal daily wages which have been deflated by a price index which sets the price index for "all urban" Japan in 1950–1951 = 100.

[d] Based on 1970 census data, this is the difference between proportion of persons completing some schooling aged 30–34 who have graduated from a school above a postwar junior high school minus the proportion aged 55–64 completing some schooling who graduated from a school above a prewar elementary school.

[e] Significant at the 1 percent level.

[f] Significant at the 5 percent level.

TABLE 7.15

Trends[a] in Marital Fertility and the Diffusion of Parity-Specific Control: Prefectures of Japan, 1930–1950

			Demographic variable	Labor force variables			Education			
							Proportion of children receiving higher education[c]			
Trend period	Dependent variable	Constant	Infant mortality rate *IMR*	Proportion of male labor in primary industry *PPIM*	Real male wage *RWM*[b]	Real female wage *RWF*[b]	Males	Females	R^2	Adjusted R^2
Linear specification										
1930–1950	m	.13	−1.50	.27	.16	−.09	−.15	1.29[d]	.32	.22
1930–1950	I_g	−.39	.41	.24[e]	−.03	.02	−.09	−.15	.71	.66
Logarithmic specification										
1930–1950	m	.82[e]	−.04	−.87[d]	.36	−.76	−.47	.96[d]	.38	.28
1930–1950	I_g	−.04	.11	.18[e]	−.17	.01	−.06	−.04	.63	.57

[a] Trends in each variable are computed as $(X_{t_2} - X_{t_1})$, where X_{t_1} and X_{t_2} are the values of variable X_t in the year $t = t_1$ and $t_2, t_2 > t_1$. All variables have been entered as trends in the regressions in linear specification; their logarithms are entered in logarithmic specification. All tests are one tailed.

[b] Trends in nominal daily wages that have been deflated by a price index that sets the price index for "all urban" Japan in 1950–1951 = 100.

[c] Based on 1970 census data, this is the difference between proportion of persons completing some schooling aged 30–34 who have graduated from a school above a postwar junior high school minus the proportion aged 55–64 completing some schooling who graduated from a school above a prewar elementary school.

[d] Significant at the 1 percent level.

[e] Significant at the 5 percent level.

concerning male and female wages are erratic, and we found them difficult to interpret in a satisfactory manner. Further work must be done with these trends before a fully satisfactory interpretation of them is possible, and so we present these results in a very tentative manner.

It is now possible to tie these results and those in Chapter 5 together and suggest their implications for the dynamics of the Japanese transition. What we shown is that the structure of the premodern demographic regime persisted for a long time in Japan, and, ignoring the question of natural fertility for a moment, that the relationship between natural fertility, infant mortality, and nuptiality continues into the 1950s, when the patriarchal stem family system finally gives way to modernization in labor markets (especially with regard to education) and technology. Moreover, these same variables appear to play a crucial role in accounting for the diffusion of parity-specific control and the decline in marital fertility. The speed of the upward surge in *m* after the war, however, is not really explicable in these terms because the erosion of the patriarchal stem family system appears to have been a very gradual process. In accounting for the speed of the decline, four factors come to mind. First, there are the legal changes associated with the National Eugenics Law, which reduced the costs of controlling births. Second, there is the reduction of income in the late 1940s and early 1950s relative to the late 1930s. We have seen that the income constraint is important empirically and the depressed early postwar income levels were probably important in encouraging control. Third, education was rendered compulsory for both sexes through middle school, perhaps reducing further in some quarters the economic benefits parents could expect to secure from the offspring (this is undoubtedly a minor factor in light of the already declining leverage of parents over children). Fourth, the new family code enhanced the relative legal and social position of women within the *ie*, facilitating her right to divorce her husband and secure property and income in a divorce settlement. Thus the quantifiable variables introduced into the analysis and discussed in Tables 7.6 – 7.15 explain only part, if albeit a very crucial part, of our story. The institutional changes associated with the American occupation also played a part—especially in producing a *swift* drop in marital fertility during the decade of the 1950s. In short, the implication of the analysis is that the downward trend in marital fertility occasioned by the changes we pinpointed was well underway prior to 1940, and the specific institutional developments associated with the United States' control over Japan only served to accelerate the long-term movements.

Finally, in closing this discussion, mention must be made of developments concerning nuptiality. Insofar as the trends through the mid-1950s are concerned, the analysis carried out in Chapter 5 applies. By the late

1950s, however, a new phenomenon appears to emerge, one whose traces we can detect in Table 5.8 in the regression for 1960. Here we see that *m* has begun to emerge as a determinant of the age of marriage. This suggests that as the patriarchal control over nuptiality finally came to an end as it had in Sweden over half a century earlier, the ability to effectively control reproduction (i.e., the ease at which a married woman could stay in the labor force before, and reenter after, having children) was becoming a factor in determining nuptiality patterns. We have already discussed in some detail in Chapter 6 how nuptiality adjusts in such an environment, and we shall return to this issue at much greater length in Chapter 8, where we examine Swedish nuptiality patterns during and after the Swedish fertility transition.

Now we would like to turn to an exploratory analysis of the relationship between social status and marital fertility. Although the theoretical chapter does not touch directly on these issues, there are some implications of the approach that bear on the question of social status, and we would like to consider briefly their theoretical and empirical nature in the next section.

7.5. Social Status and the Fertility Transition: The Rural and Urban Sectors of the Prefectures, 1925–1960

In examining data for the rural and urban sector of the Japanese prefectures we had in mind two goals, which the previous exploration of this material in Chapter 5 motivated. The principal goal was to probe the relationships between social status and the fertility transition. In particular, we wished to explore two facets of this connection. First, there is the question of whether groups enjoying higher status tended, *ceteris paribus,* to adopt practices of control earlier than others. The logic of the argument is that children wish to be placed in positions with comparable (or higher) status from that of the parents. Because education serves initially as a screening device for jobs that carry status, parents of these children lose leverage over their offspring comparatively quickly. Second, social status is a factor insofar as the distribution of assets and income, which helps fashion the status, in communities (especially agricultural villages) conditions the labor market and, in particular, the facility with which higher income groups can secure hired labor as substitutes for their own family labor. This elasticity of supply of hired labor, remember, is important in shaping the response of demand for child labor to increases in the standard of living—the more elastic the supply, the more rapidly does the demand for labor services from one's children fall off. The second goal is to more fully develop some of the empirical relationships developed in the previous section.

We shall commence the investigations with the rural districts, because,

TABLE 7.16

Means and Standard Deviations[a] for Measures of Marital Fertility and Nuptiality and Urban–Rural Relatives, 1930–1960, for Groups of Prefectures Defined in Terms of Percentage Occupied Male Labor Force in Primary Industry (*PPIM*) in 1930

	Marital fertility								Nuptiality							
	Hutterite index I_g						Urban I_g divided by rural I_g		Hutterite index I_m						Urban I_m divided by rural I_m	
	Rural			Urban					Rural			Urban				
Group	1930	1950	1960	1930	1950	1960	1950	1960	1930	1950	1960	1930	1950	1960	1950	1960
$PPIM \leq 29.9\%$	.52	.50	.30	.43	.44	.28	.88	.94	.67	.57	.56	.63	.58	.54	1.00	.97
	(.06)	(.05)	(.02)	(.02)	(.04)	(.01)	(.07)	(.06)	(.02)	(.02)	(.05)	(.06)	(.02)	(.04)	(.47)	(.13)
$30\% \leq PPIM \leq 49.9\%$	.54	.50	.29	.43	.45	.28	.89	.96	.71	.61	.63	.64	.58	.58	.95	.92
	(.05)	(.07)	(.04)	(.05)	(.06)	(.03)	(.04)	(.06)	(.03)	(.03)	(.04)	(.03)	(.03)	(.03)	(.34)	(.03)
$50\% \leq PPIM \leq 54.9\%$	.57	.50	.28	.46	.44	.28	.88	.98	.70	.61	.63	.60	.56	.58	.92	.93
	(.05)	(.05)	(.04)	(.04)	(.04)	(.03)	(.03)	(.04)	(.04)	(.03)	(.03)	(.05)	(.06)	(.04)	(.05)	(.04)
$55\% \leq PPIM \leq 59.9\%$	.58	.53	.30	.48	.45	.28	.85	.95	.69	.59	.63	.59	.57	.57	.96	.91
	(.07)	(.05)	(.03)	(.07)	(.04)	(.02)	(.04)	(.05)	(.05)	(.04)	(.04)	(.03)	(.02)	(.03)	(.04)	(.02)
$60\% \leq PPIM$	.60	.56	.42	.50	.49	.29	.88	.95	.73	.62	.66	.59	.56	.59	.91	.90
	(.06)	(.04)	(.05)	(.05)	(.04)	(.03)	(.02)	(.04)	(.04)	(.03)	(.02)	(.04)	(.02)	(.02)	(.04)	(.02)

[a] The standard deviations are in parenthesis under the means for the variables.

owing to the richness of quantifiable material available for rural districts, they reveal the most useful information about these issues. Table 7.16 provides us with a perspective on rural fertility. It demonstrates two points that will be useful in what follows. First, it shows that up until the close of the fertility transition, the rural value of marital fertility fell but remained *slightly* higher than that obtaining in the corresponding urban area (on this point see Mosk, 1977, 1979a, and 1980b). This testifies to two assertions maintained in the analysis. First, rural marital fertility is higher than that in the urban areas during the transition because the occupational structure of the cities tends to discourage the utilization of child labor and encourages the wife to seek employment outside her home. The importance of education is felt more keenly in the cities than the villages at any given time because placement in urban jobs is generally required for *all* male children (not just second and third sons, etc.) and this works to weaken the urban patriarch's position more rapidly than is the case in the village. But the comparatively *tiny* gap between rural and urban marital fertility is intriguing for another reason. In light of the substantial variation in rural fertility across the prefectures, the slightness of the margin suggests that urban and rural marital fertility within each prefecture must have influenced each other through migration and information flows. As we have argued previously, frequency of contact with controllers reduces the costs of regulation. Thus if urban populations initiate the transition within a prefecture, because the gap between desired fertility and natural fertility is wider for them than for rural populations surrounding them, their practices tend to reduce the costs of control for the villagers who subsequently follow them through the transition. Here we would expect the influence to flow from the cities to the countryside. However, because many residents of the cities in a prefecture are migrants from the neighboring villages and towns and tend to emulate (because of the social and psychological conditioning, the noneconomic costs of regulation) the reproductive behavior characteristic of their home districts (with some modification), the influence presumably runs the other way as well. That is, the costs of regulation deter rural to urban migrants from cutting back on their reproductive performance as rapidly as those born and raised in cities. The second facet of this table worthy of note concerns the nuptiality differentiations. The persistence of the pattern we observed for Japan in 1925 (see Chapter 5 and the contrast to the Swedish patterns noted in Chapter 6) bolsters the contention, elaborated in the previous section, that the influence of the patriarchal stem family system over nuptiality was being dissipated only gradually.[10] In short, the linkage of rural and urban natality is seen in both marital fertility and nuptiality during Japan's fertility transition.

Now let us turn to a detailed analysis of rural fertility to ferret out those determinants that are characteristic of the rural communities themselves. Table 7.17 contains the relevant results for the prewar period in the form of cross-sectional regressions for 1925 and 1930. As before, we attempt to capture both the distribution of assets and income and social status with two variables: the proportion of cultivable hectares owned (*PCHO*) and the proportion of occupied women who are domestic servants (*PDSF*). The latter variable may also measure, in part, the standard of living, but we have tried to capture this variable separately with the variable for real male agricultural wages. The variables that measure structure of the labor force (*PPIM*) and dependence on silk raising (*PCHM*) are meant to be proxies for the demand for child labor. Finally, the infant mortality rate and the stillbirth rate are designed to capture factors that hold down natural fertility.

The findings concerning the demographic variables confirm what we have already learned from the prefectural regressions on *M* for 1925 and 1930, namely, that there were still significant constraints on natural fertility during the interwar period, and they involved infant mortality, a point central to the model of the evolution of the premodern demographic regime. The coefficients of the variables that stand for the demand for labor services from children also have the expected signs whenever they are significant. Moreover, the measures of social structure also are consistent with the theoretical analysis. Higher social status is associated with lower fertility (note the negative coefficient on the variable measuring the degree of landownership). Moreover, the coefficients on the proportion of occupied women who are servants and real male agricultural wages are also negative, supporting the notion that a skewed distribution of assets and improvements in the standard of living work to reduce overall dependence on child labor.[11] These results all come through very robustly. However, the most tantalizing finding concerns female wages. The coefficient on this variable is always *positive* and significant in the prewar cross sections. This result, which runs exactly counter to the "cost of time" hypothesis, is easily explicable in terms of the model of the patriarchal stem family system. For, as previously argued, those influences that enhance the absolute and relative economic value of girls as compared with boys tend to encourage couples to keep female babies when they are born rather than dispose of them through acts of infanticide. This, of course, presumes that the patriarch can secure rents from his daughters through his control of the arrangement of the marriages of daughters, and it also assumes that infanticide was sex specific, a point we have advanced evidence on previously.

Findings for the postwar period, 1950 and 1960, given in Table 7.18, are also worthy of examination here. They demonstrate a reversal of the role of the labor force variables, real wages, as compared with the prewar cross sections. The variable expressing the product of male and female wages is

TABLE 7.17

Labor Force, Wages, Status, and Marital Fertility in Rural Japan: Cross Sections, 1925 and 1930

			Demographic variables		Structural variables				Labor force variables			
Year	Dependent variable	Constant	Infant mortality rate *IMR*	Still-birth rate *SBR*	Proportion of cultivable hectares owned *PCHO*	Proportion of cultivable hectares in mulberry production *PCHM*	Proportion of male labor force in primary industry *PPIM*[a]	Proportion of occupied women who are domestic servants *PDSF*	Real male agricultural wages *RAWM*[b]	Real female agricultural wages *RAWF*[b]	R^2	Adjusted R^2
Linear specification												
1925	I_g	.59[c]	−.01	−1.11[d]	−.16[d]	.02	.16[d]	−.03[d]	−.13[c]	.23[c]	.63	.55
1930	I_g	.35[d]	.10	−1.81[d]	−.06	.01	.34[c]	.35	−.18[c]	.33[c]	.66	.58
Logarithmic specification												
1925	I_g	−12.4[d]	−.02	−.09[d]	−.12[d]	−.01	.15[d]	−.05[d]	−.41[c]	.56[c]	.66	.58
1930	I_g	−.85[c]	−.01	−.18[c]	−.04	−.0003	.18[c]	.01	−.68[c]	.83[c]	.67	.60

[a] For the 1925 regression these variables are computed from 1920 census data and entered into the equations. In the 1920 case, *PPIM* is percentage labor force in agriculture, not primary industry (i.e., it excludes fishing and forestry, both categories of which are very small.)

[b] Estimated nominal daily agricultural wages deflated by a rural price index based on rural and urban prices that sets equal to 100 the price index for these goods in "all urban" Japan for 1950–1951. See Appendix 3.

[c] Significant at the 1 percent level. All are one-tailed tests except for tests on *RAWM* and *RAWF*.

[d] Significant at the 5 percent level.

TABLE 7.18

Labor Force, Wages, and Marital Fertility in Rural Japan: Cross Sections and Trends[a], 1950 and 1960

					Labor force variables				
Year or trend period	Dependent variable	Constant	Infant mortality rate *IMR*	Male labor force in primary industry *PPIM*	Real male agricultural wages *RAWM*[b]	Real female agricultural wages *RAWF*[b]	Product of real male and female agricultural wages *RAWP*[c]	R^2	Adjusted R^2
1950	I_g	1.08[d]	−.37	.14	−.27[f]	−.27	.11[g]	.24	.14
1960	I_g	.85[d]	−.95	−.02	−.21[d]	−.19[d]	.08[d]	.44	.37
1950–1960	I_g	−.23[d]	.67	−.26[e]	−.13[e]	−.25[d]	.08[d]	.45	.38

[a] Regression on absolute trends in all variables where the absolute trend in variable x_t between time t_1 and t_2, $t_1 < t_2$, is $X_{t_2} - X_{t_1}$.

[b] Estimated nominal daily agricultural wages deflated by a rural price index based on rural and urban prices that sets equal to 100 the price index for these goods in "all urban" Japan for 1950–1951. See Appendix 3.

[c] $RAWP = RAWM \cdot RAWF$.

[d] Significant at the 1 percent level (two-tailed test).

[e] Significant at the 5 percent level (two-tailed test).

[f] Significant at the 10 percent level (two-tailed test).

[g] Significant at the 15 percent level (two-tailed test).

TABLE 7.19

Wages, Labor Force, and Marital Fertility in Urban Sectors of the Prefectures of Japan: Cross Sections, 1925 and 1930

Year	Dependent variable	Constant	Demographic variables: Infant mortality rate IMR	Demographic variables: Still-birth rate SBR	Structural variables[a]: Proportion male labor force in manufacturing $PMAM$	Structural variables[a]: Proportion occupied women who are domestic servants $PDSF$	Labor force variables[b]: Real male manufacturing wages $RNAWM$	Labor force variables[b]: Real female manufacturing wages $RNAWF$	R^2	Adjusted R^2
Linear specification										
1925	I_g	.9[c]	−.7[d]	−1.3[d]	−.01	1.1	−.03[e]	−.1[d]	.47	.38
1930	I_g	.9[c]	−1.1[c]	−1.4[c]	−.1	.1	−.02	−.1[c]	.50	.43
Logarithmic specification										
1925	I_g	−1.3[c]	−.16[d]	−.19[d]	.15	.003	−.16	−.34[c]	.43	.34
1930	I_g	−1.7[c]	−.31[c]	−.18[d]	−.07	.03	−.12	−.29[c]	.50	.43

[a] For the 1925 regression these variables are calculated from 1920 census data.

[b] Estimated nominal daily factory wages deflated by price index with all urban Japan in 1950–1951 = 100 for the prefectures in which the urban area is located for 1930 in the 1925 and 1930 regressions.

[c] Significant at the 1 percent level. All are one-tailed tests except for the *RNAWM* and *RNAWF* variables.

[d] Significant at the 5 percent level.

[e] Significant at the 15 percent level.

significant here, and it points to the nonlinearities in the relationship between income and fertility mentioned previously. This is in keeping with conclusions reached in Chapter 5. With the collapse of the patriarchal stem family system and the premodern demographic regime during the decade of the 1950s, children no longer offered a net economic advantage and were valued primarily for their contributions to parental satisfaction in the sense of consumption. Moreover, women were less entrammeled by the patriarchal system. Thus the coefficients on the real wage variables for 1960 are consistent with the "income constraint" and "cost of time" hypotheses.

Finally, the results concerning trends over the period 1950–1960 (also given in Table 7.18 along with the cross sections) bolster these points in a slightly different fashion. The results for the short trend period 1950–1960 testify to the new role male and female wages play in the determination of marital fertility, once the patriarchal stem family system and the dependence on the family labor have given way.

Now let us turn our attention to the data for urban areas. Consider Table 7.19, which provides the principal analytical findings for the urban districts of prewar Japan. The variables are self-explanatory except for the measure of male labor force composition. Here we use the proportion of males in manufacturing as a proxy, albeit a crude one, for the preponderance of modern factory work in which the worker serves as an employee and not as self-employed. Retail and wholesale trades are dominated by self-employed workers who commonly utilized family labor in running their operations.

The results seem relatively clear, particularly when read in conjunction with the previous analysis. During the period 1925–1930, when natural fertility still dominated marital fertility in most urban areas, the demographic variables that represent constraints on natural fertility play the role we expect. So does the rural marital fertility rate. The proxies for (inverse) demand for child labor and the income constraint, the variable measuring the incidence of domestic service being a proxy for both income and perhaps the demand for child labor, are not significant in any of these equations, so inferences about them are difficult to draw. However, the real wage variables, especially female wages, behave in general as we would expect. For the results concerning these variables suggest, as the model implies, that in urban areas, once modern economic growth is well underway, the functioning of the patriarchal stem family system is eroded relatively quickly, and married women actually begin to seek work in the labor market outside the home. In general, the operation of urban labor markets—with regard to opportunities for the patriarch's children and his wife—undercuts the natural fertility strategy of the patriarchal stem family system. These points can also be seen in the postwar cross sections (for 1950 and 1960) given in Table 7.20. The variable giving the product of male and female wages turned out to be significant in 1960 as did female wages.

TABLE 7.20

Wages, Labor Force, and Marital Fertility in Urban Sectors of the Prefectures of Japan: Cross Sections, 1950 and 1960

					Labor force variables[a]				
Year	Dependent variable	Constant	Infant mortality rate *IMR*	Proportion male labor force in manufacturing *PMAM*	Real male manufacturing wages *RNAWM*	Real female manufacturing wages *RNAWF*	Product of real male and female manufacturing wages *RNAWP*	R^2	Adjusted R^2
1950	I_g	.5[b]	.4	−.4[b]	−.04[b]	−.07[c]	n.e.	.28	.21
1950	I_g	.5[b]	.5	−.4[b]	.03	−.10	.08	.29	.20
1960	I_g	.3[b]	−1.1	−.08	.01	−.01	n.e.	.06	.00
1960	I_g	.7[b]	−1.0	−.06	−.05	−.15[d]	.25[e]	.12	.01

[a] Estimated nominal daily wages in manufacturing for the prefecture in which the urban area is located deflated by price index with all urban Japan in 1950–1951 = 100 for the prefectures in which the urban area is located in 1950 and 1960. $RNAWP = RNAWM \cdot RNAWF$.

[b] Significant at the 1 percent level. All are two-tailed tests. n.e. = Not entered into the regression as an independent variable.

[c] Significant at the 5 percent level.

[d] Significant at the 10 percent level.

[e] Significant at the 15 percent level.

By way of closing this discussion of the marital fertility of rural and urban sectors, it is useful to consider estimates we have worked out of the Coale–Trussell parameters M and m for a group of cities and the corresponding "rural" hinterlands in 1930.[12] The results bear directly on our previous discussion concerning Table 7.1 and are presented in Table 7.21. What is striking about these figures is that the rural–urban differential in marital fertility for the prewar years appears to largely stem from differentials in

TABLE 7.21

Rural–Urban Differentials in M and m, 1930

Prefecture, city, or rural sector	M	m	m 25–29	30–34	35–39	40–44	45–49
Hokkaidō							
Sapporo	.74	.24	.25	.41	.35	.35	.09
Otaru	.64	.15	.08	.21	.37	.32	−.07
Hakodate	.69	.35	.49	.32	.39	.40	.30
Rural	.75	.10	.13	.13	.12	.12	.06
Miyagi							
Sendai	.67	.10	.10	.15	.20	.29	−.08
Rural	.80	.17	.24	.16	.14	.19	.18
Tokyo							
Tokyo	.59	.29	.27	.33	.35	.39	.20
Rural	.60	.12	.04	.16	.20	.24	.01
Kanagawa							
Yokohama	.59	.13	.07	.19	.25	.29	−.04
Rural	.69	.02	−.02	.06	.07	.09	−.05
Niigata							
Niigata	.77	.39	.26	.42	.34	.52	.30
Rural	.88	.41	.53	.30	.26	.29	.57
Ishikawa							
Kanazawa	.61	.49	.60	.52	.37	.50	.52
Rural	.70	.39	.54	.34	.23	.31	.52
Aichi							
Nagoya	.67	.42	.44	.42	.39	.44	.41
Rural	.78	.45	.61	.39	.33	.33	.58
Kyōto							
Kyōto	.60	.23	.45	.03	.18	.33	.21
Rural	.70	.46	.51	.43	.36	.44	.52
Ōsaka							
Ōsaka	.82	.35	.24	.33	.40	.49	.24
Sakai	.53	.25	.11	.26	.39	.42	.08
Rural	.63	.43	.50	.31	.29	.36	.55
Hyōgo							
Kobe	.54	.29	.17	.32	.41	.42	.15
Rural	.63	.29	.40	.27	.27	.29	.30

Table 7.21 continues

TABLE 7.21 (Cont.)

Prefecture, city, or rural sector	M	m	m 25–29	30–34	35–39	40–44	45–49
Okayama							
Okayama	.49	.24	.03	.45	.38	.61	−.12
Rural	.60	.40	.35	.39	.42	.47	.35
Hiroshima							
Hiroshima	.51	.23	.25	.29	.38	.44	.00
Kure	.53	.19	.08	.26	.23	.33	.07
Rural	.69	.31	.39	.26	.30	.36	.29
Fukuoka							
Fukuoka	.55	.02	−.11	.13	.19	.27	−.23
Yawata	.54	.18	.14	.12	.21	.37	.04
Rural	.62	.04	−.06	.08	.12	.18	−.09
Nagasaki							
Nagasaki	.54	.17	.11	.21	.18	.26	.09
Rural	.64	−.13	−.23	−.03	−.01	.05	−.32
Kumamoto							
Kumamoto	.53	−.13	−.41	−.06	.13	.10	−.39
Rural	.71	−.03	.03	−.14	.06	.09	.15
Kagoshima							
Kagoshima	.53	−.09	−.10	−.12	.00	−.00	−.18
Rural	.74	−.17	−.28	−.03	.03	.03	−.40

natural fertility M. This confirms the idea presented at several points preceding that, during the prewar period, urban populations faced considerably greater costs to reducing natality than the rural populations that entered the transitions later, and, consequently, city dwellers favored a strategy of lengthening birth intervals. More importantly the narrowness in rural–urban differences in values of m taken in conjunction with the gaps in M bolsters a contention made previously when we were analyzing the regressions with M as dependent variable reported on Table 7.6. Namely, rural populations, especially farmers, were reluctant to reduce M below that constrained by environmental conditions like infant mortality and health because M was crucial to the life-cycle demographic strategy.[13] By contrast, city dwellers, and other populations for whom the life-cycle strategy was of minimal consequence, were perfectly willing to manipulate natural fertility to reduce overall reproduction. This means that by 1930 M was being determined by two sets of factors: natural limits and adjustments to those limits that were fashioned to *maximize* surviving family size, and which almost wholly fixed its level in the agricultural districts; and efforts consciously designed to reduce total fertility and surviving family size that, together with natural limits, conditioned natural fertility in industrial districts.

To summarize: In this section we examined a wide variety of evidence concerning the determinants of rural and urban marital fertility in Japan. As a whole, it does yield considerable support for the theoretical approach and sheds interesting light on many facets of the dynamics of the Japanese fertility transition.

7.6. Conclusions

In this chapter we continued and concluded the empirical testing of the model for Japan begun in Chapter 5. The primary findings presented in this chapter bear on the importance of education in the fertility transition and the movement toward a situation in which labor markets affect marital fertility along the lines of the "cost of time" hypothesis. The task that remains before us, and which will occupy our attention in the next chapter, is verifying that the model also explains the fertility transition in Sweden. Once we have accomplished this, we can fairly claim that the model is not only consistent with observed Japanese patterns, but also reasonable and plausible. Moreover, we can also argue that the model can explain at least some of the diversity in fertility transitions that we noted in Chapter 1.

Notes to Chapter 7

1. See, among others, Hashimoto (1974), Ohbuchi (1976), Tsubouchi (1970), and Yamamura and Hanley (1975). The list of studies referred to here is hardly complete. It does include, however, the major writings concerning the Japanese transition that utilize systematically worked out analytical theory and econometrical testing of that theory. For a discussion of some of the literature on this subject, which does not deal with formal models, see Taeuber (1958).

2. However, the ban did not apply to private consultation between a doctor and a patient. For pamphlets issued by doctors in which contraceptive devices are discussed, see Ōta (1969). Margaret Sanger describes how the police governor in Tokyo refused to permit her to speak about birth control during her trip to Japan in 1921 because contraception was a dangerous thought covered by the Dangerous Thought Law. See Sanger (1938:318–328).

3. As mentioned in Chapter 5, we cannot definitely establish when the Japanese transition commenced. From the data on m for 1925 it would appear that it was just getting started after World War I.

4. In Mosk (1979a:28), using slightly different estimates of M and m, we show that the linear correlation between the two variables is negative (−.48).

5. It should be noted that Japan experienced an influenza epidemic just prior to 1920, and it may have had some ramifications on the 1920 figures. These figures are not out of line with those for the prewar period in general, however, because the recorded infant mortality rates around the turn of the century appear somewhat to exceed those for 1920 (and it should be stressed that the figures around 1900 are probably still substantially biased downward because

of underregistration of infant deaths and births, a problem that had assuredly diminished by the 1920s) and because the rates throughout the interwar period reveal a gradual uninterrupted downward trend from the levels obtaining around 1920. See Chapter xiv of Taeuber (1958) regarding the mortality decline in Japan.

6. This is less true after the 1960s than it was prior to the 1960s, though it still remains an important factor in the labor market of Japan, as well as in Europe. It has been customary for Japanese firms to grant a woman a substantial "retirement" bonus when she leaves work to get married, but more recently many married women have stayed on to work, so this practice, reflective of the ideology of the patriarchal stem family system, has diminished in importance.

7. It should be noted that migration affects these averages, and perhaps biases the figures upward for the industrial prefectures and downward for the agricultural zones because the census data are for those resident in the prefecture as of October 1, 1970. Presumably many such residents in the five industrial prefectures migrated from rural areas to the industrial regions. The issue is as follows: Were they the best educated within their generation of those growing up in their places of origin? And, were children actually born and raised within the industrial prefectures securing a more advanced schooling than the immigrants, on average? The 1970 census data do not give us definitive answers to these problems. See Thomas (1938) for a discussion of some of the general issues raised here.

8. In previous versions of this work, we experimented with a variable calculated by taking the average value for m for the prefectures contiguous to the prefecture for which the observation is taken. The idea behind this variable is that it is a proxy for the costs of regulating marital fertility. The notion is that information about, and social approval of, birth control techniques is diffused through individual contact. Thus if m is high in the districts immediately surrounding a population, one would assume contact with controllers would also be frequent. This would stand in contrast to a prefecture where average m is the dependent variable. However, the contiguous prefecture m variable probably also captures unspecified regional effects not picked up by the other independent variables and, as a consequence, is difficult to interpret. For this reason we decided to omit this variable in the final presentation of the findings, even though it is an interesting proxy for the costs of controlling fertility within marriage.

A similar though slightly more rigorous approach to capturing this "cost of controlling" variable would be to use a "gravity model" (i.e., to calculate the proxy with values of m for every other prefecture in the country divided through by the square of its mean distance away from the prefecture under observation). I am grateful to Ronald Lee for suggesting these two approaches.

9. "Advanced" or "higher" education here refers to schooling completed beyond that stipulated in the compulsory legal requirements (i.e., beyond the legal minimum).

10. The proportions married (I_m) may also reflect migration of females for jobs as well as age structure.

11. That is, the effect of the income constraint (which would render a positive association between income and marital fertility) is dominated by the reduced demand for labor services stemming from the conditions in the labor market and the standard of living. We would expect the pure "income constraint" effect to be more pervasive in urban and industrial populations where the demand for child labor services are relatively slight to begin with. This probably explains why, when we analyze prefectural data that includes a great mix of occupational structures as in Table 7.6, the two effects tend to cancel out (because one dominates in the agricultural districts and the other in the industrial zones) whereas analysis of rural areas alone reveals one dominant association.

12. The special volumes that give age-specific fertility rates for the prefectures in 1925 and 1930 also provide figures for the cities with populations of 100,000 or over as of the previous

census. The term "rural" here refers to the remainder of the prefecture (i.e., that outside the city or cities with 100,000 persons or more).

13. To the extent that infant mortality rates soar and health is generally poor in cities because of poor sanitation, overcrowding, and the like, natural fertility in cities may on those grounds alone fall short of that characteristic of the surrounding agricultural communities. It is unlikely, however, that this argument can account for the entire spread in natural fertility observed for most of these prefectures.

CHAPTER 8

Comparison with the Fertility Transition in Sweden

8.1. Introduction

In the last chapter we analyzed the Japanese transition. In this chapter we continue the comparisons with the history of Swedish fertility begun in Chapter 6, concentrating here on the Swedish fertility decline. As with the findings for Japan previously discussed, we have been forced to work with data that are far from perfect. Proxies for the variables concerned with in the theory are far from ideal, and for this reason the results must be interpreted with caution and delicacy. Nevertheless, the statistical analysis and the related discussion of qualitative material lends important support for the views discussed here.

Again, as mentioned in Chapter 7, the interpretations and quantitative results do not necessarily agree with earlier studies. It should be emphasized, however, that although this is perhaps partly because of the methodological approach we adopt, it probably stems primarily from the nature of the data we worked with as compared with the materials others worked with. As the reader can ascertain from Appendix 6, a detailed set of figures for the counties of Sweden have been assembled, and the rural and urban sectors of these counties, that cover the years 1880, 1890, 1900, 1910, 1920, 1930, 1940, 1950, and 1960. Previous studies have tended to concentrate on cross sections for one or two years during the fertility transition in Sweden (e.g.,

TABLE 8.1

Means and Standard Deviations[a] for the Coale–Trussell Parameters of Natural Fertility and Parity-Specific Control (Average and for Individual Age Groups) for Groups of the Prefectures of Japan Defined in Terms of Percentage Occupied Male Labor Force (*PPIM*) in 1930: 1900, 1920, and 1960

			1900 *m*						1920 *m*						1960 *m*			
Group	*M*	*m*	25–29	30–34	35–39	40–44	*M*	*m*	25–29	30–34	35–39	40–44	*M*	*m*	25–29	30–34	35–39	40–44
PPIM ≤ 39.9%	.89	.36	.47	.46	.38	.32	.69	.64	.89	.78	.66	.58	.63	1.56	1.59	1.42	1.54	1.60
	(.07)	(.16)	(.12)	(.14)	(.15)	(.17)	(.10)	(.24)	(.27)	(.21)	(.22)	(.25)	(.01)	(.05)	(.05)	(.05)	(.04)	(.08)
40% ≤ *PPIM* ≤ 59.9%	.91	.20	.29	.30	.24	.16	.74	.40	.58	.53	.43	.35	.60	1.42	1.47	1.35	1.43	1.43
	(.08)	(.09)	(.11)	(.13)	(.10)	(.08)	(.09)	(.11)	(.13)	(.10)	(.11)	(.12)	(.03)	(.14)	(.12)	(.10)	(.12)	(.17)
60% ≤ *PPIM*	.96	.18	.33	.27	.23	.14	.84	.38	.52	.49	.41	.33	.61	1.32	1.41	1.28	1.32	1.33
	(.05)	(.15)	(.20)	(.11)	(.15)	(.15)	(.04)	(.15)	(.16)	(.14)	(.11)	(.18)	(.03)	(.11)	(.14)	(.09)	(.09)	(.13)

[a] The standard deviations are in parenthesis below the mean of the variable.

Edin and Hutchinson, 1935) or on the postwar period after the transition was completed (e.g., Bernhardt, 1971). Wilkinson (1973), working with the "cost of time" model, tests his model over the period 1870–1965, but only on national time series, whose interpretation (particularly in the case of fertility, where observations from one year to the next are so close) is problematic to say the least. In any event, it should be pointed out that we incorporate almost all the variables other scholars have selected for study and include a number hitherto unutilized. So we are confident that the tests performed are very comprehensive, and the differences that arise between the empirical observations we make and those advanced by others do not stem from serious oversight on our part.

The organization of this chapter roughly parallels that of Chapter 7. In the next section we briefly touch on the most salient features of the Swedish transition and some of the major issues surrounding its interpretation. Then in Sections 8.2 and 8.3 the principal statistical findings that we have arrived at are laid out.

8.2. Fertility Transition in Sweden: Timing and Speed

In this section we discuss the dating of the inception of Sweden's transition, the speed of the drop in marital fertility, and the implications of these facts for the interpretation of the reasons underlying the Swedish fertility decline. We shall set forth an interpretation and suggest why an alternative view, although plausible, is less persuasive.

Let us begin our discussion by returning to Table 6.3. As the reader will recall with regard to the analysis of the figures displayed, the data demonstrate that the Swedish transition was commencing in the 1880s, and was making only very gradual progress through the period before the turn of the century. Only Stockholm Stad (City) appears to have made significant headway in the fertility decline before 1880. Table 8.1 provides us with the continuation of this series of indicators for the period 1900–1960.[1] Four points can be made on the basis of the figures reported here. First, the rise in m was not extremely rapid for the counties of Sweden. Even in 1900, the values of m tend to be substantially less than .40. Second, the prewar Swedish transition (which in terms of I_g [see Tables 3.8 and 8.7] was substantially over by 1930) was accomplished almost as much with the deliberate lengthening of birth intervals, that is, the reduction in M, as it was with the diffusion of parity-specific control. During the postwar period 1950–1960, the introduction of contraceptive devices, by substantially lowering the costs of control, changed this situation rather dramatically; but for the period of the transition proper (1880–1930 or so), the conscious manipulation of the interbirth interval seems to have been crucial to the fertility decline in Sweden. As argued in Chapter 7, this testifies to the importance of the high costs of regulating natality before World War II in determining the speed of the fertility decline. Third, the age-specific values of m point to the same conclusion. Their tendency to diminish with the age of the mother is absent in the data for 1960 but salient in the figures for 1900 and 1930, and this result is in accord with the "cost of control" hypothesis. Fourth, it is noteworthy that the figures show that M falls substantially even in the rural agricultural counties of Sweden between 1900 and 1930, strengthening the argument made in Chapter 6 that there was an early demise of the premodern demographic regime in Sweden. In short, Table 8.1 accords well with the position concerning the speed of transitions and the relationship of the speed to the costs of regulating reproduction within marriage.

The thrust of Table 8.1 is that the means and acceptability of controlling natality were important in the Swedish case. The question that this observation naturally raises is how crucial were these costs? For example, would it be possible to take the extreme view that Swedish marital fertility commenced its decline in the 1880s because birth control had become a subject of public debate and attention throughout Europe in the 1870s, as a result of the spread of neo-Malthusian ideology? (Bradlaugh and Besant were tried for disseminating literature advocating birth control, and their trial gave them a forum for stating their views with great publicity.) That is, can we explain the timing of the Swedish transition—if not its ultimate causes—in terms of Sweden being located in Western Europe where the idea of restricting births within marriage had probably been spreading slowly but inexorably since the late eighteenth century in France? That the late 1870s and early 1880s appear to have constituted a watershed in the history of fertility everywhere in Western Europe seemingly fits in neatly with this view.

We would suggest another interpretation. Before laying out the argument, however, it would be well briefly to make mention of the early history of the neo-Malthusian movement in Sweden to see how readily it can be understood in the light of the pure "cost of control" thesis. Swedish historians customarily date the beginning of neo-Malthusianism in Sweden with the famous speech of the economist Knut Wicksell delivered on February 19, 1880 in the Lutheran Mission Hall in Uppsala.[2] In that lecture, Wicksell created a public furor, and stimulated discussion of the question of birth control, by arguing, in his talk entitled "The Most Common Causes of Habitual Drunkenness and How to Remove Them," that poverty was the cause of drunkenness and the cause of poverty was excessive population. By "poverty" Wicksell did not merely mean hunger or starvation, although he argued that even this existed among certain strata of the Swedish populace, but also the condition when "a man . . . does not possess, and has no reasonable hope of acquiring, what he desperately needs" (Gårland, 1958:49). By this latter object of desire, Wicksell meant "to live together with a family and have children" (Gårland, 1958:50). In short, Wicksell was arguing that prior population growth had so diminished the job opportunities for young men that they were forced to postpone matrimony for many years, or forego it altogether, because they faced a life of inferior social status relative to their parents' positions if they married and began to have children youthfully (in the absence of birth control). Thus, Wicksell maintained, these men were attracted to prostitutes and drunkenness as an outlet for their repressed sexual energies. Wicksell then concluded that the practice of birth control would remove these obstacles to marriage, because couples could now effectively restrict their reproduction, and alleviate the associated social problems, of which drunkenness was the most salient example. Finally, Wicksell pleaded for the creation of societies for limiting the procreation of children, modelled after temperance associations: "Each member of such a society would have to pledge himself, as long as he remained a member, not to increase his present or future family above three children" (Gårland, 1958:52). Wicksell continued to write and speak out on these issues for many years after the delivery of this controversial address, and his public utterances helped stimulate others to write about these matters. For instance, his ideas frequently appeared in the novels of authors from the Eighties School: two famous examples being Strindberg's *On the General Discount,* penned in the 1880s, and the collection of short stories titled *Married,* which gives a grim account of how large family size leads to marital unhappiness. Another example is Anne Edgren's *A Summer Saga,* which describes "birth control as a solution to the problem of 'truth' in marriage" (Gårland, 1958:96).

This discussion raises two questions: Was Wicksell completely influenced by the neo-Malthusian movement in delivering this talk and establishing a public debate? And how influential were Wicksell and his colleagues in encouraging the control of fertility among the general populace? Kock (1945:83), who had studied the first question extensively, gives the following answer: "It is hardly believable that Wicksell was familiar with the details of the Bradlaugh-Besant trial when he delivered his lecture . . . He gives a German Book published in 1880 as his source. . . ." Kock concludes that Wicksell pretty much arrived at his views on the basis of his own reasoning. Moreover, Kock (1945) argues that the immediate stimuli for Wicksell's thoughts were twofold: the great wave of emigration from Sweden to the United States that characterized the period around 1880 and the belated industrialization of Sweden, which meant her standard of living was lagging considerably behind that of the industrial heartland of Western Europe and the United States. That Wicksell was concerned about emigration with regard to the question of fertility is of interest because it points directly toward the concerns that are crucial to the origins of the Swedish transition.

Some figures on emigration will assist us in establishing the background for this argument. First, it should be noted that migration of Swedes to the United States was not a major movement until the last forty years of the nineteenth century. The estimates shown in the accompanying tabulation, worked up by Hofsten and Lundström (1976:66), make this clear.

Years	Estimated net emigration
1851–1860	30,575
1861–1870	146,327
1871–1880	138,754
1881–1890	347,285
1891–1900	180,340

Especially noteworthy is the peak around the 1880s. Thomas (1941:28) researched the question of Swedish emigration with considerable care, and she calculated from vital rates both estimated net emigrants per 100,000 population and percentage deviations away from trends over the period of intense emigration 1861–1908. These are, for selected years, as shown in Table 8.2. Thomas's series clearly shows that the period around 1880 marked a peak in the Swedish emigration experience. Why did the peak occur at this particular juncture? On the basis of detailed periodization of Swedish and American business conditions, Thomas (1941:169) concludes ". . . that prosperity in America was highly important as a stimulus to emigration from Sweden, but that cyclical upswings in Sweden were a far more powerful counterstimulant than is generally recognized. In prosperous years, Swedish industry was able to compete successfully with the lure of America. . . ." Thomas argues that the push from Swedish agriculture was constant throughout this period, but that the real wages to be earned in Swedish industry relative to those obtaining in the United States determined the direction of the flow out of the Swedish countryside. She also points out that the fall in transportation costs between Europe and the United States around the early 1860s encouraged the general trend across the period 1861–1908.

What connection does this have to fertility? Recall that the thesis concerning the net economic value of children hinges on the demand and supply of labor services and income flow that the patriarch can secure from his offspring. In the case of Western Europe around 1850, the standard of

TABLE 8.2

Year	Emigration per 100,000 population	Percentage deviations from trend (1861 – 1908)
1861	70	– 56.6
1865	208	– 32.0
1871	306	3.7
1876	167	– 62.1
1881	1043	70.1
1886	599	– 17.6
1891	779	26.2
1896	272	– 18.6
1901	379	6.3
1906	333	– 2.4

living was sufficiently high that labor markets in which youths could secure employment at relatively early ages existed. So children often left home at young ages and worked elsewhere. They might not provide services for many years on the patriarch's farm, but they remained in the locality and could be asked to support the patriarch or his wife, or take over the farm or croft, should the inheriting son die or prove incompetent. The spread of compulsory education in Western Europe was gradual throughout the nineteenth century, but it left in its wake an important consequence: it constrained parents, by law, to rear and care for their children until they were a certain age. This not only cut into the services children could perform on the patriarch's farm or in his shop, but it also increased the age at which children could leave the patriarch's care. However, as long as the patriarch retained some leverage over job placement and marriage, he could continue to extract services from his offspring after he bore the costs of raising them during the time they were being educated. This was particularly important for the patriarch as he and his wife reached old age, for if the inheriting son proved deficient or perished, it would be difficult economically to manage the household production unit. The growth of rural labor markets certainly eased this problem for the patriarch, but the considerations that encouraged natural fertility remained valid, despite compulsory education, as long as the patriarch retained some leverage over jobs.

However, the reduction in transportation costs across the Atlantic, the flooding of Western European markets with cheap American grain, and the encouragement that this agricultural crisis gave to emigration to the United States dramatically reduced the patriarch's position. For sons could now remain at home until they had secured education and then, given the cheap fares required for Atlantic travel, leave for the United States where they could secure employment on their own. Nor, given the relatively higher

TABLE 8.3

Means and Standard Deviations[a] for Measure of Nuptiality for Groups of the Counties of Sweden Defined in Terms of the Percentage Adult Male Labor Force in Primary Industry (*PPIM*) for 1900: 1910–1960

Group	Hutterite index I_m 1910	1930	1960	Singulate mean age at marriage, females 1930	1960
PPIM ≤ 39.9%	.43	.42	.62	26.5	22.9
	(.05)	(.05)	(.04)	(.7)	(.4)
40% ≤ *PPIM* ≤ 59.9	.44	.44	.64	26.5	22.8
	(.03)	(.02)	(.02)	(.4)	(.3)
60% ≤ *PPIM*	.40	.42	.62	26.8	23.1
	(.03)	(.03)	(.02)	(.5)	(.6)

[a] The standard deviations are in parenthesis below the mean of the variable.

standard of living in the United States (and even in Swedish industry), was there any guarantee they could be enticed to return to help with the farm in the future, or even that an inherited son or son-in-law could be found. Moreover, the supply of local hired labor was also threatened by the growth of markets at home and abroad, rural youth were entering these markets and abandoning farming altogether. In short, the 1870s and 1880s marked a watershed in Western Europe in terms of the operation of the patriarchal stem family system. A shock was sent into those populations that, by dint of geography and language, were already supplying the United States with its immigrants.[3] This explains the coincidence of timing of fertility declines in most of Western Europe.[4]

To summarize: We have argued here that the timing of the Swedish fertility decline can be understood in terms of a particular shock to the operation of the Swedish patriarchal stem family system—one Wicksell himself was concerned with—a shock whose impact continued to be felt over the next several decades and the cumulated effect of which (working both through emigration and the functioning of the domestic Swedish labor market) encouraged the relatively rapid decline of the premodern demographic regime and the fertility transition in Sweden. Moreover, we have also shown that the evidence does not lend itself to an interpretation in terms of the impact of British Neomalthusianism.

Now let us turn to the evolution in nuptiality that accompanied the Swedish transition in marital fertility. Table 8.3 contains the relevant figures. It clearly shows that the consequence Wicksell desired of birth control—the reduction in the age at marriage—was slow to come in Sweden. It is obvious from the table that the revolution in nuptiality that Wicksell advocated did finally come, but only after World War II. However, given the costs of control that are emphasized at several points in the preceding discussion, this is not surprising nor, indeed, is this inconsistent with Wicksell's arguments. We shall return to this issue at the end of the next section for it bears on our general analysis.

8.3. Education and the Fertility Transition in Sweden: Cross Tabulations and Regressions for the Counties, 1880–1960

As noted at a number of points in the analysis, the Swedish fertility transition (in terms of a decline in I_g) was virtually complete by 1930. The dramatic rise in m occurred primarily in the postwar period with the international diffusion of contraceptives and birth control methods, so M played a major role in the prewar Swedish transition. Because the principal interest is in pinpointing the social and economic changes lying behind the transition (and not the factors affecting the costs of contraception), we shall concentrate on the study of cross sections and trends in natality between 1880 and 1930, for it is during this half century that Swedish marital fertility plummeted from high to low levels.

That Sweden experienced a profound economic and social transformation on the national level between 1880 and 1930 has already been discussed in Chapter 2. That this set of changes characterized all the counties of Sweden is logical given the operation of national labor markets and governmental programs designed to improve public health, and, as Table 8.4 shows, the modernization of Swedish society did, in fact, take place in all locales, although at different speed and with different timing depending on the county. Let us first consider infant mortality. The column for 1880 suggests that infant mortality varied considerably across Sweden in the nineteenth century. For instance, the level for Stockholm City is 195.7 and for Vasternorrland it is 145.6 but the level in Jönköping is only 83.2. Moreover, *within* each of the three groups of counties, as classified by labor force composition in 1900, infant mortality varied substantially. There is no simple association between the composition of labor force and infant mortality evident in the column for 1880. Finally, the declines in infant mortality between 1880 and 1930 are across-the-board, and by 1930 the absolute geographical differentials are much smaller than they were in 1880. The uniformity of improvements in the standard of living and public health that shaped mortality apparently cut across the counties and produced the

TABLE 8.4

Means and Standard Deviations[a] for Various Aspects of Economic and Social Development for Groups of the Counties of Sweden Defined in Terms of Percentage Male Labor Force in Primary Industry (*PPIM*) in 1900: 1880–1930

	Demographic			Labor force characteristics												
	Infant mortality rate, *IMR*			Real male wages[b]			Real female wages[b]			Female–Male wage differential[c]		Female employment ratio, E_f			Education (proportion pupils in primary school who are full time, 1920)
Group	1880	1900	1930	1880	1900	1930	1880	1900	1930	1880	1930	1880	1900	1930	
PPIM ≤ 39.9%	132.1	76.0	51.2	3.15	4.96	6.80	1.53	2.51	4.69	.49	.69	.44	.50	.88	.89
	(43.1)	(4.0)	(5.9)	(.64)	(.63)	(.78)	(.27)	(.47)	(.33)	(.01)	(.04)	(.04)	(.08)	(.20)	(.15)
40% ≤ *PPIM* ≤ 59.9%	116.4	87.6	57.0	2.69	4.28	6.15	1.30	2.17	4.10	.49	.67	.38	.41	.62	.76
	(20.6)	(17.8)	(11.6)	(.21)	(.32)	(.35)	(.15)	(.28)	(.26)	(.06)	(.05)	(.08)	(.09)	(.11)	(.16)
60% ≤ *PPIM*	100.1	74.5	51.3	2.55	3.91	5.42	1.30	2.13	3.76	.51	.69	.34	.39	.58	.70
	(12.0)	(11.9)	(5.3)	(.33)	(.33)	(.24)	(.14)	(.18)	(.27)	(.04)	(.03)	(.04)	(.05)	(.11)	(.23)

[a] The standard deviation is in parenthesis below the mean of the variable.
[b] Estimated nominal daily wages deflated by a price index, which equals 100 for Stockholm City in 1915. See Appendix 6. Thus measured in 1915 kroner per day.
[c] Estimated female wage divided by estimated male wage.

dramatic convergence in rates revealed in Table 8.4. The interested reader should consult Norman (1977) for further details concerning areal variations in infant mortality in Sweden during this period.

Also uniform were improvements in the standard of living and changes in the relative position of women in the labor market, as the figures on real daily wages and female–male wage differentials indicate. The contraction in female–male wage differentials is especially striking and merits special attention here. Some might be tempted to associate this rather dramatic contraction with the "solidaristic wage policy" that trade unions in Sweden began to adopt in the interwar period as part of their collective bargaining strategy. The idea behind the "solidaristic wage policy" is simple: the union movement pledges itself to support the workers in the lowest-paid industries, with the aim of reducing the differentials in wages between the various industries. The Swedish Federation of Trade Unions (*Landsorganisationen i Sverige*) has in principle subscribed to this policy for a long time and passed a resolution formally going on record in support of it in its congress of 1922. Nevertheless, it is unlikely that this policy explains the contraction we observe, in light of the expansion of interindustry differentials and "wage drift" that apparently has become characteristic of the postwar economy. It is more likely that the movements in the wage differential reflect worker productivities in the industries, which in turn hinge quite importantly on the conditions surrounding demand.[5] Male workers have tended to be concentrated in export-oriented heavy industries—forestry, iron and steel, and machinery—and women have tended to find employment in industries such as textiles that depend, in main, on the domestic market for total demand. Thus the contraction in international demand for Swedish exports, which came with especial force in the late 1920s and the 1930s, reduced prices for Swedish export products and, consequently, had a major impact on productivity in the industries in which males were concentrated. The light industries, which responded more to domestic aggregate demand, were less drastically hurt by this state of affairs (though the general reduction in aggregate income during the period did, of course, have an impact on them as well), and as a result the wage differential contracted sharply. This, of course, is not the entire story, for the improvements in education for women, the opening up of positions in professional activity and government, and the "solidaristic wage policy" also help explain the contraction. The rise in female employment ratios (E_f) in all the counties of Sweden, especially evident in the period 1900–1930, testifies to this expansion of job opportunities for women outside agriculture.

It is noteworthy in passing that the E_f ratios for the Swedish counties in 1880 are already, in comparison to the Japanese figures for the 1920s and 1930s, very large in magnitude, as a comparison with Table 7.3 shows. It is

TABLE 8.5

Diffusion of Parity-Specific Control and the Spacing of Births for the Counties of Sweden (Cross Sections), 1900–1920[a]

Year	Dependent variable	Constant	Demographic variable (legitimate infant mortality rate), *IMRL*	Structural variable (proportion male labor force dependent on primary industry), *PPIM*	Labor force variables: Real male wage, *RWM*	Labor force variables: Real female wage, *RWF*	Education (proportion pupils in primary school who are full time, 1920) *PFTES*	R^2	Adjusted R^2
Linear specification									
1910	*m*	−1.48	−.005[c]	.56	.23	.15	.41[b]	.54	.41
1910	*M*	.94[d]	.003	.16	−.04	−.02	−.11[d]	.46	.31
1920	*m*	−.37	−.003	.40	−.03	.25	.27[d]	.58	.47
1920	*M*	2.26[e]	.003	−1.09	−.19	−.13	−.04	.48	.33
Logarithmic specification[f]									
1910	*m*	−.73	−1.09[c]	.25	2.58	.38	.82[c]	.49	.35
1910	*M*	−.22	.19	.03	−.32	−.07	−.11[c]	.44	.29
1920	*m*	.37	−.42	.19	−.39	1.31[c]	.42[c]	.59	.48
1920	*M*	.36	.15	−.56	−.72	−.44[d]	−.01	.52	.38

[a] Significant intercorrelations between the independent variables (1910 values given here) are: *PPIM* and *RWF* (−.74); *PPIM* and *RWM* (−.90); *RWM* and *RWF* (−.52). (All are one-tailed tests except for coefficients on *IMRL* in regression on *m*).

[b] Significant at the 1% level.

[c] Significant at the 5% level.

[d] Significant at the 10% level.

[e] Significant at the 15% level.

[f] Logarithms of all variables (dependent and independent) were entered in the regression.

necessary to emphasize this point because people often form the false impression that, because the textile industry was more crucial to Japanese than to Swedish modern economic growth up to 1930, and because female workers tended to dominate employment in that industry in the two countries, the female employment ratio in Japan must have exceeded that in Sweden. Table 7.3 and Table 8.4 refute that view.

Finally, the figures in Table 8.4 shed some light on the modernization of Swedish education. It is unfortunate that the only proxy that we can use for the counties during this period is both crude and only available for one census year, 1920.[6] That variable measures the proportion of pupils in primary school who are full-time students. Because full-time attendance was a virtual prerequisite for continuation on to more advanced education, this variable, albeit somewhat crudely, measures the degree to which children were able to advance past the lowest level of compulsory schooling into schools from which graduation would strongly affect their ability to secure good jobs and positions in the labor market. In short, it is a measure of the costs patriarchs were incurring in maintaining leverage over their children. In any case, the column concerning education clearly shows that, although educational achievement was considerable everywhere in Sweden by 1920, differentials still persisted during this period. These differentials do reflect, although only in part, the industrial composition of the economically active population. In general, as the reader can see, the districts that depend more heavily on primary industry reveal lower levels of educational attainment.

In sum, the figures in Table 8.4 indicate forcibly that the modernization of Swedish economy and society between 1880 and 1930 was thoroughgoing and its influence was evident in every county, regardless of geographical locality.

Now we can turn our attention to the analytical results concerning the determinants of marital fertility during the Swedish transition. Because the transition was basically complete by 1930, and because useable county educational data are only available for 1920, this means we must focus our attention primarily on the cross sections for 1910 and 1920. We begin our examination of the evidence with Table 8.5, which contains the results of regressions with the Coale–Trussell parameters M and m as the dependent variables.[7] It should be noted that, as with the Japanese regressions discussed in the previous chapter, both standard linear and log–linear specifications are used, and there are some problems of multicollinearity evident in the regressions. (See the footnotes to Tables 8.5 for the significant cases of this for 1910.) As for our expectations for the coefficients on the variables, these coincide with those for Japan given in Section 7.3. It should be noted, however, that we lack figures on educational attainment for each sex separately, so the coefficient on the educational variable most closely captures the effect of female education, that is, it should be positive when m is

TABLE 8.6

Regression on Marital Fertility for the Swedish Counties, 1910 and 1920: Hutterite Index I_g as Dependent Variable

			Independent variables						
					Labor force variables				
Year	Dependent variable	Constant	Legitimate infant mortality rate, *IMRL*	Proportion male labor force dependent on primary industry, *PPIM*	Real male wages[a] *RWM*	Real female wages[a] *RWF*	Proportion pupils in primary school who are full time, 1920	R^2	Adjusted R^2
Linear Specification									
1910	I_g	1.04[d]	.004[d]	.002	−.08	−.07	−.20[d]	.57	.45
1920	I_g	1.64[e]	.003[c]	−.81	−.13	−.15[c]	−.10	.68	.59
Logarithmic Specification[b]									
1910	I_g	−.54	.38[c]	−.10	−.71	−.37	−.24[c]	.57	.45
1920	I_g	1.29	.25[c]	−.23	−.44	−.52[d]	−.17[d]	.69	.61

[a] Estimated daily wages deflated by a price index for county that sets Stockholm City in 1915 = 100. See Appendix 6.
[b] Logarithms of all variables were entered into the regression (dependent and independent).
[c] Significant at the 1% level (one-tailed test).
[d] Significant at the 5% level (one-tailed test).
[e] Significant at the 10% level (one-tailed test).

the dependent variable and negative when M is the dependent variable. This is reasonable because the supposition is that the income effect would be weak compared with the impact of a decline in parental leverage. The cross sections show relatively clearly that educational attainment of the children is positively associated with the index of parity-specific control m. This shows up in both the regressions using simple linear, and logarithmic, forms.

Somewhat different findings were obtained by using I_g as the dependent variable. These results are laid out in Table 8.6. Note that a larger class of variables appear to be statistically significant in these regressions. Particularly noteworthy is the finding that infant mortality rates are positively associated with levels of marital fertility. Because the signs in the infant mortality rate in the regressions on M and m revealed in Table 8.5 are consistent with this finding (but the coefficients are not significant), the overall evidence suggests that the decline of Swedish infant mortality was an important factor in the Swedish fertility transition. That this was not so in the Japanese case is perhaps owing to the persistence of the structure of the premodern demographic regime in Japan until the mid-1950s, households primarily reacting to infant mortality declines in terms of rising ages at marriage and improvements in natural fertility. Equally worthy of mention is that the female wage variable emerges with a significant and negative coefficient in 1920, implying that "cost of time" considerations were operative in Sweden at the close of the transition, as in Japan.

Now let us turn to the evolution of Swedish nuptiality. The gradualness of the downward trend in age at marriage for women and men can, by and large, be explained in terms of the slow rise in m and the very sluggish diminution in the costs of controlling fertility. By the same token, the sharp postwar trends imply that with the introduction of contraceptives and the greater social approval of controlling natality within marriage that obtained once the transition in I_g had been fully completed, the age at marriage for females fell sharply. This accords with our previous arguments and Wicksell's polemical position. Although it is difficult to give a rigorous demonstration of these assertions, the following results lend credence to this view. Absolute trends between 1950 and 1960 were calculated for the following variables: the Coale–Trussell indices (ΔM and Δm), the legitimate infant mortality rate ($\Delta IMRL$), the proportion males engaged in primary industry ($\Delta PPIM$), and the singulate mean age at marriage for females ($\Delta SMAMF$). Finally, treating $\Delta SMAMF$ as the dependent variable, we regressed it against the trends in the other variables and the *level* of parity-specific control for 1950 (*m1950*), a measure of the costs of contraception for the beginning of the decade. The result was

$$\Delta SMAMF = (.63)\Delta m + (.02)(\Delta IMRL) + (3.71)(\Delta M) + (.63)(\Delta PPIM) - (1.52)(m1950), \qquad R^2 = .29$$

TABLE 8.7

Means and Standard Deviations[a] for Measures of Marital Fertility and Nuptiality, and Urban–Rural Relatives, 1900–1960, for Groups of Counties Defined in Terms of Percentage Occupied Male Labor Force in Primary Industry (*PPIM*) in 1900

	Marital fertility[b]								Nuptiality							
	I_g						Urban I_g divided by rural I_g		I_m						Urban I_m divided by rural I_m	
	Rural			Urban					Rural			Urban				
Group	1900	1930	1960	1900	1930	1960	1930	1960	1900	1930	1960	1900	1930	1960	1930	1960
PPIM ≤ 39.9%	.64	.33	.25	.54	.20	.25	.65	1.01	.46	.48	.65	.36	.40	.62	.87	.98
	(.08)	(.04)	(.01)	(.08)	(.03)	(.01)	(.01)	(.03)	(.05)	(.03)	(.01)	(.05)	(.04)	(.04)	(.03)	(.01)
40% ≤ *PPIM* ≤ 59.9%	.67	.34	.25	.57	.23	.23	.70	.92	.47	.46	.65	.37	.39	.63	.86	.96
	(.09)	(.09)	(.02)	(.07)	(.05)	(.03)	(.08)	(.09)	(.04)	(.03)	(.02)	(.04)	(.03)	(.02)	(.09)	(.05)
60%	.70	.39	.26	.59	.27	.21	.71	.79	.41	.43	.63	.33	.38	.60	.89	.96
	(.10)	(.04)	(.02)	(.05)	(.02)	(.03)	(.05)	(.09)	(.04)	(.03)	(.02)	(.03)	(.03)	(.03)	(.08)	(.04)

[a] The standard deviations are in parenthesis below the mean of the variable.
[b] Based on averages of births for five years about census date.

Only the variable "$m1950$" proved to be significant in this regression (at the 5 percent level in a one-tailed test), implying that the costs of control were indeed important in shaping Swedish nuptiality after World War II.[8]

This concludes our discussion of the findings for the aggregate counties of Sweden. Now let us proceed to an examination of material for the rural and urban sectors of the Swedish counties to shed light on some aspects of the connection between social status and the fertility transition in Sweden.

8.4. Social Structure, Wages, and the Fertility Decline in Sweden: The Rural and Urban Sectors of the Counties, 1900–1960

The long term drop in Swedish marital fertility, for both the rural sectors of each county and the urban sectors, is chronicled in Table 8.7. The table shows that in a few counties, rural marital fertility was still substantial in 1930 and in these counties it dropped off to low levels by 1960 (actually by 1950, as figures for 1950 demonstrate). As with the Japanese figures on rural I_g and relatives to urban I_g, the narrowness of the rural–urban differentials are noteworthy. The relevance of these results for the Japanese figures was discussed in Chapter 7, and no further treatment of that issue is needed here.

Now let us consider the analytical results for the rural districts. Table 8.8 contains the principal findings for 1900. Because the richest and most accurate data for the rural sectors are available for the year 1900, we concentrate on this cross section only. The results closely parallel those for Japan. Here we find the wage pattern characteristic of rural districts of Japan in 1925, a finding that played an important role in the interpretation of the dynamics of the early Japanese transition in agricultural zones. The patriarchal stem family system with household production still continued to be important, although with diminished force, in rural Sweden around 1900, so the result can be interpreted along the same lines with which we have explained the Japanese results. From the point of view of social structure, the variables for estate owners and *statare* capture the proportions in the highest and lowest status groups, respectively, and the negative signs on the coefficients for these variables are consistent with the arguments (laid out in Section 7.5) concerning the especially high costs of retaining patriarchal leverage that the modernization of labor markets imposes on the groups in the extremes of social status (i.e., those of very high and very low social position).

Finally, we turn our attention to the Swedish cities. Table 8.7 provides us with the values of I_g for the urban sectors of the counties during the transition and the relatives to the rural values. The low values of I_g for *all* the

TABLE 8.8

Social Structure and Marital Fertility, 1900: The Rural Sectors of the Swedish Counties

				Labor force variables		Social structure			
Trend or dependent variable	Constant	Legitimate infant mortality rate, *IMRL*	Proportion population dependent on primary industry, *PPIM*	Real male agricultural wages *RAWM*[a]	Real female agricultural wages *RAWF*[a]	Percentage farming population who are farm and estate owners, 1910, *PFE*	Percentage farming population who are *statare*, 1910, *STAT*	R^2	Adjusted R^2
Linear specification									
I_g	.96[b]	.003[c]	−.39	−.13[c]	.11[c]	−.01[c]	−.03[b]	.68	.57
β coefficients for regression in row 1	n.e.[d]	.46	−.09	−.73	.39	−.58	−1.09	n.e.	n.e.
Mean of variable	n.e.	76.6	.63	3.22	1.80	23.5	3.70	n.e.	n.e.
Standard deviation of variable	n.e.	16.2	.10	.55	.32	7.2	3.76	n.e.	n.e.
Logarithmic specification[e]									
I_g	.56	.12	.001	−.72[b]	.23	−.16[c]	−.14[b]	.71	.60

[a] Estimated daily wages deflated by price index for county with Stockholm City in 1915 = 100.
[b] Significant at the 1% level (two-tailed tests except for coefficient on *PPIM*).
[c] Significant at the 5% level (two-tailed tests except for coefficient on *PPIM*).
[d] n.e. indicates that the variable was not entered into the regression.
[e] Logarithms of all variables were entered into the regression (dependent and independent).

TABLE 8.9

Male and Female Wages and Marital Fertility: The Urban Sectors of Swedish Ccunties, Cross Section and Trends[a]

Year or trend period	Dependent variable	Constant	Legitimate infant mortality rate, *IMRL*	Labor market variables: Real male nonagricultural wages[b], *RNAWM*	Labor market variables: Real female nonagricultural wages[b], *RNAWF*	R^2	Adjusted R^2
Linear specification							
1900	I_g	1.15[d]	.0003	.10	−.36[e]	.16	.04
1900/1920	I_g	−.02	.0006[d]	−.02	−.23[d]	.23	.23
1900/1930	I_g	−.06	.008[c]	.04	−.20[c]	.52	.45
Logarithmic specification[f]							
1900	I_g	.24	.02	.85	−1.83[e]	.16	.03
1900/1920	I_g	−.10	.05[d]	−.36	−.94	.23	.12
1900/1930	I_g	−.23	.15[c]	.36	−1.24[d]	.47	.40

[a] Regression on absolute trends in all variables where the absolute trend in variable X_t between time t_1 and t_2, $t_1 < t_2$, is $X_{t_2} - X_{t_1}$.

[b] Nominal wages for selected sectors outside of agriculture deflated by a price index which sets Stockholm City in 1915 = 100. See Appendix 6.

[c] Significant at the 1% level (two-tailed test).

[d] Significant at the 5% level (two-tailed test).

[e] Signigicant at the 10% level (two-tailed test).

[f] Logarithms of all variables (dependent and independent) were entered into the regression.

urban sectors show that by 1930 the regulation of reproduction within marriage had reached a high level in the cities of Sweden. This stands in contrast to the rural findings mentioned previously, for Table 8.7 also shows that rural I_g in certain counties was still substantial in 1930.

The analytical findings for the urban districts of Sweden, summarized in Table 8.9, run parallel to those for the Japanese cities, just as the two sets of rural results display marked similarities. For here real wages play the role we would expect for populations in which the "cost of time" hypothesis is reasonable, that is, for populations in which the patriarchal system and household production are of slight importance as far as fertility is concerned.

In sum, the findings for rural and urban Sweden parallel nicely those we have secured for Japan, and as a whole they are consistent with the results for Japan reported in Chapter 7. This replication of Swedish data similar to the previous results for Japan lends important support, indeed, to the assertion that the theoretical framework, which predicts similar findings for the two nations, is reasonable.

8.5. Conclusions

In this chapter we have demonstrated that there is an empirical basis for the theories in the materials concerning the Swedish fertility transition. Education, real wages, and the costs of controlling fertility all emerge as important in explaining the Swedish transition in marital fertility. Moreover, and this is what is especially crucial for this study, the findings show that there is a strong and consistent similarity between the results for Japan and those for Sweden. To document this, indeed, is the main point of this chapter. Having done this, we have advanced a goodly amount of evidence in support of the applicability of the theoretical framework. And so with this empirical discussion completed, we can now turn to the broader implications and conclusions of this study, our goal in the final chapter of this book.

Notes to Chapter 8

1. Also see Table 8.7 concerning the Hutterite index I_g. (The county values can be easily estimated from the levels of the rural [or urban] values and the figures on the relatives to the county level.) See Appendix 7 for a discussion of the methodological issues surrounding the Coale–Trussell measures, which is of especial relevance to the values reported in Table 8.1.

2. See Gårland (1958) and Kock (1945). I am grateful to Christina Tweedie for translating the article by Kock for me. See Kälvemark (1980a, 1980b) for a related discussion concerning the ideological debates about birth control in Sweden.

3. Marvin McInnis has hinted at an argument along these lines (but one that is not thoroughly worked out). See Carlsson (1968, 1969) on Swedish emigration and Tederbrand (1972) for information on reimmigration from the United States to Sweden.

4. It is critical to the thesis that the patriarch is placed in a position where he must support his children while they are receiving an education (or provide them with an inheritance later on) either because he must educate his children to secure future income flow and services from them (because education becomes crucial for job placement and this affects his bargaining position) or because it becomes a legal requirement. In the British case, for instance, the expansion of the labor market in manufacturing weakened the patriarch's leverage well before the 1870s but rearing children still involved relatively small net economic costs because they left home at early ages and could be brought back to help the parents if the inheriting son was unable to care for the parents. This may help explain why the British fertility decline begins around 1880, after the introduction of compulsory education. In the French case the Napoleonic code required equal division of the property, regardless of what the individual children did, so it drastically reduced the patriarch's leverage because he was now required, by law, to provide his children with shares of his estate, regardless of whether they performed labor services for him or not. This may help account for the early French decline, beginning around the time of the French Revolution. The critical point is that the costs of maintaining leverage over the children are now raised so high relative to the benefits to be secured from the leverage that children cease to hold a net economic advantage to the patriarch. Conversations with David Weir were useful to the author in working out this point.

5. I am grateful to Bent Hansen for suggesting this point to me.

6. There is a good deal of material for the national level, but the source, Sweden. Statistiska centralbyrån (1974). *Pupils in Compulsory Schools in Sweden 1847–1962* only gives one table, for 1920, which contains a reasonable proxy for county indicators of educational attainment.

7. See Appendix 7 for a discussion of the problems encountered in estimating M and m, problems that are especially relevant for the Swedish data given the relatively poor fit of the Coale–Trussell model to the Swedish data between 1900 and 1930. The reader should note that the regressions with I_g as dependent variable avoid the problems of estimation of the dependent variable that those with M and m involve.

8. Since 1960 the proportion of women never marrying in Sweden has increased rather dramatically, along with the divorce rate and the level of illegitimacy. With the rather thoroughgoing dismantling of the legal and institutional bases of the patriarchal system in Sweden, and the vigorous role women play in the labor market as a result of these changes, trends probably should be interpreted as illustrative of the almost total demise of the patriarchal system insofar as is affects Swedish demographic behavior.

CHAPTER 9

Conclusions

9.1. Introduction

The arguments and the presentation of evidence in support of the theses of this book have now been presented, and it is time to stand back and take stock of what we have learned from the work as a whole. The most useful means of highlighting the salient lessons of this study is to consider the implications of the theory, and the empirical results that buttress it, for the various fields of academic inquiry that the research directly bears on. Six areas of study seem particularly relevant with regard to the implications of this study: the literature concerning theories of the household, theories of the fertility transition, demographic history, the economic history of Japan, comparative history, and the study of empirical determinants of fertility in the world today. Before turning our attention to each of these areas of concern, however, it is useful to review briefly the main theoretical arguments and findings of this study.

The theoretical core of this study is a model of the peasant household in which the household practices a maximizing behavior subject to environmental and institutional constraints. The institutional rules dealt with are those governing a patriarchal stem family system. The patriarch has leverage over his children, and with this leverage he secures labor services from his offspring. A stylized representation of household maximizing behavior is laid out in the basic equation of Section 2.3, which relates household reproduction to the future labor supply for the household. The point of the model is that the household develops a demographic strategy to satisfy certain economic constraints. That is, the life cycle of the household is determined by maximizing behavior subject to economic constraints.

With this model of the household, we turn to the problem of explaining levels and trends in natality, and in particular, we attempt to explain the behavior of the two major components of fertility, nuptiality and marital fertility. The main thesis is that as the operation of labor markets changes, the costs of and benefits for leverage over children are transformed and a natural fertility strategy becomes disadvantageous. This leads to the fertility transition. But prior to this structural transformation, the household pursues a natural fertility strategy, with nuptiality adjusting to natural fertility and mortality. In Chapter 2 we demonstrate that the demographic adjustment mechanism, according to which the age at marriage of females adjusts to natural fertility and mortality, can be generalized from household behavior to a model of behavior for aggregate populations. Finally, we suggest how this theory can be utilized in explaining why there is marked diversity in the evolution of natality for some populations that have experienced, or are experiencing, economic modernization in the nineteenth and twentieth centuries.

Employing four major data sets, we have empirically explored the validity of this theory and its quantitative ramifications for Japan and Sweden, 1880–1960. The major empirical findings involve six issues: the importance of education of children in explaining the fertility decline, the timing of the disappearance of the premodern demographic regime, the role of the index of natural fertility M in accounting for the fall in marital fertility during the transition, the reversal in the impact of real wages in rural districts, the early development of an environment in cities in which real wages take on the role we are accustomed to observing after or toward the close of the fertility transition, and the response of nuptiality to increases and levels in the index of parity-specific control m. In Chapters 5–8 the evidence involving these points is presented, and in addition a number of other related, but more minor, issues are touched on.

With this as background, let us now turn to the implications of these results for the five areas of research mentioned previously.

9.2. Implications for the Economic Theory of the Household

As noted in Section 2.7, there is considerable literature concerning the economic theory of the household. Almost all of this literature treats the demography of the peasant household as exogenous and its economic behavior as endogenous. The model of the household reverses this implicit direction of causation and treats the demography of the household as a function of economic considerations. A few other scholars in this area of research have recognized the potential gain from doing this, and it is hoped that the research in this area discussed in this book will stimulate other researchers to work on this problem.

Although a number of economists have noted that institutional constraints may be important in shaping household behavior, little work of a concrete nature has actually been accomplished in this area. It is again hoped that the attempt made here in this study of integrating certain specific institutional rules into a theory of the household will encourage related research concerning the impact of other institutional rules in cultural settings different from the ones looked at here (e.g., cultures in which all sons coreside and farm the land as a group).

9.3. Implications for the Theory of the Fertility Transition

In Section 2.7, a few of the most prominent economic and sociological theories of the fertility transition are noted. As a whole, the approach used in this book supports the notion advanced by the classical theories of the transition (e.g., Notestein) that the "traditional" family system discourages fertility control. But the results disclosed here go much further than the classical school in pinpointing the precise mechanisms that explain this association; moreover, the rationality of the behavior discussed regarding the premodern demographic regime is largely inconsistent with the view that the "traditional" family system is inflexible. By the same token, the findings do not support Davis's theory of challenge and response, which was partially a critique of the classical view, precisely because they lend credence to the importance of the premodern family system. In addition, Davis puts great emphasis on infant mortality in accounting for the transition, whereas we do not find this factor to be of serious consequence to the decline in marital fertility.

However, portions of the findings *do* lend support to some of the sociological theories discussed in Chapter 2. For we do argue along the lines proposed by Caldwell that the reversal of intergenerational flows of income and wealth transfers is crucial to the fertility decline. However, it should be emphasized that our interpretation is very different in terms of specifying the rationale and mechanisms underlying the reversal of these flows and transfers and their specific connection to natality.

The study also bears on the economic theories discussed in Chapter 2. Most notably, it calls into question the applicability of the "cost of time" hypothesis as a theory of fertility decline or a universal theory of natality per se. The results concerning the reversal in the impact of wages are noteworthy in this regard, as are the arguments concerning leverage and family decision making as the result of a bargaining process within the household. Our results do tend to support Leibenstein's emphasis on the contributions of labor services and support for the old age security of parents that children make, although, of course, our approach in terms of patriarchal leverage differs rather strongly from that of Leibenstein's. Finally, a good deal of support for Easterlin's theory of the costs of fertility regulation was found, but we do not find that the dynamics of the transition that he outlines (the shift from excess demand to excess supply of number of surviving children) captures the main aspects of the actual process of the transition very closely.

9.4. Implications for Demographic History

The principal implication of the research for demographic history lies in the issues it raises for the European Fertility Project. It raises two particular problems. First, it calls into question the notion that "culture" as a diffuse and ill-specified concept should be used as an explanation of differences in premodern demographic regimes in Europe and Asia. Some scholars may wish to interpret the variations in natural fertility and infant mortality for the premodern populations we focus attention on as reflecting differences in cultural attitudes toward breast feeding; if so, we have no great quarrel with this view, although we do not subscribe to it. The point, however, is that breast feeding practices are not vague, but specific, concrete manifestations of culture, and it is these, after all, that we should pinpoint clearly. Second, the relative success of the study in statistically finding important factors underlying the transitions in Japan and Sweden calls into question the rather skeptical conclusions of the European Fertility Project. The authors of the country studies for the Project find little empirical support for the notion that changes in wages, income, labor markets, education, and the like actually set off the transitions in the European case, but it should be noted that they have not, as a whole, attempted to assemble rich data sets with many social and economic variables, as we have done for Japan and Sweden. In short, one implication of the study is that further research must be done on the European countries examined in the Project; and especially, much more economic and social data must be gathered and utilized in the analysis of levels and trends in natality before we conclude that the determinants of the European transition are virtually impossible to ascertain.

In sum, because we have demonstrated in this work that it is possible to construct an empirically viable model of the premodern demographic regime and the fertility transition—at least empirically viable for two countries, Japan and Sweden, which entered their transitions before World War II—it is reasonable to expect that other scholars may be able to secure equally useful results for the other European countries. In this regard, the emphasis on the agricultural sector, and the hypothesis developed in Chapter 8 concerning the shock delivered to Western European farming by American grain exports, should be kept in mind.

Finally we have taken an initial step to developing a general explanation for why there is diversity in fertility transitions, a puzzle posed at the inception of this work.

9.5. Implications for Japanese Economic History

There are at least four major problems concerning the economic history of Japan that the research here bears on: Tokugawa development, the labor market, the economic behavior of farm families, and savings and consumption.

With regard to the Tokugawa economy, the discussion in Chapters 3, 4, and 5 makes the issues evident. Per capita output and consumption did not necessarily improve to any *marked* degree during the Tokugawa period, although population increase during the seventeenth century may have encouraged institutional and technological changes that raised productivity *per hectare* and the expansion of markets for the sale and purchase of output (especially in the most densely inhabited districts of Japan). The demographic data assembled for the Tokugawa and Meiji periods is consistent with the hypothesis that the standard of living was relatively low during the Tokugawa era and improved considerably after the Meiji restoration principally because of the abolition of Tokugawa policies concerning feudal class structure, the relative isolation of the *han* (fiefdom) populations from one another, and international trade.

Second, the theory advanced here bears on the question of how Japanese labor markets functioned historically and how they have changed. The gradual but definite shift from job placement through family connections and the patriarch's intervention, to screening via educational achievement, which we document, is certainly important to an understanding of the history of Japanese labor.

Third, we have developed a model of household behavior that is applicable to Japanese farm families, a result that is of importance to the modeling of Japanese agriculture during the nineteenth and twentieth centuries. The theory also bears directly on the question of differentials in productivity between the agricultural and industrial sectors, and explains, in part, why patriarchal leverage in farming tended to drive average and marginal labor productivities to considerably lower levels than obtained in manufacturing and services (with the exception of family-run firms in these latter sectors).

Finally, the life-cycle model advanced here, and the analysis of its modification under the impetus of a secular advance in the standard of living, bears on the question of how households allocated their incomes between savings and consumption. The long-term secular increase in the Japanese savings rate during the nineteenth and twentieth centuries is well known, and our work raises some intriguing possibilities about how this advance may, at least partially, be explained.

In sum, the research touches on a number of topics crucial to an understanding of Japanese economic growth, and it is hoped that other scholars will be stimulated to explore these issues more thoroughly on the basis of the results and theories presented here.

9.6. Implications for Comparative History

The systematic, quantitative analysis of two societies during an historical period is a relatively new field, and it is hoped that work in this area will demonstrate the fruitfulness of such an approach. Indeed, one of the themes in this book is that the exploration of an hypothesis, advanced for one country then applied to another country sheds important light both on the applicability of the thesis and on its limitations, especially on its implicit assumptions. That it is possible to assemble rich data sets for two nations and carry out a detailed, systematic, quantitative analysis that bears very directly on the validity and appropriateness of theoretical arguments that one tests the data with, is one of the most useful general implications to emerge from the research.

9.7. Implications for Fertility in the Current Period

The sixth area in which the study has important implications is the analysis of natality in nations today. In this regard, three points are especially worth noting: the importance of the type of family system, the importance of education and its relationship to job markets, and the related general issue of institutions and culture raised in Chapter 1.

Let us consider the issue of the family system first. One important conclusion of the approach used here is that cultural and institutional factors directly affect fertility and its evolution through their molding of the family system. For instance, changes in the institutional settings of the family, specifically the forging of the legal underpinning of the patriarchal stem family system in the Meiji Civil Code and its dismantling during the American occupation, undoubtedly played some role in the Japanese transition. More generally, the institutional framework for the family as codified in law (e.g., inheritance, property rights of spouses, and freedom to marry without parental permission) appears to have been important in both Sweden and Japan in determining how economic and social changes affected fertility. Although it is difficult to disentangle the purely institutional (e.g., legal) aspects from the cultural and economic aspects surrounding the family system, the point is that the institutions of the family system may make a difference in the timing of fertility transitions. Moreover, the importance of the family system in general must be recognized in evaluating the relevance of the European and Japanese experience for less developed countries today, in which birth rates are often substantial. For the channeling of economic and social changes into decisions about regulating marital fertility may be very different in nations in which extended joint family systems, for example, prevail as opposed to a stem family system. This must be kept in mind in any attempt to draw inferences about the future course of natality in high fertility nations today from the histories of European nations, the United States, Australia, Canada, and Japan.

The second area in which the question about the relevance of institutions arises is that of education. The finding that education is important must be understood in terms of its implications for patriarchal leverage over children. It would be a misleading generalization to draw from the study that a program of compulsory education will automatically encourage parity-specific control in countries with high birth rates. Such programs may have this impact, but only when the environment surrounding education (e.g., the labor market) is conducive to this effect. Indeed, under some circumstances an educational program may actually raise marital fertility because of its possible influence on natural fertility and conditions of public health and sanitation.

Thus the question arises: Can governments wishing to encourage parity-specific control manipulate, through legal changes in institutions, the decision making of households to achieve this end? For although we must grant that *culture* itself (as opposed to institutions) is exceedingly difficult to transform through such legizlation and related policies, it may be possible to transform relatively quickly institutions with such methods; so the issue is whether the type of institutional modifications pointed to previously can serve as a vehicle for population policies. Although it is impossible to definitively address such a sweeping issue, it would appear that the answer is a qualified "yes"; a combination of policies designed to tackle the problem of parental leverage may well have the desired impact (and here the type of family system of the specific population under consideration is assuredly an issue). Indeed, the postwar occupation reforms in Japan, which reshaped both education and family law, undoubtedly did contribute to the Japanese fertility decline (at any rate they certainly sped it up). However, the point that must be emphasized is that the institutional changes that policy attempts to utilize must be understood in terms of parental leverage over, and the related total costs and benefits from, children of higher parity.

9.8. For the Future

These, then, are the main implications of this study. At least, these seem to be the most important problems for future research to have emerged from this study of the household and the evolution of natality in Japan and Sweden. It is a fervent hope that other scholars will tackle these issues, for it does seem that the results discussed here raise serious questions about each of these areas of scholarly endeavor.

PART IV

Appendixes

APPENDIX 1

Geographical Regions of Japan

Beginning with the 1930 census, the prefectures of Japan were listed in an order running from the Northeast (Hokkaidō) to the Southwest (Kagoshima). This ordering naturally places the prefectures into geographical groups that correspond broadly to cultural zones, each region being uniquely defined by climate, dialect, local craft specialities, soil, strains of rice, etc. For example, the districts of Hokkaidō and Tōhoku are known for their harsh climate and short growing season; Kyūshū and Shikoku for their relatively mild winters and protracted growing season that permits double cropping of rice in some areas; and Tōsan and Tōkai for silk raising and related textiles. Figure A1.1 shows the prefectures grouped into regions and numbered according to the 1930 census numbering (a numbering that remains in effect today).

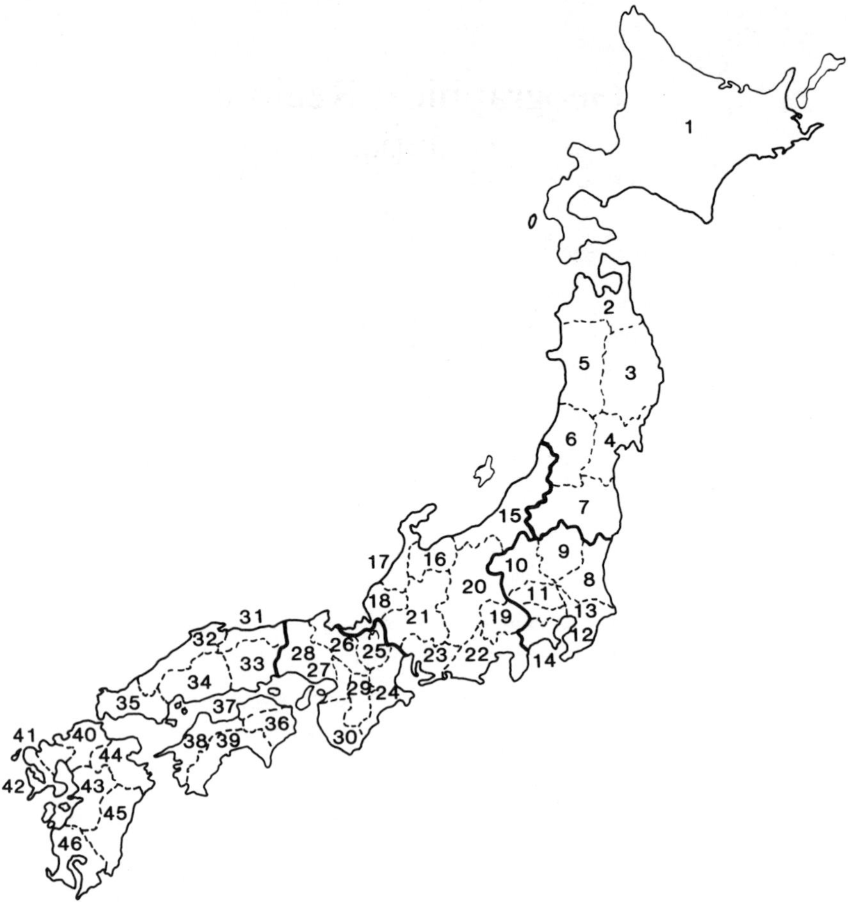

Fig. A1.1. The regions (unnumbered) and prefectures (numbered) of Japan. *Hokkaidō,* Hokkaidō (1); *Tōhoku,* Aomori (2), Iwate (3), Miyagi (4), Akita (5), Yamagata (6), and Fukushima (7); *Kantō,* Ibaraki (8), Tochigi (9), Gumma (10), Saitama (11), Chiba (12), Tokyo (13), and Kanagawa (14); *Hokuriku,* Niigata (15), Toyama (16), Ishikawa (17), and Fukui (18); *Tōsan,* Yamanashi (19), Nagano (20), and Gifu (21); *Tōkai,* Shizuoka (22), Aichi (23), and Mie (24); *Kinki,* Shiga (25), Kyōto (26), Ōsaka (27), Hyōgo (28), Nara (29), and Wakayama (30); *Chūgoku,* Tottori (31), Shimane (32), Okayama (33), Hiroshima (34), and Yamaguchi (35); *Shikoku,* Tokushima (36), Kagawa (37), Ehime (38), and Kōchi (39); *Kyūshū,* Fukuoka (40), Saga (41), Nagasaki (42), Kumamoto (43), Ōita (44), Miyazaki (45), and Kagoshima (46).

APPENDIX 2

Geographical Regions of Sweden

There are 24 counties in Sweden, or, counting Stockholm City (Stockholm Stad) as a county, 25 counties. These are traditionally put into seven groups (or eight, if one includes Stockholm City, which constitutes group 8). These contiguous county groups correspond roughly to regions that are similar in terms of natural resources and climate. For example, the North (North and South Norrlan) is rich in forests and the agricultural population commonly worked seasonally in forestry, cutting trees and pulling the felled trees to the rivers for subsequent transportation. The lake Mälar and Hjälmar district (most of East Sweden) contains several wide plains, but the soil is hard, which has made cultivation difficult. Iron ore deposits are primarily located in the old Bergslagen district (in Central Sweden) and because the ore is easily accessible in many of these locales, the region has been known as a center for mining since the Middle Ages. Figure A2.1 shows the regions and the counties numbered by the typical numbering system used in government publications.

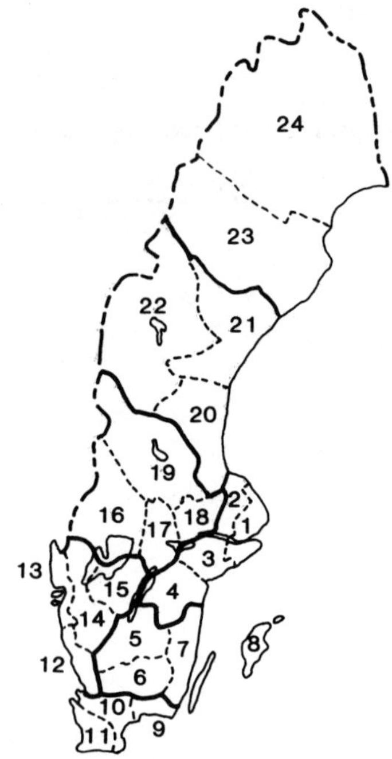

Fig. A2.1. Regions (unnumbered) and counties (numbered) of Sweden. *East Sweden,* Stockholm (1), Uppsala (2), Södermanland (3), and Östergötland (4); *Smaland,* Jönköping (5), Kronoberg (6), Kalmar (7), and Gotland (8); *South Sweden,* Blekinge (9), Kristianstad (10), and Malmöhus (11); *West Sweden,* Halland (12), Gothenburg and Bohus (13), Alvsborg (14), and Skaraborg (15); *Central Sweden,* Värmland (16), Örebro (17), Vastmanland (18), and Kopparberg (19); *South Norrlan,* Gälveborg (20), Vasternorrland (21), and Jämtland (22); *North Norrlan,* Vasterbotten (23) and Norrbotten (24).

APPENDIX 3

Data for the Prefectures of Japan

It is unnecessary to provide an elaborate discussion of the data assembled for the Japanese prefectures (and their rural and urban sectors) because the interested reader can secure from Mosk, on request, a copy of the paper by Mosk *et al.* (1980), which describes in great detail the data tape we have prepared containing all of the figures. Persons interested in obtaining a copy of the tape should contact the author, and a copy of the working paper and an estimate of the charges involved in duplicating, checking, and shipping the tape will be sent. The approximately 5000 variables entered on the tape fall into four categories: demographic; labor force and agriculture; education; and wage, price, and income variables, and so each set will be discussed separately.

A3.1. Demographic Figures

The variables in this file consist of raw data concerning population (classified by characteristics such as age group, sex, marital status, etc.) and vital events (births, deaths, infant deaths, etc.), and of various measures calculated from these raw data (e.g., Coale–Trussell parameters, Hutterite indices, etc.). The sources—primarily censuses and vital statistics—for these figures are given in the "Official Japanese Sources" section of the bibliography. As noted in Chapter 6 of the text, the figures on Japanese births are adjusted by estimating births from figures on children aged 0 and infant deaths. Only for the year 1960, when preliminary calculations showed registration was highly accurate, was this adjustment eschewed.

A3.2. Labor Force and Agriculture

The labor force data was secured from the censuses for 1920, 1930, 1950, and 1960, or the variables were calculated from these raw figures. The figures for 1930, 1950, and 1960 consisted of data on *both* employed persons classified by occupation and employed persons classified by industry. In 1920 no distinction was made between the two categories. It should also be noted that the prewar censuses asked persons what they "customarily did during the year" and not specifically what they did on October 1st, the date set for the Japanese census. The postwar censuses asked persons what they did on October 1st. October 1st was chosen as the date for the implementation of the Japanese census because most farmers bring in the harvest around that time and have not yet left for seasonal work in the cities, a practice (called *dekasegi*) common to a number of regions of Japan, especially the Northeast. The sources for these data appear in the "Official Japanese Sources" section of the bibliography.

The agricultural figures were taken from the special agricultural census of 1929 noted in the "Official Japanese Sources" section of the bibliography.

A3.3. Education

The data on education were secured from the 1970 census of Japan (see Nihon. Sōrifu Tōkeikyoku [various years] in "Official Japanese Sources"). It consists of figures for persons simultaneously classified by sex, age group (there are eight age classes: 15–19, 20–24, 25–29, 30–34, 35–44, 45–54, 55–64, and 65+), and educational attainment. There are eight categories of educational achievement listed, these groups are "have completed school," "have completed elementary school," etc., "have completed training school," etc., "have completed middle school," "have completed junior college, higher professional school," etc., "have completed college," etc., "are currently in school," and "never completed any schooling." The precise definition of some of these categories varies from cohort to cohort because of the various educational reforms. The postwar reforms of the late 1940s and early 1950s are especially important with regard to this point. Interested users of these data should consult the 1970 Japanese census (which like all censuses since 1955 has both English and Japanese throughout) before actually using the data.

A3.4. Prices, Wages, and Income

The data on prices, wages, and income were secured from various titles listed in the "Official Japanese Sources" section of the bibliography. Specifically, the volumes listed there that concern prefectural income, labor statistics, agricultural statistics, and prices yielded most of these figures. In addition figures worked up by Cleaver (1970) were used for some of the income data.

The raw data were all entered onto the tape as were all variables calculated from them. In a number of cases figures were unavailable and we had to "fill them in" by various techniques, methods that are described in Mosk *et al.* (1980). Moreover, calculating the price indices that we used in deflating nominal wages and income involved a number of strong working assumptions, and again the potential user of this material is encouraged to consult Mosk *et al.* (1980) with regard to these assumptions and the precise methodology employed.

APPENDIX 4

Data for the *Shi* (Cities) and *Gun* (Counties) of Japan

We prepared a data tape that consists of figures for each of the major subdivisions of each prefecture of Japan: the *shi* (cities) and *gun* (counties) for the years 1925–1938. Each prefecture (*ken*) is broken down into cities and counties that have jurisdiction independent of each other in the sense that counties do not contain cities within their boundaries. There were approximately 550 counties in interwar Japan and about 100 cities. The sources for these data are the same sources used to obtain the interwar prefectural data discussed in Sections A3.1 and A3.2 (the labor force data were only available for 1930). Potential users of this material should consult the working paper by Mosk and Faris (1979), and can inquire about obtaining copies of the tape from the author.

The figures for the cities consist of demographic data (for 1925, detailed census figures on population by sex, age, and marital status, etc.; and general vital statistics for 1925, 1930, and 1935), occupational and industrial data for 1930, agricultural data for 1929, and the results of a special official survey of infant mortality conducted in 1938. As noted, detailed census demographic data for the *shi* and *gun* are only available for 1925, although some population totals also exist for 1930 and 1935.

It is virtually impossible to utilize the *shi* and *gun* data for the postwar period in conjunction with these figures because of the myriad of administrative changes involving jurisdiction of *shi* and *gun* that were carried out soon after the war. Even during the period 1925 – 1938 some *shi* grew solely by incorporation of neighboring *gun* or portions of *gun,* and some *gun* ceased to exist for this or other reasons. However, these changes were minor and infrequent compared with the wholesale reorganization of the postwar period.

The reader of this study should note that m was estimated for each *shi* and *gun* for 1925 by assuming that the prefectural value of M was equal to the M value for each *shi* and *gun* in that prefecture and employing the data on married women in the quinquennial age classes. For the precise estimation procedure that involves approximating the solution to a nonlinear homogeneous equation, see Mosk and Faris (1979).

APPENDIX 5

Data for the Farm Households of Japan

The Japanese government began publishing, on an annual basis, detailed survey data on farm households during the interwar period. The data consist primarily of economic figures: budget figures on expenditures, income, labor, and capital inputs, etc., but also include demographic measures (e.g., age and sex structure of households) and some material concerning social status (tenancy class). In 1929 the survey involved 219 families, about equally divided between the three tenancy classes: owners, part-owners and part-tenants, and tenants. Because the 1929 data are especially rich, because 1929 was also the date for the agricultural census (see Appendixes 3 and 4), and because during the period after 1935 or so there were substantial distortions in the farmers' use of capital owing to the shortage of fertilizer and the like (attributable to the military circumstances of the time), it was decided to concentrate the analysis of farm household data on that one year. The source for the figures is given in the "Official Japanese Sources" section of the bibliography.

Mosk and Stoft (1979) provide a detailed discussion of the figures and the calculations employed to secure variables from the raw data. It also provides a glossary of the Japanese terms used in the survey. Persons interested in securing a copy of the data tape we created from these materials should contact the author for details concerning costs of duplication, checking, and related expenses that will be incurred in securing the tape. The potential user should also consult Mosk and Stoft (1979) for the precise details about the tape and the figures underlying it.

APPENDIX 6

Data for the Counties of Sweden

As with the Japanese prefectural tape described in Appendix 3, the Swedish county tape (also containing figures for the rural and urban sectors of the counties) that we created consists of data that captures aspects of demographic history, as well as circumstances surrounding labor force, education, prices, income, and wages. Potential users of the data tape interested in details should consult Mosk *et al.* (1980) and write to Mosk for information about securing a copy of the tape. In the working paper noted previously we describe the tape in terms of three categories of data and we discuss it briefly here with the same groupings (the data on education was added to the tape after the working paper by Mosk *et al.* [1980] was written and so it is not described there): demographic data, special figures on social and economic status, and estimates of wages, prices, and income.

A6.1. Demographic Variables

The raw data for these figures are taken from the census and vital statistics listed in the "Official Swedish Sources" section of the Bibliography, and from Hofsten and Lundström (1976). The demographic files on the tape consist of the raw figures on population structure (age, sex, marital status, etc.), and vital events (births, deaths, etc.). The variables we estimated from these numbers include Hutterite indices, the Coale–Trussell parameters, the singulate mean age at marriage, etc. The reader should note that the

Hutterite indices for each census year are calculated by averaging together births for a five-year period centered about that census date (e.g., 1878–1882 for the 1880 figure). This procedure reduces possible errors owing to special circumstances that might obtain during the census year under consideration. We were unable to utilize this technique with the Japanese prefectural data because we had to adjust the Japanese birth figures with figures on children aged 0, and the latter are only available for census years.

A6.2. Special Socioeconomic Variables

These figures include figures on income, social structure (e.g., types of landholdings and landless classes in rural areas, farm sizes, etc.), and population that were published by Stockholm University staff of the Institute for Social Sciences (1941) and variables we calculated from these. Related files involve figures on composition of the labor force (by sex) secured from sources given in the "Official Swedish Sources" portion of the bibliography.

A6.3. Wages, Prices, and Income

As with the Japanese prefectural estimates of wages, prices, and income (nominal and "real" [i.e., deflated]), the estimation of Swedish real and nominal wages and income was rather complicated, and the potential user of this material is urged to read carefully through the relevant sections of Mosk *et al.* (1980) before actually employing any of the figures. Discussion of how the estimates were obtained would take us too far afield here, except to note that the price indices we constructed are based on an extensive list of 45 commodities. In addition, it should be noted that Swedish counties had gathered figures on nominal wages (and prices), even prior to 1880, for administrative purposes (e.g., to help determine the wages that were to be paid out by the county authorities). Although certain scholars have criticized some of these figures, particularly for the nineteenth century, a detailed study by Jörberg (1972) provides a spirited and thorough defense of their basic accuracy.

APPENDIX 7

The Coale–Trussell Parameters of Natural Fertility and Parity-Specific Control[1]

As noted in Chapter 3, Ansley Coale and T. James Trussell have developed measures of aspects of marital fertility that they label M (the index of natural fertility) and m (the index of parity-specific control). Actually m is the average of age-specific values $m(a)$, where a represents the age or age group. The indices have received wide attention and have been used by many scholars in the analysis of natality. There is no doubt that the Coale–Trussell parameters are useful, indeed, we have utilized them at many points in this study as the reader can see, but it is also the case that they must be used and interpreted with great care. The purpose of this appendix is to describe briefly the methodology underlying the Coale–Trussell measures and then suggest the type of problems that the techniques they have developed produce. As we shall show, the issues that emerge from a discussion of the difficulties encountered in the estimation of the Coale–Trussell parameters do not lead to the conclusion that the method is invalid, but rather to the conclusion that the estimates one derives from the application of the technique must be treated and interpreted with care and caution.

A7.1. The Original Coale–Trussell Formulation and Its Modification

The intellectual origins of the Coale–Trussell methodology is the well-known paper by Henry (1961). In this paper Henry was concerned with variations in marital fertility among populations who apparently were not practicing fertility control *in the sense that couples were not changing their practices concerning reproduction as they moved from a given parity to the next.* That is, whatever practices they adopted concerning reproduction (e.g., postpartum sexual taboos, lactation customs, seasonal avoidance of intercourse, etc.) remained unchanged regardless of the number of children they had already given birth to (i.e., reproduction was parity independent). Henry called this type of reproduction "natural fertility." By contrast, Henry argued, populations that showed strong evidence of birth control in the sense that couples ceased having offspring altogether after they had given birth to a certain specified number (or stopped and then, after a sustained interval, started reproduction again, after which they stopped altogether, etc.) were not practicing natural fertility because their behavior was parity dependent. He called this type of parity-dependent control "parity-specific control." It should be emphasized that Henry was concerned with describing natural fertility in populations showing no evidence of parity-specific control. This must be emphasized because Coale and Trussell unfortunately choose Henry's terms to describe the parameters of marital fertility they developed estimation techniques for and, in general, the parameters M and m that one secures do *not* have the simple meaning Henry intended them to have, for his goal was simply to *define* and measure natural fertility (as reproduction in the absence of parity-specific control) in populations not practicing parity-dependent control and *not* to measure it in populations practicing parity-specific control.

Coale (1971) commenced his investigations concerning the empirical decomposition of fertility schedules with the observation, noted by Henry (1961), that natural fertility populations show a characteristic pattern of marital fertility with respect to the age of women, regardless of the level of marital fertility at each age. This, it should be stressed, was the germ of Henry's idea, in the sense that he made this point the empirical basis, the justification, for his definition. The shape of the curve traced out by the age-specific marital fertility rates when natural fertility obtains is convex to the origin (i.e., "bowed outward" away from the origin). This is well illustrated by the schedule for Miyagi Prefecture in 1925 as pictured in Fig. A7.1. The *shape* primarily reflects the biological conditioning of reproductive capacity associated with age: relatively rapid improvement in reproductive capacity from menarche until a peak (plateau) is reached, and then

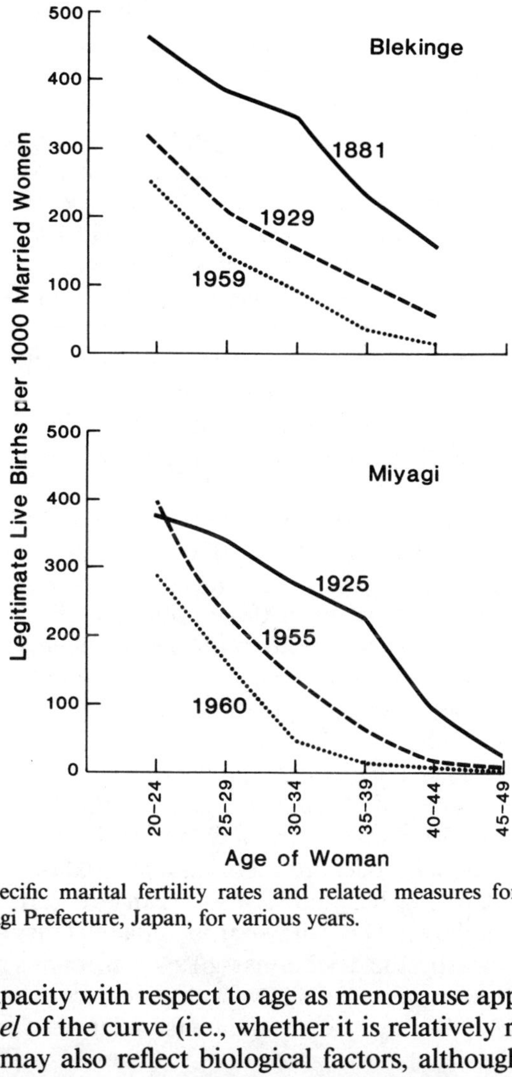

Fig. A7.1. Age-specific marital fertility rates and related measures for Blekinge County, Sweden, and Miyagi Prefecture, Japan, for various years.

falling off of capacity with respect to age as menopause approaches. Variations in the *level* of the curve (i.e., whether it is relatively remote from the origin or not) may also reflect biological factors, although breast feeding practices and postpartum sexual taboos undoubtedly also determine the level of natural fertility (see the arguments in Chapters 3 and 4). The point is that, in the absence of parity-specific control, the fertility schedule tends to take on a characteristic shape, although its level (i.e., distance from the origin) varies depending on biological and behavioral practices that affect the length of interbirth intervals.[2] The idea behind the Coale–Trussell technique is to capture the *level* of age-specific marital fertility with the index M and the shape of the schedule by m [and the age-specific values of

m, $m(a)$]. Specifically, a "pure" natural fertility population would be described by a value of M (its level) and the condition that the shape conformed to the characteristic curvature (i.e., $m = m(a) = 0$, for all a). The index of parity-specific control m then would measure the deviation away from the characteristic natural fertility shape, the idea being that the greater the distortion (i.e., deviation away from the characteristic shape) the greater would be the overall index of parity-specific control m. The values of age-specific marital fertility for Blekinge and Miyagi in 1960 (see Fig. A7.1) correspond to populations in which m is substantial. Note that they are concave ("bowed in") to the origin, suggesting, along the lines sketched out by Henry in his original formulation, that parity-specific control involves the cessation of reproduction at the higher ages (i.e., after couples have achieved a certain parity). In short, the original Coale–Trussell model is based solely on the *age*-specific characteristics of marital fertility, i.e., the level of the rates and their relative deviation away from the "natural fertility" shape implicit in the schedule.

The concrete problem solved by Coale (1971), a solution that was later modified somewhat in Coale and Trussell (1974), was how to actually estimate M, m, and the $m(a)$. The procedures they adopted are ad hoc in the sense that they are not based on a theory about natural fertility (i.e., a mathematical model of reproduction), but rather involve an application of standard curve fitting techniques, under the assumptions [which Trussell (1979) shows to be robust] that natural fertility populations have a characteristic shape in their schedule of age-specific marital fertility, and as parity-specific control develops, the distortion in the shape of the schedule (i.e., its tendency to become "bowed in") is *also* regular, in the sense that fertility at the higher ages (over 30) falls to extremely low levels.

Coale's (1971) original procedure was to assume that one level of natural fertility (the "standard" for his model, $M = 1$) can be described by a specific schedule of age-specific rates $n(a)$ drawn from data in Henry (1961). He also assumed that the age-specific deviations $v(a)$ away from this natural fertility schedule observed for an average of low fertility modern populations for the postwar period, describe the second standard (standardized as $m = 1$). Thus the original schedule $n(a)$ corresponds to $m = 0$ and $M = 1$, and a population having age-specific rates that were a constant multiple (the same multiple for each age) of those used to calculate the $v(a)$ would have $m = 1$. To calculate M, m, and the $m(a)$ Coale (1971) proceeded as follows. Let $f(a)$ be the age-specific marital fertility rate for age group a. Then he wrote

$$f(a) = Mn(a)e^{m(a)v(a)} \tag{A7.1}$$

and he estimated M (denoting $\hat{M}$ as the estimator of M) on data for women aged 20–24 as

$$\hat{M} = f(20\text{–}24)/n(20\text{–}24) \tag{A7.2}$$

From this the estimate of $m(a)$, $\hat{m}(a)$, can be calculated as

$$\hat{m}(a) = \{\log[f(a)/\hat{M}n(a)]\}/v(a) \qquad \text{(A7.3)}$$

Therefore

$$\hat{m} = \left[\sum_{a=25-29}^{40-44} \hat{m}(a)\right] \Big/ 4$$

gives the estimate of m, where there are four age groups for which the $m(a)$ are estimated.[3] The $n(a)$ and $v(a)$ used are shown in the accompanying tabulation.

	20–24	25–29	30–34	35–39	40–44
$n(a)$	460	431	395	322	167
$v(a)$	0	–.279	–.667	–1.042	–1.414

Coale and Trussell (1974, 1978) modified the original procedure by simultaneously estimating M and m [rather than sequentially estimating them as Coale (1971) does] with the following equation, which is estimated by ordinary least squares:

$$\log[f(a)/n(a)] = \log(M^*) + m^*v(a) + \epsilon \qquad \text{(A7.4)}$$

where M^* and m^* are the estimates of M and m, respectively, as obtained in this approach. The mean square error of the regression Eq. (4) is used as a measure of the goodness of fit of the schedule. It should be emphasized that either approach involves curve fitting in the sense that the curves are embodied in the $n(a)$ and $v(a)$, which are then used to obtain the estimates of M and m.

Page (1977), working within the general framework developed by Coale–Trussell, has attempted to refine the estimates to take into account duration of marriage as well as age, noting that a number of studies of modern populations show coitus decreases with the number of years of marriage.[4] She arrives at a four parameter model that accomplishes this. Unfortunately her estimation of the model requires data on age-specific legitimate births classified by age of mother and duration of marriage. This data is rarely available for aggregate populations, although it often can be worked up for populations studied by family reconstitution methods (but see Note 2 of this appendix on the problems often plaguing application of these techniques to family reconstitution figures).

Before we proceed to systematically discuss the problems that arise with this methodology, let us emphasize that (in the absence of data on marital duration) its application hinges solely on the *age*-specific nature of marital fertility. Everything is inferred from data classified by age, which is, after all, the basis of the curve fitting used in the Coale (1971) and Coale–Trussell (1974, 1978) models. It is precisely this feature that causes the most problems for the estimation and interpretation of the empirical parameters, as we shall see.

To systematically carry out the discussion of the methodological problems, we shall group these into two types and take up each group separately. The first relates to the problems of interpretation of M and m; the second to the problems of measurement. Although related—in the sense that the meaning one wishes to give to the parameters is obviously intimately bound up with the question of how one attempts to statistically capture the parameters—the two issues are best discussed separately.

A7.2. Problems in the Interpretation of the Coale–Trussell Parameters

Perhaps the greatest difficulty with interpreting the indices involves the very names Coale assigned to them—a decision that reflects their intellectual origins in the work of Henry (1961). When the estimated value of $m \simeq 0$ and the mean square error on the regression used to estimate M and m is small, it is a relatively safe conclusion that M measures natural fertility. But when parity-specific control is clearly present, this is not necessarily the case. As the discussion in Chapters 7 and 8 indicates, and as one can see from the Blekinge data in Fig. A7.1, M often falls during the initial phase of the fertility transition. What is clearly at work is a deliberate lengthening of birth intervals for the purpose of restricting overall number of births and surviving family size, the opposite type of behavior from that in which couples deliberately stretch out the birth interval to maximize the number of surviving offspring (see the discussion in Chapters 4, 5, and 6 on this point). Thus the estimate of M obtained no longer has the simple interpretation it does when $m \simeq 0$ as a measure of reproductive capacity modified only by practices like postpartum sexual taboos, which are *not* designed to limit overall surviving family size. For manipulation of M as well as m may well have become part of the strategy of reducing fertility (i.e., lengthening interbirth intervals as well as terminating reproduction). In such a case it is better to think of M as a measure of level (and not of natural fertility), that is, a parameter that roughly corresponds to interbirth intervals. Thus the names "natural fertility" and "parity-specific control" are undoubtedly inappropriate in such a context, if we invest them with the meaning that Henry (1961) originally wished to give them. Trussell (1979:47–48) has conceded this point:

> Something, therefore, is wrong with the interpretation that the level parameter represents the level at which natural fertility is experienced, since there is no reason to suppose that in general the level of natural fertility shall fall as control is increased . . . A more reasonable interpretation would be that the level parameter is composed of several factors, only one of which is the level of underlying natural fertility . . . Unfortunately, further separation of the level parameter cannot be accomplished and we conclude that, in the presence of control, discovery of the underlying level of natural fertility from existing models of age-specific (marital) fertility rates is not possible.

In short, the labels given to M and m by Coale and Trussell are often misleading when $m > 0$ (e.g., $m > .2$). And for this reason one must be very careful in interpreting them.

A7.3. Problems in the Estimation of the Coale–Trussell Parameters

The basic problem in estimating M and m arises from the rigid curve fitting that underlies the estimation procedure, that is, from the failure to take into account other things besides the rates of reproduction by age of mother. Even a model that, like Page's (1977), takes into account marital duration, will not address the problem raised here. Consider the following possibility. There are two populations and married women have on average two children in both populations, spaced about 3 years apart, but in the first population on average women begin childbearing at age 22 and in the second they on average begin childbearing at age 32 (ignore mortality here). Then a consideration of the Coale–Trussell methodology, which measures basically the existence or nonexistence of childbearing after age 30 (the concaveness of the curve) suggests that if we estimate m in the first population we will get a higher value than in the second. But the total marital fertility rate (the sum of the age-specific rates) is the same in the two populations, so this means the estimate of M must be *higher* in the first than in the second population. (Intuitively this can be seen from the formulae discussed in Section A7.1. The idea is that the greater m is, the greater M must be, because they "multiply" out, after some functional transformation, to the total marital fertillity rate.) Specifically, Weir (1980) has employed methods of numerical approximation on empirical data to develop the following approximate functional relationship:

$$M = TMFR(.11361 + .0607m) \qquad \text{(mean squared error} = .0000329) \qquad \text{(A7.5)}$$

where the $TMFR$ is the total marital fertility rate. In short, the timing of reproduction (when control occurs)—whether it comes early or late in the woman's reproductive years—obviously can be a factor in determining the estimates of M and m that one obtains. For this reason the age at marriage may be a factor in determining the levels of M and m one estimates. Figure A7.1 illustrates this. One reason why both m and M are so much higher in Miyagi in 1960 than in Blekinge in 1960 is because at that time Japanese women typically had children in their early or middle 20s and then stopped reproducing altogether whereas many women in Sweden postponed child-bearing until their late 20s or early 30s. As a result, we tend to inflate M and m in the Coale–Trussle estimation procedures for Miyagi as compared with Blekinge, both populations of which had low overall total marital fertility rates.

Notes to Appendix 7

1. I am grateful to Kenneth Wachter and David Weir for their assistance in developing the arguments presented in this appendix. In particular Weir (1980) contains an extremely detailed and useful discussion of a number of the points noted here, and of related issues.

2. In small populations the variance in the age-specific rates one secures is often very great, and the observed schedules are not quite shifts of the characteristic (standard) schedule selected by Coale (1971) and Coale and Trussell (1974).

This is especially the case for the schedules secured from parish or village figures resulting from family reconstitution studies, for which estimates for age-specific marital fertility are usually based on very small samples. For aggregate data this is not such an issue. Trussell (1979), using principal components factor analysis to decompose the thirteen schedules for natural fertility populations presented by Henry (1961) in his original article, concludes that the basic idea of assuming a characteristic shape to natural fertility is valid. For instance, Trussell (1979:38–39) concludes:

> These general findings support the hypotheses made by Henry. First an underlying pattern is evident, and the major variation is one of level. A second source of variation is one which acts to decrease the standardized rates at low ages and increase the rates increasingly at higher ages. This factor may be interpreted as the inverse of the rate at which sterility occurs. The small contribution given by the third factor, which acts upon the extremes, may indicate that age at menarche, adolescent sterility, and age at menopause are the source of small variations in natural fertility.

3. Because of the substantial variability in the marital fertility rate for the age groups 45–49, the figures for this group are usually not included in making the estimates of M and m.

4. In natural fertility populations this may or may not occur. It is not at all clear. Insofar as it does, it may lead to a positive correlation between M and the age at marriage for females, although Weir (1980) suggests that this factor is *not* important in his data for French villages. For this reason we place greater weight on the infant mortality rate than the index of natural fertility in claiming empirical support for the model of the premodern demographic regime (see Chapters 5 and 6). It should be pointed out, moreover, that the relationship between the *SMAMF* and M is not significant everywhere, and that Weir (1980) does not find it to have any empirical foundation in his data.

APPENDIX 8

The Determinants of Natural Fertility[1]

In Section 2.3, we present a behavioral model concerning the determination of natural fertility; and in Section 2.5, we indicated that one would expect a direct relationship between natural fertility levels and the standard of living. When there is little or no parity-specific control, so that we can approximate natural fertility levels relatively accurately with the Coale–Trussell parameter M, we would expect M to be positively related to per capital income. Table 3.10 is consistent with this thesis. The question arises, however, as to why this association exists. Is it attributable at least in part to the behavioral mechanisms suggested, or is it primarily owing to something else? The point of this appendix is to argue that the association between natural fertility and the standard of living is not spurious, there are two plausible interpretations of this association: one biological and the other behavioral; and behavioral mechanisms probably dominate.

To coherently organize this discussion first consider Table A7.1. The table lists the possible interactions between the components of the two major categories of determinants of natural fertility and natural fertility itself. Let us begin with the biological connections first.

A8.1. Biological: Mother's Condition

In numerous articles and papers Frisch and her co-authors have advanced the argument that age at menarche (and the length of postpartum amenor-

TABLE A8.1

Possible Avenues Through Which the Standard of Living Can Influence Natural Fertility

Biological

(1) Mother's Condition[a]

(a) Direct physiological connection (e.g., body fatness, effects of lactation when nutritional intake is low, etc.) between nutrition and natural fertility. Main direct effect of body fatness is on age at menarche and in consequence it probably does not have a great impact on overall fertility. Effect of interaction of lactation with nutrition on birth intervals is known to exist but probably is not great.

(b) Morbidity (e.g., temporary or permanent sterility owing to diseases whose incidence is related to the standard of living such as tuberculosis, libido, etc.).

(2) Father's condition

morbidity (e.g., libido).

(3) Childrens' Condition

Risks of infant mortality.

Behavioral

(1) Lactation and Sexual Practices

Lactation practices and postpartum sexual taboos attributable to behavior designed to maximize number of surviving children (as health conditions improve this artificial spacing of births presumably declines in length, seasonality of intercourse related directly to harvest cycle, etc.).

(2) Separation of Spouses

Out migration of husbands owing to poor harvest in locale, etc.

[a] The terms "mother's" and "father's" are used although to be precise the terms "woman's" and "man's" should be used to make the distinction with "children's" condition. Thus under "mother's condition" menarche, sterility, etc., are included.

rhea periods) depends on the body's storing a critical minimum level of fatness [see Frisch (1978, 1979)]. The reasoning is simple and appealing. Pregnancy and lactation demand considerable amounts of energy, and hence they drain away calories stored in the body. If fat reserves are insufficient to supply these requisite calories, fecundity is hampered. Frisch's work has been controversial and has been criticized on two grounds: (i) because there are deficiencies in her statistical methodology [see Trussell (1978)] and (ii) because field studies of various populations indicate that various anthropometric measures of fatness do not appear to be related to the reproductive performance of women [see Chowdhury (1978) and Bongaarts and Delgado (1979) for this evidence]. Although no scholar working in this area claims a definitive conclusion has been reached on the fatness hypothesis, the general thrust of the literature appears to run counter to it.

In contrast, there is considerable evidence that supports the view that nutritional deficiencies prolong the periods of postpartum amenorrhea and anovulatory cycles following the resumption of menstruation. All field studies in the two volumes considered here support this generalization as do the reviews of the medical literature.[2] It has been suggested that the nutritional status of the mother influences the volume of milk produced (but not its quality, its nutritional composition), and this in turn determines the infant's suckling time. Suckling causes prolactin to be released, which inhibits the release of gonadotrophins that cause the menstrual cycle to resume. It should be emphasized that we are only concerned with the biological impact of nutrition on the effects of lactation here, the decision to breast feed and its possible relation to nutrition is a separate issue involving behavioral mechanisms. What is plausible is that in societies in which women practice prolonged breast feeding, good nutrition improves natural fertility.

As suggested in the chart, another possible biological link between the standard of living and reproductive performance runs through the effects of food intake on morbidity, and morbidity on reproduction. Although it is difficult to accept a connection between venereal diseases and the standard of living, there is evidence that suggests diet and household resources have an impact on the incidence and effective treatment of tuberculosis (this is a more reasonable conclusion for the period prior to World War II). One form of tuberculosis is genital tuberculosis, and it is possible that some of the involuntary sterility of European and Japanese women in the period prior to World War I was owing to this disease, see Gray (1979), also see McFalls (1981). Finally, libido may respond to nutritional circumstances.

A8.2. Biological: Father's Condition

The factor usually cited is loss of libido. There is some evidence that associates this with dearth of food, or at least particular nutrients.[3]

A8.3. Biological: Children's Condition

There is substantial data that favors the view that maternal nutrition and food intake of the infant affect the infant's survival chances. If a woman breast feeds, the survival of an infant affects her chances of becoming pregnant because, as we have already noted, lactation stretches out birth intervals [see Knodel (1979)]. In this instance the effects of nutrition run in both directions. To the extent better nutrition enhances the survivorship of children already born, natural fertility will be reduced. However, to the extent better food intake reduces the lactation effect, natural fertility increases.

A8.4. Behavioral: Lactation and Sexual Practices

At this juncture we enter a gray area where culture and rational behavior reponding to nutrition commingle. A number of papers point out that breast feeding has an economic cost associated with it, and that women respond to job opportunities and the availability of foodstuffs in deciding how long to breast feed.[4] When alternative sources of healthful foods are scarce, breast feeding is a rational response to the problem posed by infant mortality. But culture may play a role independently of these considerations, and it is difficult to draw a clear distinction. (However, it should be pointed out that cultures tend to make a virtue out of necessity.)

There is a considerable body of descriptive material that supports the notion that, in a natural fertility setting, couples practice postpartum and lactation sexual taboos as a means of stretching out interbirth intervals, to protect the health of the mother and the infant.[5] That is, a strategy of maximizing the number of surviving offspring may dictate a low natural fertility strategy, in conditions of poor nutrition.

A8.5. Behavioral: Separation of Spouses

Finally, in periods of famine or poor harvest (when nutritional input is typically impaired), husbands or wives may migrate away from their homes in search of employment in more prosperous districts. This tends to reduce natural fertility.

In sum, what can we say about this literature? The following points seem to be reasonable:

(1) There is some definite connection between the standard of living and average levels of natural fertility for populations. This does not mean that culture does not matter but only that, given a cultural regime, we would expect variations in the standard of living to be positively associated with variations in levels of natural fertility.

(2) The direct biological connection between the standard of living and natural fertility is not especially strong, the most important linkage probably running through genital tuberculosis.

(3) There do appear to be important behavioral linkages between the standard of living and natural fertility.

The general conclusion, then, is that the literature in this area does tend to support the theoretical approach as laid out in Sections 2.3 and 2.5.

Notes to Appendix 8

1. This section rests heavily on four publications: Leridon and Menken (1979), Mosley (1978), Page and Lesthaeghe (1981), and Mosk (1981c).

2. For the medical literature see Tyson and Perez (1978), Van Ginneken (1978), and Wray (1978). For field studies see Caraël (1978); Delgado *et al.* (1978); Osteria (1978); Hull (1978); and Jain *et al.* (1979).

3. See Stein and Susser (1978). They discuss the Dutch famine of 1944–1945.

4. See Butz (1978), Popkin (1978), Corsini (1979), and Caldwell (1979). In a number of papers Bongaarts [see for instance, Bongaarts (1980a, 1980b)] has argued that breast feeding practices account for an extremely large percentage of the variation of natural fertility within populations that do not practice parity-specific control. It should be noted, however, that the data (for samples of women in various countries) from which he derives his estimates do not allow Bongaarts to deal with the possible coexistence of postpartum sexual taboos with breast feeding in these populations. This is an important point because some of the contribution in reducing natural fertility that he assigns to breast feeding may be owing to low levels of coital frequency involving postpartum sexual taboos. It should also be emphasized that findings that point to breast feeding as a major factor in shaping natural fertility do not mean—as some enthusiasts of this position seem to imply—that nutrition does not matter in determining natural fertility. It only means, as Bongaarts himself concedes, that nutrition may be having an indirect (via the behavior practice of breast feeding) influence on natural fertility rather than a direct, physiological influence of the sort Frisch (1978, 1979) has in mind. See Lithell (1981a) for a discussion of breast feeding practices on historical populations in Sweden.

5. See Corsini (1979) and Caldwell (1979) and Caldwell and Caldwell (1981). In Chapter 5 we present evidence for Japan that supports this point for the Japanese case.

PART V

References

References

This bibliography is divided into three sections: (*a*) Official Japanese Statistics, (*b*) Official Swedish Statistics, and (*c*) Other Sources.

Official Japanese Sources

Japan. Bank of Japan (1938). *Economic Statistics of Japan,* 1937 (Tokyo).

Nihon. Eiseikyoku (various years). [Japan. Health Bureau]. *Eiseikyoku nenkan* [Yearbook of the Health Bureau.] Tokyo.

Nihon. Keizai Kikakuchō. [Japan. Economic Planning Agency] (various years). *Chiiki kankei tōkei yōran* [Survey of Regional Statistics.] Tokyo.

Nihon. Keizai Kikakuchō Shotokubu Kanshū [Japan. Economic Planning Agency, Office of Income]. (1963). *Kenmin shotoku tōkei* [Statistics of Prefectural Income.] Tokyo.

Nihon. Kōseishō Eiseikyoku. [Japan. Health Bureau of Ministry of Health and Welfare]. (1938–present). *Eisei nenpō.* [Annual Health Report.] Tokyo.

Nihon. Kōseishō. Jinkō Mondai Kenkyūjo (1966). *Standardized birth rates by prefectures, 1930, 1950, 1955 and 1960.* Tokyo.

Nihon. Kōseishō. Jinkō Mondai Kenkyūjo (1967). [Japan. Ministry of Health and Welfare. Office of Population Problems]. *Standardized vital rates by prefectures,* 1925. Tokyo.

Nihon. Kōseishō Eiseitōkeikyoku [Japan. Ministry of Health and Welfare, Health Department Statistics] (various years). *Jinkō dōtai tōkei.* [Vital statistics.] (1946–present). Tokyo.

Nihon. Kōseisho Shakaikyoku [Japan. Ministry of Health and Welfare, Bureau of Social Affairs]. (1941). *Shōwa jūsannen tenkoku dō, fu, ken, shi, ku, chō, son betsu shussan, shussei, shisan oyobi nyūyoji shibō tōkei* [Statistics on births, live births, stillbirths, and infant and child deaths for the whole country, the prefectures, cities, wards, towns, and villages in 1938.] Tokyo.

Nihon. Naikaku Tōkeikyoku [Japan. Cabinet Bureau of Statistics] (1927). *Fubo no nenrei to shussei to no kankei.* [Births in relation to ages of parents.] (For 1925; for 1930, a similar volume was published.) Tokyo.

Nihon. Naikaku Tōkeikyoku [Japan. Cabinet Bureau of Statistics] (various years). *Jinkō dōtai tōkei.* [Vital Statistics.] (For 1899–1942). Tokyo.

Nihon. Naikaku Tōkeikyoku [Japan. Cabinet Bureau of Statistics] (various years). *Kokusei chōsa hōksho.* [Report of the Population Census.] (For 1920, 1925, 1930, and 1935.) Tokyo.

Nihon. Naikaku Tōkeikyoku [Japan. Cabinet Bureau of Statistics] (various years). *Nihon teikoku jinkō seitai tōkei.* [Statistics of the State of Population.] (For 1898, 1903, 1908, 1913, and 1918.) Tokyo.

Nihon. Naikaku Tōkeikyoku [Japan. Cabinet Bureau of Statistics] (1911). *Nihon teikoku shiin tōkei, Meiji yon-jū-ichi-nen.* [Statistics on the causes of death in the Empire of Japan, 1908.] Tokyo.

Nihon. Naikaku Tōkeikyoku [Japan. Cabinet Bureau of Statistics] (various years). *Nihon teikoku tōkei nenkan.* [Statistical Yearbook of the Empire of Japan.] Tokyo.

Nihon. Naikaku Tōkeikyoku [Japan. Cabinet Bureau of Statistics] (1932). *Nōgyō chōsa kekka.* [Report of the results of the Agricultural Census] (For 1929). Tokyo.

Nihon. Naikaku Tōkeikyoku [Japan. Cabinet Bureau of Statistics] (various years). *Rōdō tōkei jicchi chōsa hōkusho.* [Report on the Statistics of the on-site survey of labor.] Tokyo.

Nihon. Naikaku Tōkeikyoku [Japan. Cabinet Bureau of Statistics] (1927, 1932, 1938). *Shi, chō, son betsu jinkō dōtai tōkei.* [Vital Statistics for cities, towns and villages.] Tokyo.

Nihon. Nōrinshō. [Japan. Ministry of Agriculture and Forestry] (various years). *Nōsaku yatoi chingin tōkeihyō.* [Statistical tables on the wages of agricultural workers.] Tokyo.

Nihon. Nōrinshō Nōmukyoku. [Japan. Ministry of Agriculture and Forestry Agricultural Bureau] (various years). *Nōka keizai chōsa.* [Survey on Economy of Agricultural Families.] Tokyo.

Nihon. Nōrinshō. Nōrin Keizaikyoku Tōkeichōsabu. [Japan. Ministry of Agriculture and Forestry. Agricultural Economic Bureau. Statistics and Survey Division] (various years). *Nōrin tōkeihyō* [Statistical tables on agriculture and forestry.] Tokyo.

Nihon. Rōdōshō. Daijin Kanbō Rōdō Tōkei Chōsabu. [Japan. Ministry of Labor. Minister's Office. Labor Statistics and Survey Division] (various years). *Rōdō tōkei chōsa geppo.* [Monthly Labor Statistics and Research Bulletin.] Tokyo.

Nihon. Rōdōshō Daijin Kanbō Tōkei Chōsabu. [Japan. Ministry of Labor. Minister's Office. Statistics and Survey Division] (various years). *Rōdō tōkei nenpō.* [Yearbook of Labor Statistics].

Nihon. Sōrifu Tōkeikyoku. [Japan. Prime Ministers' Statistical Bureau.] (various years). *Kokusei chōsa hōkusho.* [Report of the Population Census.] (For 1950, 1955, 1960, and 1970). Tokyo.

——— (1962) *Retail Price in Japan, 1950–1960.* Tokyo.

Nihon. Tōkeiin (1882). *Kai* (*no*) *Kuni Meiji 12-nen Jimbetsu* (*no*) *Shirabe.* [Census of individuals in the province of Kai.] Tokyo.

Official Swedish Sources

Sweden. Socialstyrelsen. [Sweden. Social Welfare Board]. (various years). *Lönestatistisk årsbok for Sveriges* [Yearbook of Labor Statistics for Sweden]. Stockholm.

Sweden. Statistiska centralbyrån. [Sweden. Central Statistical Office]. (various years). *Bidrag till Sveriges officiella statistik.* [Supplement to official Swedish statistics.] A. *Befolkningsstatistik Ny följd.* [Population Statistics. New Series] (for 1900 to 1910). Stockholm.

——— (1974). *Elever i Obligatoriska Skolor 1847–1962.* [Pupils in Compulsory Schools in Sweden, 1847–1962.] Stockholm.

——— (various years). *Sveriges officiella statistik.* [Official Swedish statistics]. *Befolkningsrörelsen* [Population Movements] (for 1911–1960). Stockholm.

——— (various years). *Sveriges officiella statistik* [Official Swedish statistics]. *Folkmängdens förändringar.* [Changes in Population Size.] (For 1961–1966). Stockholm.

——— (1959). *Historical Statistics of Sweden,* II (1955) (Stockholm).

——— (1969). *Historisk statistik för Sverige Del. I: Befolkning. Andra upplagan 1720–1967.* [Historical statistics of Sweden. Part I. Population. Second Edition, 1720–1967.] Stockholm.

Other sources

Åberg, Y. (1969). *Produktion och produktivitet i Sverige, 1861–1965.* Stockholm: Almquist and Wiksell.

Åkerman, S. (1978). A demographic study of a pre-transitional society. In *Chance and change: social and economic studies in historical demography in the baltic area* (S. Åkerman, H. C. Johansen, and D. Gaunt, eds), pp. 33–48. Odense: Odense University Press.

Akimoto, H. (1981). Capital formation and economic growth in mid-19th century Japan. *Explorations in Economic History* **18**(1):40–59.

Ariga, Kizaemon (1968). *Ariga Kizaemon Sakushū.* [Collected Works of Ariga Kizaemon], Vol. VI. Tokyo: Miraisha.

Barnum, H. N., and Squire, L. (1979). An econometric application of the theory of the farm-household. *Journal of Development Economics* **6**:79–102.

Beardsley, R.; Hall, J.; and Ward, R. (1959). *Village Japan.* Chicago: University of Chicago Press.

Becker, G. (1976). *The economic approach to human behavior.* Chicago: University of Chicago Press.

Becker, G. (1981). *A treatise on the family.* Cambridge, Massachusetts: Harvard University Press.

Berent, J. (1970). Causes of fertility decline in Eastern Europe and the Soviet Union, Part I. *Population Studies* **24**:35–38.

Bernhardt, E. (1971). *Trends and variations in Swedish fertility: A cohort study.* Stockholm: Statistiska Centralbyran.

Bongaarts, J. (1980a). Does malnutrition affect fecundity: A summary of evidence. *Science* **208; 209**:564–569.

Bongaarts, J. (1980b). The fertility-inhibiting effects of the intermediate fertility variables. Population Council. Center for Policy Studies. Working Paper No. 57.

Bongaarts, J., and Delgado, H. (1979). Effects of nutritional status on fertility in rural Guatemala. In *Natural Fertility* (H. Leridon and J. Menken, eds.), pp. 107–134. Leige: Ordina Editions, for the International Union for the Scientific Study of Population.

Butz, W. (1978). Economic Aspects of Breast-Feeding. In *Nutrition and Human reproduction* (W. H. Mosley, ed.), pp. 231–255. New York/London: Plenum Press.

Caldwell, J. (1976). Toward a restatement of demographic transition theory. *Population and Development Review* **2–4**:321–366.

Caldwell, J. (1978). A theory of fertility: from high plateau to destabilization. *Population and Development Review* **4**(4):553–577.

Caldwell, J. (1979). Variations in the incidence of sexual abstinence and the duration of postnatal abstinence among the Yoruba of Nigeria. In *Natural Fertility* (H. Leridon and

J. Menken, eds.), pp. 397–407. Leige: Ordina Editions for the International Union for the Scientific Study of Population.

Caldwell, J. (1980). Mass education as a determinant of the timing of fertility decline. *Population and Development Review* **6**(2):225–255.

Caldwell, P., and Caldwell, J. C. (1981). The function of child-spacing in traditional societies and the direction of change. In *Child-spacing in tropical Africa: traditions and change* (H. Page and R. Lesthaeghe, eds.), pp. 73–92. New York: Academic Press.

Caraël, M. (1978). Relations between birth intervals and nutrition in three Central African populations (Zaire). In *Nutrition and human reproduction* (W. H. Mosley, ed.), pp. 365–384. New York/London: Plenum Press.

Carlsson, S. (1968). *Från Familjeutvandring till Ensamutvandring. En Utvecklingslinjen i den Svenska Emigrationens Historia.* [From Family Emigration to Individual Emigration. A Line of Development in the History of Swedish Emigration]. In *Emigrationer. En Bok till Vilhelm Moberg,* pp. 101–122. Stockholm: Almquist and Wiksell.

Carlsson, S. (1969). Some aspects of the Swedish emigration to the United States. *SPHQ* **20**(4):192–203.

Carlsson, S. (1978). Unmarried women in the Swedish society of estates. In *Chance and change: social and economic studies in historical demography in the baltic area* (S. Åkerman, H. C. Johansen, and D. Gaunt, eds.) pp. 220–226. Odense: Odense University Press.

Chayanov, A. V. (1966). *The theory of peasant economy.* Homewood: R. D. Irwin. (Reprint and translation for the American Economic Association).

Cho, Lee-Jay and Kobayashi, K., editors (1979). *Fertility transition of the East Asian populations.* Honolulu: The University Press of Hawaii.

Chowdhury, A. K. M. A. (1978). Effect of maternal nutrition on fertility in rural Bangladesh. In *Nutrition and human reproduction* (W. H. Mosley, ed.), pp. 401–410. New York/London: Plenum Press.

Cipolla, C. (1969). *Literacy and development in the West.* Baltimore: Penguin Books.

Cleaver, T. (1970). Regional income differentials in Japanese economic growth. Ph.D. dissertation, Harvard University.

Coale, A. (1965). Factors associated with the development of low fertility: An historic survey. *United Nations World Population Conference* **2**:205–209.

Coale, A. (1971). Age patterns of marriage. *Population Studies* **25**(2):193–214.

Coale, A. (1973). The demographic transition reconsidered. In *International union for scientific study of population. International Population Conference,* Vol. 1 pp. 53–72. Leige: I.U.S.S.P.

Coale, A. (1979). The demographic transition: A summary, some lessons, and some observations, edited by L. J. Cho and K. Kobayashi. *Fertility transition of the East Asian populations.* Honolulu: The University Press of Hawaii.

Coale, A.; Anderson, B. A.; and Harm, E. (1979). *Human fertility in Russia since the nineteenth century.* Princeton: Princeton University Press.

Coale, A., and Trussell, J. (1974). Model fertility schedules: variations in the age structure of childbearing in human populations. *Population Index* **40**:185–258.

Coale A., and Trussell, T. J. (1978). A new procedure for fitting optimal values of the parameters of a model schedule of marital fertility rates. *Population Index* **4**:211–213.

Cornell, J. (1956). Matsunagi: A Japanese mountain community. In *Two Japanese Villages.* (J. Cornell and R. Smith, eds.), Ann Arbor: University of Michigan Press. Center for Japanese Studies, *Occasional Papers* No. 5.

Corsini, C. A. (1979). Is fertility-reducing effect of lactation really substantial? In *Natural Fertility* (H. Leridon and J. Menken, eds.), pp. 195–215. Leige: Ordina Editions for the International Union for the Scientific Study of Population.

Davis, K. (1963). The theory of change and response in modern demographic history. *Population Index* **29**(4):345–366.

Delgado, H.; Lechtig, A.; Brineman, E.; Martorell, R.; Yarbrough, C.; and Klein, R. (1978). Nutrition and birth interval components: The guatemalan experience. In *Nutrition and human reproduction* (W. H. Mosley, ed.), pp. 385–400. New York/London: Plenum Press.

Demeny, P. (1968). Early fertility decline in Austria-Hungary: A lesson in demographic transition. *Daedalus* **97**(2):502–521.

Dixon, W. (1965). *Society, schools and progress in scandinavia.* New York: Pergamon Press.

Dore, R. P. (1959). *Land reform in Japan.* New York: Oxford University Press.

Dore, R. P. (1965). *Education in Tokugawa Japan.* Berkeley: University of California Press.

Dore, R. P. (1978). *Shinohata: A portrait of a Japanese village.* New York: Pantheon Books.

Drake, M. (1969). *Population and society in Norway, 1735–1865.* Cambridge: Cambridge University Press.

Easterlin, R. (1978). The economics and sociology of fertility: A synthesis. In *Historical studies of changing fertility,* edited by C. Tilly. Princeton: Princeton University Press.

Easterlin, R; Pollak, R.; and Wachter, M. (1980). Toward a more general economic model of fertility determination: endogenous preferences and natural fertility. In Population and economic change in developing countries (R. Easterlin, ed.), pp. 81–149. Chicago: University of Chicago Press.

Edin, K. A., and Huchinson, E. (1935). *Studies of differential fertility in Sweden.* London: P. S. King and Son.

Embree, J. (1939). *Suye Mura: A Japanese village.* Chicago: University of Chicago Press.

Eriksson, I., and Rogers, J. (1978). *Rural labor and population change: social and demographic developments in East-Central Sweden during the nineteenth century.* Uppsala: Almquist and Wiksell.

Fernando, D. (1972) Recent fertility decline in Ceylon. *Population Studies* **26**:445–453.

Fridlizius, G. (1975). Some new aspects on Swedish population growth. II: A study at parish level. *Economy and History* **18**(2):126–154.

Friedlander, D. (1969). Demographic responses and population Change. *Demography* **6**:359–381.

Frisch, R. (1965). *Theory of Production.* Chicago: Rand McNally and Co.

Frisch, R. (1978). Nutrition, fatness and fertility: The effect of food intake on reproductive ability, edited by Mosley, pp. 91–122.

Frisch, R. (1979). Some further notes on population, food intake and natural fertility, edited by Leridon and Menken, pp. 135–148.

Gårlund, T. (1958). *The life of Knut Wicksell.* Stockholm: Almquist and Wiksell.

Gaunt, D. (1973). Family planning and the pre-industrial society: Some Swedish evidence. In *Aristocratis, farmers and proletarions: Essays in Swedish demographic history* (K. Ågren, D. Gaunt, I. Eriksson, J. Rogers, and S. Åkerman, eds.), pp. 28–59. Uppsala: Studia Historica Upsaliensia.

Gaunt, D. (1978). Household typology: problems—methods—results. In *Chance and change: Social and economic studies in historical demography in the baltic area* (S. Akerman, H. C. Johansen, and D. Gaunt, eds.), pp. 69–83. Odense: Odense University Press.

Goody, J. (1976). Inheritance, property and women: some comparative considerations. In *Family and inheritance: rural society in western Europe, 1200–1800,* edited by Goody, J.; Thirsk, J.; and Thompson, E. P. Cambridge: Cambridge University Press.

Gray, R. H. (1979). Biological factors other than nutrition and lactation which may influence natural fertility: A review. In *Natural Fertility* (H. Leridon and J. Menken, eds.), pp. 217–251. Leige: Ordina Editions for the International Union for the Scientific Study of Population.

Haines, Michael (1978). Recent developments in historical demography: A review of the european fertility project with some comparisons from Japan. *Historical Methods* II, **4**:162–173.

Hanley, S. B., and Yamamura, K. (1977). *Economic and demographic change in preindustrial Japan, 1600–1868.* Princeton: Princeton University Press.

Härm, E. (1976). Asian population data on magnetic tape. *Population Index* **42**(4):636–652.

Hashimoto, M. (1974) Economics of postwar fertility in Japan. In *Economics of the family: marriage, children and human capital,* edited by T. Schultz, pp. 225–249. Chicago: University of Chicago Press.

Hayami, A. (1968). The demographic analysis of a village in Tokugawa Japan: Kando-Shinden of Owari Province, 1778–1871. *Keio Economic Studies* **5**:50–88.

Hayami, A. (1973). *Kinsei nōson no rekishi jinkō gakuteki kenkyū* [A demographic historical study of a Tokugawa village]. Tokyo: Tōyō Keizai Shinpōsha.

Hayami, A. (1980). Illegitimacy in Japan. In *Bastardry and its comparative history,* edited by P. Laslett, K. Oosterveen, and R. M. Smith. Cambridge, Massachusetts: Harvard University Press.

Hayami, Y.; Akino, M.; Shintani, M.; and Yamada, S. (1975). *A century of agricultural growth in Japan: its reference to Asian development.* Minneapolis: University of Minnesota Press.

Hayami, Y., and Ruttan, V. (1971). *Agricultural development: An international perspective.* Baltimore: Johns Hopkins Press.

Hayami, Y.; Ruttan, V.; and Southworth, H. M. (1979). *Agricultural growth in Japan, Taiwan, Korea, and the Philippines.* Honolulu: University Press of Hawaii.

Hayami, Y., and Yamada, S. (1970). Agricultural productivity at the beginning of industrialization. In *Agriculture and economic growth: Japan's experience,* edited by K. Ohkawa, B. Johnston, and H. Kaneda. Princeton: Princeton University Press.

Heckscher, E. (1954). *An economic history of Sweden.* Cambridge: Harvard University Press. (Translated by Göran Ohlin.)

Henry, L. (1961). Some Data on Natural Fertility. *Eugenics Quarterly* **8**(8):81–91.

Hofsten, E., and Lundstrom, H. (1976). *Swedish population history: main trends from 1750 to 1970.* Stockholm: Norstedts Tryckeri.

Hull, V. J. (1978). A study of birth interval dynamics in rural Java. In *Nutrition and human reproduction* (W. H. Mosley, ed.), pp. 433–460. New York/London: Plenum Press.

Husén, T. (1962). *Problems of differentiation in Swedish compulsory schools.* Stockholm: Svenska Bokforlaget.

Institut International de Statistique (1916). *Annuaire International de Statistique.* Le Haye.

Johansson, Ö. (1967). *The gross domestic product of Sweden and its composition, 1861–1955.* Stockholm: Almquist and Wiksell.

Jain, A. K.; Hermalin, A. J.; and Sun, T. H. (1979). Lactation and Natural Fertility, edited by Leridon and Menken, pp. 149–194.

Jones, E. L. (1981). *The European miracle: environments, economies and geopolitics in the history of Europe and Asia.* Cambridge, England: Cambridge University Press.

Jörberg, L. (1972). *A history of prices in Sweden, 1732–1914.* 2 Volumes. Lund: CWK Gleerup.

Jorgenson, D., and Lau, L. (1969). An economic theory or agricultural household behavior. A paper presented at the Far Eastern Meeting of the Econometric Society. Tokyo, Japan.

Kälvemark, A. S. (1977–1978). Äkerskap och familj i Sverige i historiskt perspektiv. [Marriage and family in Sweden in an historical perspective.] *Historielärarnas Förenings Årsskrift.*

Kälvemark, A. S. (1980a). Malthus and Neo-Malthusianism in Sweden. A paper delivered to the conference Malthus hier et aujourd'hui, Congres International de Demographie Historique, Paris-UNESCO, May 27–29.

Kälvemark, A. S. (1980b). *More children of better quality? aspects on Swedish population policy in the 1930s.* Stockholm: Almqvist & Wiksell.

King, M. (1978). *Sweden: educational data.* Washington: U.S. Department of Health, Education and Welfare.

Knodel, J. (1974). *The Decline of Fertility in Germany, 1871–1939.* Princeton: Princeton University Press.

Knodel, J. (1979). The influence of child mortality in a natural fertility setting: An analysis of German villages, edited by Leridon and Menken, pp. 273–284.

Kobayashi, K., and Tsubouchi, Y. (1979). Recent Trends and Regional Variations in Japanese Marital Fertility. In *Fertility transition of the East Asian Populations,* edited by Lee–Jay Cho and K. Kobayashi. Honolulu: University Press of Hawaii.

Kock, K. (1945). Nymalthusianismens Genombrott i Sverige. [Neo-Malthusianism's breakthrough in Sweden], edited by K. Kock, pp. 73–88. *Studier i Ekonomi och Historia. Tillägnde Eli Heckscher* [Studies in economics and history: dedicated to Eli F. Heckscher].

Koyama, T. (1961). *The changing social position of women in Japan.* Geneva: UNESCO.

Krantz, O., and Nilsson, C. A. (1975). *Swedish national product, 1861–1970: new aspects on methods and measurement.* Lund: CWK Gleerup.

Kuczynski, R. (1935). *The measurement of population growth: methods and results.* London: Sidgwick and Jackson, Ltd.

Kuznets, S. (1966). *Modern economic growth: rate, structure and spread.* New Haven and London: Yale University Press.

Kuznets, S. (1971), *Economic growth of nations: total output and production structure.* Cambridge, Massachusetts: Harvard University Press.

Lau, L. J.; Lin Wuu–Long; and Yotopoulos, P. (1978). The linear logarithmic expenditure system: an application to consumption–leisure choice. *Econometrica* **46**(4):843–868.

Lau, L. J., and Mitchell, B. (1970). A linear logarithmic expenditure system: an application to U.S. data. Paper presented at the Second World Congress of the Econometric Society, Cambridge.

Lau, L. J.; Yotopoulos, P.; Chou, E.; and Lin, Wuu–Long (1981). The Microeconomics of Distribution: A Simulation of the Farm Economy. *Journal of Policy Modeling* **3**(2):175–206.

Leasure, W. (1963). Factors involved in the decline of fertility in Spain, 1900–1950. *Population Studies* **17**:271–285.

Lee, R. (1980). Age structure, intergenerational transfers and economic growth: An overview. Démographie économique **31**(6):1129–1156.

Leibenstein, H. (1975). The economic theory of fertility decline. *Quarterly Journal of Economics* **84**(1):1–31.

Leibenstein, H. (1976). *Beyond economic man: A new foundation of microeconomics.* Cambridge: Harvard University Press.

Lesthaeghe, R. J. (1977). *The decline of Belgian fertility, 1800–1970.* Princeton: Princeton University Press.

Lewis, W. Arthur (1978). *Growth and fluctuations,* 1870–1913. London: George Allen and Unwin.

Lithell, U. B. (1981a). Breast-feeding habits and their relation to infant mortality and marital fertility. *Journal of Family History* **6**(2):182–194.

Lithell, U. B. (1981b). Infant mortality rate and its relation to living conditions in the past. *The Scandinavian Journal of History* **6**(4):243–260.

Livi–Bacci, M. (1971). *A century of Portuguese fertility.* Princeton: Princeton University Press.

Livi–Bacci, M. (1977). *A history of Italian fertility during the last two centuries.* Princeton: Princeton University Press.

Löfgren, O. (1974). Family and household among Scandinavian peasants: An exploratory essay. *Ethnologia Scandinavica* **3**:1–35.

Martinius, S. (1977). *Peasant destinies. The history of 552 Swedes born 1810–1812.* Stockholm: Almquist and Wiksell.

McCloskey, D. (1976). English open fields as behavior towards risk. In *Research in Economic History,* Vol. 1, edited by P. Uselding. Greenwich, Connecticut: JAI Press.

McFalls, Jr., J. (1981). Tuberculosis as a cause of subfecundity in current and historical societies, A paper presented to the Meetings of the Population Association of America, December. Washington, D.C.

McKeown, T. (1976). *The modern rise in population.* New York: Academic Press.

McNeill, W. H. (1963). *The rise of the west: A history of the human community.* Chicago: University of Chicago Press.

Mizushima, H. (1961). *A collection of prefectural life tables, Japan,* 1921–1956. Osaka: Seimei Hoken Bunka Kenkyūjo.

Montgomery, G. A. (1939). *The rise of modern industry in Sweden.* London: P. S. King & Son, Ltd.

Morris, D. and Smith, T. C. (1979). Fertility and mortality in an outcaste village in Japan, 1758–1869. A paper delivered to the Stanford-Berkeley Colloquium on Historical Demography, Fall 1979. San Francisco.

Mosk, C. (1977). Demographic transition in Japan. *Journal of Economic History* **37**(3) (September);655–674.

Mosk, C. (1978a). Demographic transition in Japan, 1920–1960 *Journal of Economic History* **38**(1) (March):285–286.

Mosk, C. (1978b). Fecundity, infanticide and food consumption in Japan. *Explorations in Economic History* **15**:269–289.

Mosk, C. (1978c). Nuptiality, Infant Mortality, and Illegitimacy in Taisho Japan. A paper presented to the Conference on Historical Dimensions of Conflict in Japan, July.

Mosk, C. (1979a). The decline of marital fertility in Japan. *Population Studies* **33**(1):19–38.

Mosk, C. (1979b). Fertility in the prefectures of Meiji Japan. Department of Economics, University of California (Berkeley), Working Paper No. 139.

Mosk, C. (1979c). Fertility transitions in Japan and Korea: A comparison. A paper delivered at a regional conference sponsored by the Committee for the Chinese Economy of the Social Science Research Council held at the Hoover Institution, Stanford University, January 26–27.

Mosk, C. (1979d). Premodern demographic regime in Sweden and Japan: A comparison. A revised version of a paper presented to the Conference on Decline of fertility in Europe by Province, July 23–27.

Mosk, C. (1979e). Scandinavian historical demography: An international perspective. A paper delivered to the panel on Scandinavian Social History of the Social Science History Association Meetings, Cambridge, Massachusetts, November 4.

Mosk, C. (1980a). Nuptiality in Meiji Japan. *Journal of Social History* **13**(3):474–489.

Mosk, C. (1980b). Rural-urban fertility differentials and the fertility transition. *'Population Studies* **34**(1):77–90.

Mosk, C. (1981a). The evolution of the premodern demographic regime in Japan. *Population Studies* **35**(1):28–52.

Mosk, C. (1981b). The evolution of premodern demographic regimes: A research note. *Explorations in Economic History* **18**:199–208.

Mosk, C. (1981c). Nutrition and fertility: A review essay. *Historical Methods* **14**(1):43–46.

Mosk, C. (1981d). Fertility and occupation: Mining districts in prewar Japan. *Social Science History* **5**(3):293–315.

Mosk, C., and Faris, J. (1979). A description of a data tape concerning the counties (*Gun*) and cities (*Shi*) of Japan, 1925–1938. Department of Economics, University of California, Berkeley, Working Paper No. 133 (October).

Mosk, C.; Faris, J.; and Mikalson, B. (1980). A description of a data tape concerning the counties of Sweden, 1880–1960. Department of Economics, University of California, Berkeley, Working Paper No. 147 (September).

Mosk, C.; Paynter, T.; and Savoca, E. (1980). A description of a data tape concerning the prefectures of Japan, 1902–1970. Department of Economics, University of California, Berkeley, Working Paper No. 148 (September).

Mosk, C., and Stoft, S. (1979). A description of a data tape concerning the farm households of Japan, 1925–1935. Department of Economics, University of California, Berkeley, Working Paper No. 134 (October).

Nakajima, C. (1969). Subsistence and commercial family farms: some theoretical models of subjective equilibrium. In *Subsistence Agriculture and Economic Development,* edited by C. Wharton, Jr. Chicago: Aldine.

Nakamura, J. (1966). *Agricultural production and the economic development of Japan, 1873–1922.* Princeton: Princeton University Press.

Nakane, Chie (1967). *Kinship and economic organization in rural Japan.* London: Athlone Press of the University of London.

Nakane, Chie (1972). Japan: The Household Over Three Centuries. In *Household and Family in Past Time,* edited by P. Laslett. Cambridge: Cambridge University Press.

Nishikawa, S. (1978). Productivity, subsistence, and by-employment in the mid-nineteenth century Choshu. *Explorations in Economic History* **15**(1):69–83.

Norman, H. (1974). *Fran Bergslagen till Nordamerika, studier i migrations-mönster, social rörlighet och demografisk struktur med utgångspunkt fran Örebro Län* 1851–1915. [From Bergslagen to North America. Studies in migration pattern, social mobility and demographic structure on the basis of Örebro County, 1851–1915]. Uppsala: Studia Historica Upsaliensia 62.

Norman, H. (1977). Den utomäktenskapliga fruktsamhetens tokala variationer, en fallstudie från Örebro Län. [Regional variations in illegitimate fertility. A case study from Örebro County]. *Historieforskning på nya Vägar.* Studier Tillagnade Sten Carlsson. Lund.

Notestein, F. (1945). Population—the long view. In *Food for the World,* edited by T. W. Schultz, pp. 36–57. Chicago: University of Chicago Press.

Ohbuchi, H. (1976). Demographic transition in the process of Japanese industrialization. In *Japanese industrialization and its social consequences,* edited by H. Patrick, pp. 329–361. Berkeley: University of California Press.

Ohkawa, K., and Rosovsky, H. (1973). *Japanese economic growth: trend acceleration in the twentieth century.* Stanford: Stanford University Press.

Ohkawa, K., and Shinohara, M; with Meissner, L. (1979). *Patterns of Japanese economic development: A quantitative appraisal.* New Haven: Yale University Press.

Ohkawa, K., in association with Shinohara, M.; Umemura, M.; Ito, M.; and Noda, T. (1957). *The growth rate of the Japanese economy since 1878.* Tokyo: Kinokuniya.

Ohkawa, K.; Takamatsu, N.; and Yamamoto, Y. (1974). *National Income.* Tokyo: Tōyō keizai Shinpōsha.

Öhngren, B. (1979). Infant Mortality in Eskilstuna 1749–1900: Social environment and Causes of Death. Paper delivered to the panel on Scandinavian Social History of the Social Science History Association Meetings, Cambridge, Massachusetts.

Olsson, L. (1980). Då barn var lönsamma. Om arbetsdelning, barnarbete och teknologiska förandringar i några Svenska Industrier Under 1800—och Borjan av 1900—talet [When children were profitable. On division of labour, child labour and technological change within some Swedish industries during the nineteenth and the beginning of the twentieth century]. Unpublished dissertation.

Orleans, L. (1976). A selective bibliography on the demography of China. *Population Index* **42**(4):653–693.

Orring, J. (1969). *School in Sweden: A survey of primary, middle and secondary education.* Stockholm: Publishing Department of the National Board of Education.

Osteria, T. S. (1978). Variations in fertility with breast-feeding and contraception in urban Filipino women: implications for a nutrition program. In *Nutrition and human reproduction* (W. H. Mosley, ed.), pp. 411–432. New York/London: Plenum Press.

Østerud, Øyvind (1978). *Agrarian structure and peasant politics in Scandinavia: A comparative study of rural response to economic change.* Oslo: Universitetsforlaget.

Ōta, Tenrei (1969). *Nihon sanji chōsetsu-shi.* [History of Japanese birth control]. Tokyo.

Page, H. (1977). Patterns underlying fertility schedules: A decomposition by both age and marital duration. *Population Studies* **31**(1):85–106.

Passin, H. (1965). *Society and education in Japan.* Bureau of Publications. Teachers College. Columbia University and East Asian Institute, Columbia University.

Popkin, B. (1978). Economic determinants of breast-feeding and contraception in urban Filipino women: implications for a nutrition program, edited by Mosley, pp. 461–497.

Population Problems Research Council, the Mainichi Newspapers Publishing Company (1952). *Family system and population of farming communities in Japan.* Tokyo: Mainichi Newspapers Publishing Company.

Preston, S. (1976). *Mortality patterns in national populations.* New York: Academic Press.

Qvist, G. (1977). Ett perspektiv på den s.k. kvinnoemancipationen i Sverige. *Historisk tidskrift utgiven av Svenska historiska föreningen* 2 [English summary: 179–180].

Rohlen, T. (1980). The *Juku* phenomenon: An exploratory essay. *The Journal of Japanese Studies* **6**(2) (Summer):207–242.

Rosenzweig, M. (1980). Neoclassical theory and the optimizing peasant: An econometric analysis of market family labor supply in a developing country. *The Quarterly Journal of Economics* **94**(1):31–55.

Samuelson, P. (1958). An exact consumption-loan model of interest with or without the social contrivance of money. *The Journal of Political Economy* **66**(6):467–482.

Sandberg, L. (1978). "The case of the impoverished sophisticate: human capital and Swedish economic growth before World War I." Ohio State University Department of Economics and the Mershon Center, Working Paper No. 134.

Sanger, M. (1938). *An autobiography.* New York: Norton and Co.

Sen, A. (1966). Peasants and dualism with or without surplus labor. *Journal of Political Economy* **74**:425–450.

Shimahara, N. (1979). *Adaptation and education in Japan.* New York: Praeger Publishers.

Shimpo, M. (1976). *Three decades in a Shiwa: economic development and social change in a Japanese farming community.* Vancouver: University of British Columbia Press.

Shorter, E. (1975). *The making of the modern family.* New York: Basic Books, Inc.

Sivesand, K. (1979). *Skifte och befolkning. Skiftenas inverkan på byar och befolkning i Mälarregionen.* Uppsala: Studia Historica Upsaliensia: 109.

Smith, R. J. (1978). *Kurusu: The price of progress in a Japanese village, 1951–1975.* Stanford: Stanford University Press.

Smith, T. C. (1966). *The Agrarian origins of modern Japan.* New York: Atheneum Press.

Smith, T. C. (1977). *Nakahara: family farming and population in a Japanese Village,* 1717–1830. Stanford: Stanford University Press.

Spence, M. (1973). *Market signaling: information transfer in hiring and related processes.* Cambridge, Massachusetts: Harvard University Press.

Stein, Z., and Susser, M. (1978). *Famine and Fertility,* edited by Mosley, pp. 123–145.
Stockholm University, Staff of the Institute for Social Sciences (1941). *Population movements and industrialization: Swedish counties, 1895–1930.* 2 Vols. London: P. S. King & Son, Ltd.
Taeuber, I. (1958). *The population of Japan.* Princeton: Princeton University Press.
Tederbrand, L. G. (1972). *Vasternorrland och Nordamerika 1875–1913. Utradring och återinvandring* [Emigration from Västernorrland County to North America and re-immigration to Västernorrland County]. Uppsala: Studia Historica Upsaliensia.
Thomas, D. S. (1938). *Research memorandum on migration differentials.* New York: Social Science Research Council.
Thomas, D. S. (1941). *Social and economic aspects of Swedish population movements,* 1750–1933. New York: Macmillan Co.
Trussell, T. J. (1978). Menarche and Fatness: Reexamination of the Critical Body Composition Hypothesis. *Science* **200**(30 June):1506–1509.
Trussell, T. J. (1979). Natural fertility: measurement and use in fertility models, edited by Leridon and Menken, pp. 29–64.
Tsubouchi, Y. (1970). Changes in fertility in Japan by region: 1920–1965. *Demography* 7(2):121–134.
Tsuchiya, K. (1976). *Productivity and technological progress in Japanese agriculture.* Tokyo: University of Tokyo Press.
Tyson, J., and Perez, A. (1978). The maintenance of infecundity in postpartum women, edited by Mosley, pp. 11–28.
United Nations (1973). *Demographic yearbook, 1972.* New York: United Nations.
United Nations, Department of Economic and Social Affairs (1958). *Recent trends in fertility in industrialized countries.* New York: United Nations.
United Nations, Statistical Office of the United Nations (1965). *Demographic yearbook, 1965.* New York: United Nations.
United Nations, Statistical Office of the United Nations (1968). *Demographic yearbook, 1968.* New York: United Nations.
Van de Walle, E. (1974). *The female population of France in the nineteenth century.* Princeton: Princeton University Press.
Van Ginneken, J. (1978). The impact of prolonged breast-feeding on birth intervals and on postpartum amenorrhea, edited by Mosley, 179–196.
Vogel, E. (1963). *Japan's new middle class: The salary man and his family in a Tokyo suburb.* Berkeley: University of California Press.
Vogel, E. (1967). Kinship structure, migration to the city, and modernization. In *Aspects of social change in modern Japan.* (R. Dore, ed.). Princeton: Princeton University Press.
Waswo, A. (1977). *Japanese landlords: The decline of rural elite.* Berkeley: University of California Press.
Weir, D. (1980). Another 'revolution au village': patterns of fertility control in 40 villages of rural France. Department of Economics, Stanford University, Stanford Project on the History of Fertility Control, Working Paper No. 8 (November).
Wilkinson, M. (1973). An Econometric Analysis of Fertility in Sweden, 1870–1965. *Econometrica* **41**(4):633–642.
Willis, R. (1980). The old age security hypothesis and population growth. In *Demographic behavior: interdisciplinary perspectives on decision-making.* (T. Burch, ed.). Boulder: Westview Press.
Willis, R. (1981). On the social and private benefits of population growth. Unpublished paper, January.
Winberg, C. (1975). *Folkökning och proletarisering. Kring den sociola strukturomvandlingen*

på Sveriges Landsbygd under den Agrara Revolutionen [*Population growth and proletarianization.* The transformation of social structures in rural Sweden during the Agrarian revolution. (*Meddelanlanden från Historiska Institutionen i Göteborg,* Nr. 10, Partille).

Winberg, C. (1978). Population growth and proletarianization, edited by Åkerman, Johansen, and Gaunt, pp. 170–184.

Wray, J. D. (1978). Maternal nutrition, breast-feeding and infant survival, edited by Mosley pp. 197–230.

Wright, G., and Kunreuther, H. (1975). Cotton, corn and risk in the nineteenth century. *Journal of Economic History* **35**:526–552.

Yamamura, K., and Hanley, S. (1975). Ichi hime, ni Tarō: education aspirations and the decline of fertility in postwar Japan. *Journal of Japanese Studies* **2**(1) (Autumn): 83–125.

Yasuba, Yasukichi (1962). *Birth rates of the white population of the United States.* Baltimore: Johns Hopkins University Press.

Yasukawa, M., and Hirooka, K. (1974). Estimates of the population size and of the birth- and death-rates in Japan, 1865–1920. *Keio Economic Studies* **11**(2):41–66.

Yotopoulos, P., and Lau, L. (1974). On modeling the agricultural sector in developing economies: An integrated approach of micro and macroeconomics. *Journal of Development Economies* **1**:105–127.

Yotopoulos, P.; Lau, L.; and Lin, Wuu-Long (1976). Microeconomics output supply and factor demand equations in the agriculture of the province of Taiwan. *American Journal of Agricultural Economics* **58**(1–3):333–340.

Index

D

E

F

G

H

I

J

O

P